Animal Biology and Care

Animal Biology and Care

Emily Jewell

Reaseheath College
Cheshire
UK

Fourth Edition

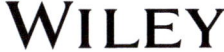

First edition published in 2000
Second edition published in 2006
Third edition published in 2014

Registered Offices
John Wiley & Sons, Inc., 111 River Street, Hoboken, NJ 07030, USA
John Wiley & Sons Ltd, New Era House, 8 Oldlands Way, Bognor Regis, West Sussex, PO22 9NQ, UK
For details of our global editorial offices, customer services, and more information about Wiley products visit us at www.wiley.com.

The manufacturer's authorized representative according to the EU General Product Safety Regulation is Wiley-VCH GmbH, Boschstr. 12, 69469 Weinheim, Germany, e-mail: Product_Safety@wiley.com.

Wiley also publishes its books in a variety of electronic formats and by print-on-demand. Some content that appears in standard print versions of this book may not be available in other formats.

Library of Congress Cataloging-in-Publication Data

Names: Jewell, Emily author | Dallas, S. E. (Sue E.) Animal biology and
    care.
Title: Animal biology and care / Emily Jewell, Reaseheath College,
    Cheshire, UK.
Description: 4th edition. | Hoboken, NJ, USA : Wiley, 2026. | Revised
    edition of: Animal biology and care / Sue Dallas, VN, Certificate in
    Education, Emily Jewell, MSc, BSc (Hons), Certificate in Education,
    Curriculum Area Manager in Animal Management, Reaseheath College,
    Nantwich, Cheshire. Third edition. Chichester, West Sussex, UK : Wiley
    Blackwell, 2014. | Includes bibliographical references and index.
Identifiers: LCCN 2025028335 | ISBN 9781394277186 paperback | ISBN
    9781394277209 adobe pdf | ISBN 9781394277193 epub
Subjects: LCSH: Veterinary medicine
Classification: LCC SF745 .J49 2026
LC record available at https://lccn.loc.gov/2025028335

Cover Design: Wiley
Cover Image: Courtesy of Emily Jewell

Printed and bound by CPI Group (UK) Ltd, Croydon, CR0 4YY

C9781394277186_021025

In memory of my uncle, John Lennox, whom I am truly blessed and eternally grateful to have had as part of my life and who will be forever missed.

"There are some who bring a light so great to the world that even after they are gone, the light remains." Unknown author

Contents

Preface

When this book was first published in 2000, it soon became an essential reference text for my students studying L2 and L3 programmes in Animal Care/Management, as well as the intended market of those studying on Animal Nursing Assistant/Veterinary Care Assistant programmes. Now updated, I have aimed to ensure that the book remains a useful study companion to those undertaking such programmes now and in the future.

This book would also be useful for those working in the animal industry who need to enhance their knowledge to better manage the animals in their care.

The format of this latest edition aims to provide a logical flow through the chapters, following a similar structural organisation of the previous editions but with some reorganisation. Additional diagrams have been included to enhance learning. Each chapter now has learning goals and a summary for readers to check their knowledge and understanding at the end of each chapter. To support the content of the book, an online website has also been developed to support learning.

Emily Jewell
MSc, BSc (Hons), Certificate in Education
Reaseheath College
Nantwich
Cheshire

Acknowledgments

I am grateful to the staff at Wiley for their help during the writing of this edition, particularly Sreemol Manikandan and Haridharini Velayoudame, whose patience have been unending and much appreciated. My thanks also go to Lisa Gee (RVN) for her guidance and advice on chapters and Kate-Marie Jeffs (RVN) for demonstrating her handling skills with her gorgeous trio.

Consideration and appreciation must be given to all the animals (past and present) for posing so well in their photographs – a clear indication that you belong to tutors involved in the delivery of animal-related courses. As always, thanks go to my family for their continuing support, patience, and encouragement. Finally, to you, the reader, I hope that this new edition remains as well used as previous ones.

Emily Jewell
MSc, BSc (Hons), Certificate in Education
Reaseheath College
Nantwich
Cheshire

About the Companion Website

This book is accompanied by a companion website:

https://www.wiley.com/go/animal/biology4e/jewell

The website includes:

- Almost 200 interactive Multiple-Choice Questions organised by chapter so that you can test your knowledge
- Chapter summaries providing learning objectives for each chapter
- PowerPoints of all figures from the book for downloading (a password is required, which can be found in the book)

Section 1

Animal Biology

1

Cells and Basic Tissues

Learning goals

In this chapter, the learning goals are:

- To identify the essential functions required to sustain life
- To identify the structure and function of animal cells and tissues
- To explain the diversity of animal cells and tissues in existence
- To explain how animal cells work in partnership to form systems

What Is Biology?

Biology is the study of life and living organisms

How do we define life?

To be considered a living organism, an organism must be able to perform all the following essential functions of life:

- *Movement* – The organism can move itself or a part of itself.
- *Reproduction* – The organism can reproduce itself so that the species doesn't die out.
- *Sensitivity* – The organism can react to stimuli in its surroundings to avoid life-threatening events in its environment.
- *Growth* – The organism can sustain growth from within itself via processes that involve taking in new materials from the outside and incorporating them into its internal structure.
- *Release of energy from respiration* – The organism can use nutritional sources to release a usable form of energy in a controlled way to sustain life.
- *Excretion* – The organism can excrete waste metabolic products from itself.
- *Nutrition* – The organism can ingest nutritional materials that provide energy to maintain life and growth.

A cell is the simplest functional unit of all tissues. Each cell can individually perform all the essential life functions identified previously. Organisms may be single-celled or multi-celled. Within multicellular organisms, the component cells show a wide range of specialisations, thereby contributing to cell diversity within an organism.

Cells can therefore be deemed to be the building blocks of the body, and therefore, the following can be stated:

Animal Biology and Care, Fourth Edition. Emily Jewell.
© 2026 John Wiley & Sons Ltd. Published 2026 by John Wiley & Sons Ltd.
Companion Website: https://www.wiley.com/go/animal/biology4e/jewell

- *Cells* form ...
- *Tissues*, and tissues form ...
- *Organs* – organs work together to form *systems* within the body.
- *Systems* have a specific function to perform in living organisms using the diverse range of cell specialisations.

Cell Diversity

Animal cells are not all identical (Figure 1.1), but they all have the same basic structure because they are all derived from a type of cell called a *Stem Cell*. Stem cells have the potential to become any type of cell within the body, and once they become specialised, they are said to have *differentiated*. Cells become specialised so that they are more efficient in the role that they have within the body. Stem cells are not only found in the embryo but can also be found in a range of locations across the adult mammalian body, e.g. bone marrow, liver, heart, brain, muscles, and skin.

Individual components of animal cells are called *organelles*, and each organelle is described in the following section:

- *Cell/Plasma membrane* – All animal cells are surrounded by a membrane which contains all the other organelles of the cell as without it, the cell contents would spill out. This membrane can be referred to as either the cell membrane or the plasma membrane.

  Cell/plasma membranes are approximately 0.00001 mm (10 nm) in thickness. The cell/plasma membrane is the boundary keeping the cytoplasm of the cell contained.

  The role of the cell/plasma membrane is to be a barrier that separates the external environment of the cell from the internal environment, along with controlling what enters/exits the cell (cell exchange). The cell/plasma membrane allows certain chemicals to pass in and out of the cell by the exchange processes of *diffusion, osmosis*, or *active transport*. The cell/plasma membrane is *selectively permeable*, i.e. it chooses what can/can't come in/out of the cell according to the needs of the cell.
- *Nucleus* – There is usually one nucleus in the cell, which is located near the centre of the cell. Its role is to be the brain of the cell and control its activities. The nucleus is surrounded

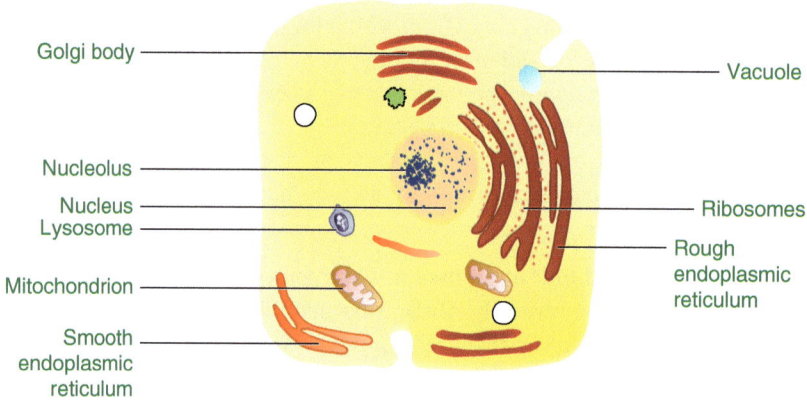

Figure 1.1   Basic cell structure.

by a double membrane called the *nuclear envelope*. Inside the nucleus is an area called the *nucleolus*, which contains the genetic material [deoxyribonucleic acid (DNA) and ribonucleic acid (RNA)] of the cell, which is important for cell reproduction. *Chromatin* is found in the nucleus and condenses to form *chromosomes*. The nuclear envelope is interspersed with *nuclear pores*, which allow material in/out of the nucleus itself. It is important to note here that red blood cells do not contain a nucleus.

- *Cytoplasm* – A gel-like material that supports the organelles within the cell between the cell/plasma membrane and the nucleus. Cytoplasm is where chemical reactions occur within the cell for metabolic purposes. Cytoplasm also allows the organelles to move around and move molecules between them.
- *Chromosomes* – These are rod-shaped components that contain the hereditary information of an organism. This hereditary material is called DNA and it controls the characteristics that an organism inherits from its parents. Chromosomes exist as thin strands of DNA and are usually found in pairs. Chromosomes are subdivided into genes.
- *Mitochondria* – These are energy-producing organelles where cell respiration takes place. Energy is generated from nutritional sources such as carbohydrates, fats, and proteins to create a usable form of energy. Mitochondria are often called the powerhouses of the cell. Mitochondria are surrounded by a double membrane. The outer membrane is the surface of the mitochondrion. The inner membrane has many folds called *cristae*, which increase the surface area to maximise the energy produced by cell respiration. Due to the energy that they need to swim, sperm cells contain many mitochondria. This is an example of cell specialisation. It is important to note that a single mitochondria is called a *mitochondrion*.
- *Endoplasmic reticulum* (ER) – ER is a series of tubules acting as a transport and packaging system in the cell. ER may be rough ER or smooth ER. Rough ER has ribosomes attached to it where proteins are synthesised. This protein can be used by the cell to synthesise enzymes, hormones, antibodies, and muscle. Smooth ER has no ribosomes and is used to synthesise and transport lipids (fats) and steroids made within the body.
- *Ribosomes* – *Ribosomes* build proteins within the cell. These proteins then join to form amino acids which are essential for growth and repair in the body. Ribosomes are found in the cell's cytoplasm. Ribosomes contain RNA.
- *Centrosome* – The centrosome is an area found near the nucleus in animal cells that helps with the ability of the cell to change its shape such as in cell division and during phagocytosis (cell eating). It is responsible for the organisation of microtubules in the cell. The centrosome is made up of two *centrioles*. Centrioles are important during cell division and the formation of the *cilia* and *flagella* of certain cells (the slender projecting hairs responsible for movement of single-celled organisms). Centrioles can only be seen during cell division; otherwise, the centrosome is seen.
- *Lysosomes* – *Lysosomes* are small vesicles (fluid-filled spheres) in cells that contain numerous types of enzymes responsible for splitting complex chemical compounds into simpler ones (known as *lysis*, meaning 'to break up') followed by digestion. They help to destroy worn-out organelles within the cell and recycle them for further use. Lysosomes are created by the *Golgi apparatus*, and the enzymes within them are produced in the endoplasmic reticulum.
- *Golgi apparatus* – The Golgi apparatus is a series of flattened sacs that extend from the endoplasmic reticulum throughout the cytoplasm of the cell. The sacs are where different chemical reactions occur. It is responsible for moving molecules from the ER to elsewhere in the cell. The Golgi apparatus is also involved in labelling some vesicles with proteins or

carbohydrates complexes so that they are transported to the correct locations. The Golgi apparatus is also referred to as the Golgi body/Golgi complex.

- *Peroxisomes* – Peroxisomes are mainly involved in breaking down lipids and toxic molecules, such as hydrogen peroxide, made during digestion into safer molecules. Peroxisomes are similar to lysosomes but have a slightly different structure and contain different lysing enzymes.
- *Cilia* – Cilia are hair-like projections on a cell, which aid absorption or movement of fluids away from a cell. Cilia are only found in animal cells and are made up of microtubules. They are usually found in groups or as a border on cell surfaces.
- *Flagella* – Flagella are long whip-like structures that can be found as part of microbial and animal cell structures. They tend to be longer and less dense than cilia. Sperm cells have a flagellum for movement.

Most of the organelles listed are common to virtually all cells, but the shape, form, and contents of individual cells be differentiated according to its intended function, as previously explained. The structural characteristics of a particular cell are closely related to its functions (Figure 1.2).

Types of cells found in the animal body

- *Epithelial cells* – These cells line the surface of the body, body organs, and cavities within it. Their shape and structural form reflect this role, e.g. tightly packed together, flattened where abrasion occurs, and ciliated where absorption occurs. Epithelial cells are often described according to their shape, e.g. squamous, cuboidal, columnar, ciliated, or stratified.
- *Endothelial cells* – These are a type of epithelial cell with a specific role to line the inside surfaces of blood vessels and lymphatic vessels.

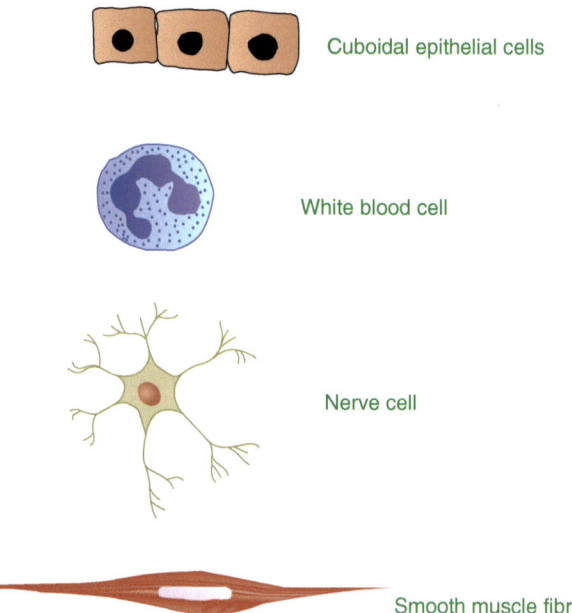

Cuboidal epithelial cells

White blood cell

Nerve cell

Smooth muscle fibre

Figure 1.2   Examples of cell diversity.

- *Glandular cells* – These are a type of epithelial cell, but they make and release secretions either inside the body or onto the body surface. They can be found in a range of locations throughout the body, and examples of secretions include sweat, saliva, enzymes, hormones, and mucus.
- *Osteoblasts* – They produce bone tissue. They form new bone and contribute to growth and repair of bone. Osteoblasts can develop into osteocytes.
- *Osteocytes* – These are mature bone cells that maintain the health of the bone. They have a role to play in maintaining calcium balance within the bone. Osteocytes have a much longer life span than osteoblasts or osteoclasts.
- *Osteoclasts* – They break down bone tissue that is old or damaged.
- *Erythrocytes (red blood cells)* – These are designed to contain the red pigment haemoglobin, which carries oxygen around the body. They have a biconcave disc shape and are one of the few cells in the body that do not have a nucleus.
- *Nerve cells* – Nerve cells or neurones have fine projections that transmit electrical impulses through the nervous system to reach the whole body.
- *Muscle cells* – These are found in cardiac muscle, smooth muscle, and skeletal muscle. They contain protein filaments that slide over each other to cause contractions once they have been stimulated by the electrical impulse from nerve cells. Muscle cells contain high numbers of mitochondria to provide energy.
- *Fat cells* – These are also called adipose cells/adipocytes. They are specialised to have a role in energy storage and metabolism. There are different types of fat cells, and they are a type of connective tissue.
- *Sperm cells* – These are the male sex cells. They have a tail for swimming and only contain half the number of chromosomes.
- *Ova* – These are the female sex cells. They contain only half the number of chromosomes of other cells in the body and once combined with a sperm cell, the resulting embryonic cell has a full set of chromosomes.
- *Stem cells* – These are cells that have not become specialised to a particular function. They are also called undifferentiated cells. Stem cells are found in early embryos following rapid division and are known as *embryonic stem cells*. They can develop into any type of cell. Stem cells can also be found throughout the adult body – *adult stem cells*. Stem cells are now used in medical treatments of certain conditions in animals such as osteoarthritis and torn ligaments. An infusion of stem cells into the affected area can improve repair and regeneration of damaged tissues. Treatments involving stem cells are known as *stem cell therapy*.
- *Cancer cells* – Cancer cells are cells that behave abnormally due to mutations in genetic DNA. These mutations can either be inherited, due to external factors (e.g. ultraviolet rays from the sun) or completely random. Cancer cells can invade surrounding healthy tissues. Cancer cells don't repair themselves or die, so they keep growing and can break off the original growth (tumour) to move to other locations in the body, known as *metastasis*. Cancer cells can be given different names according to where they are found in the body, e.g. *carcinomas* are found in epithelial tissues; *sarcomas* are found in connective tissues such as bone, fat, and muscle; and *leukaemia* and *lymphomas* are found in white blood cells.

Summary of cells

No matter what the type of cell found in an organism, cells have needs that must be met to survive:

- Food for energy
- Water (body fluid) to hydrate the cells

- Oxygen to all cells
- A suitable temperature in which to live

Cells are differentiated according to the role that they have in the body, but they are all derived from embryonic stem cells.

Animal Tissues

Tissues are a collection of cells and their products that have a common fundamental function, in which one cell type is dominant:

- *Epithelial tissue* – forms a protective layer both inside and on the surface of the body. Examples of this tissue are the skin, glands, and linings of the various body systems.
- *Connective tissue* – supports body tissues and acts as a transport system to move materials vital to tissue cells around the body. Examples of this tissue are as follows:
  - *Loose connective tissue* that surrounds organs.
  - *Dense connective tissue* that has great strength and is found as tendons and ligaments.
  - *Blood* that transports essential nutrients, gases, waste products, hormones, and enzymes to and from all body cells.
  - *Cartilage* and *bone* that provide shape and protection for organs and allow movement.
  - *Adipose* tissue is mainly found around internal organs *(visceral)* and under the surface of the skin *(subcutaneous)*. As well as storing and releasing energy, adipose tissue also plays an active part in the endocrine system to maintain homeostasis in the body.
- *Muscle/muscular tissue* – It is concerned with movement of the skeleton, the organ systems, and the heart. There are three types of muscle tissues in the body:
  - Skeletal
  - Smooth
  - Cardiac
- *Nervous tissue* – It is concerned with transporting messages to tissues and connecting body tissues for the required response.

Epithelial tissue

Epithelial tissue covers all surfaces of the body, both inside and out, whether it is a surface, a cavity, or a tube. Epithelial tissue is made up of cells arranged in a continuous sheet as either single or multiple layers. Epithelial tissues are involved in a wide range of activities, such as secretion of fluids, protection, and absorption.

Epithelial tissue varies in shape, structure, and thickness according to function and location in the body. Epithelial tissues are classified according to appearance:

- *Number of layers* – a single layer of these cells is called *simple* epithelium; more than one layer is called *stratified* epithelium.
- *Shape of the cells* involved – e.g. *squamous* (thin and flat), *columnar* (column), and *cuboidal* (cube).
- *Specialisations* – e.g. covered in tiny hairs called *cilia* or thickened surface tissue called *keratin*, which covers the nose and pads of paws/feet.
- *Glandular* – means that it is involved in secretion. Secretions that go directly into the bloodstream are called *hormones* and are produced by glands of the *endocrine* system. Some

secretions are produced by glands that have ducts onto the surface of a cell. Glands with ducts belong to the *exocrine* system, e.g. enzymes that are produced by the pancreas.

Note: Epithelial tissues always have a basement membrane as part of their structure.

Types of epithelial tissue

Epithelial tissue has many different functions, and therefore, there are different types. There are different types of epithelial tissues, which are as follows:

- *Simple squamous (Pavement epithelium)* – can be found lining the surfaces involved in the transport of gases (lungs) or fluids (walls of blood vessels) (Figure 1.3a).
- *Cuboidal* – can be found lining small ducts and tubes such as those of the kidney, pancreas, and salivary glands of the mouth (Figure 1.3b).
- *Columnar* – located on highly absorbing surfaces like the small intestine for the uptake of nutrients (Figure 1.3c).
- *Ciliated* – has tiny hair-like projections in parallel rows on the surface of the cell, which beat in a wave-like manner, moving films of mucus or fluid in a particular direction. For example, in the respiratory airway (trachea), they remove unwanted inhaled materials (Figure 1.4a).
- *Glandular* – which produce secretions containing hormones, enzymes, or sweat (Figure 1.4b).
- *Stratified* – This type of epithelium has two or more layers of cells. Its function is mostly one of protection and it is found where there is more wear on the epithelial surface, e.g. in the mouth or as skin (Figure 1.4c).
- *Pseudo-stratified* – This is only one layer in thickness but appears to be more when microscopically examined, as the nuclei of the cells are at different heights. It is found in the male reproductive system, the male urinary system, and upper respiratory tract.
- *Transitional* – This is so called as its appearance varies according to its state. It is found in the bladder and male reproductive tract. In an unstretched sample of transitional epithelium (i.e. less fluid in the bladder), the cells appear to be stratified cuboidal, but once the sample is stretched (i.e. bladder is full), the cells appear to be simple squamous.

Connective tissue

Connective tissue connects all the other body tissues together. Connective tissue comprises different cell types, which work together to provide support, bonds, and organisation to provide a matrix

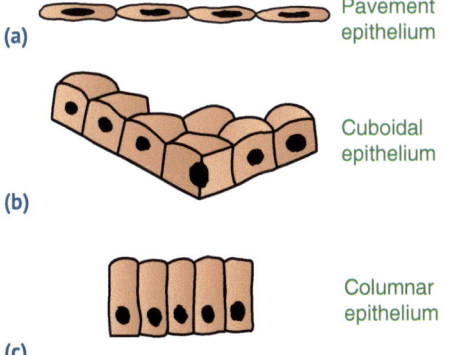

(a) Pavement epithelium

(b) Cuboidal epithelium

(c) Columnar epithelium

Figure 1.3 (a) Pavement, (b) cuboidal, and (c) columnar tissues.

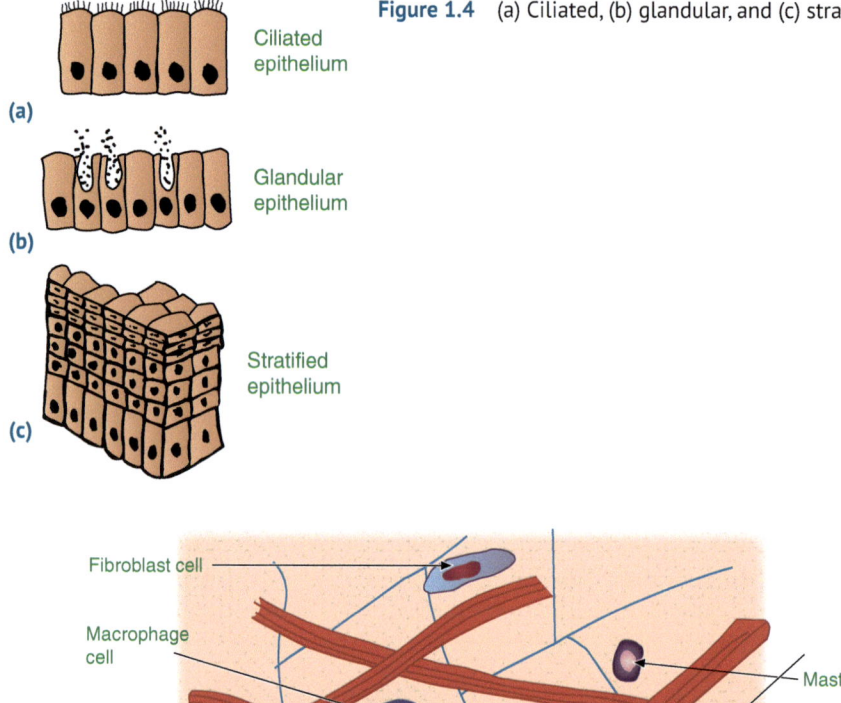

Figure 1.4 (a) Ciliated, (b) glandular, and (c) stratified tissues.

Ciliated epithelium

(a)

Glandular epithelium

(b)

Stratified epithelium

(c)

Fibroblast cell

Macrophage cell

Mast cell

Collagen fibres

Ground substance

Fat cell

Elastic fibres

Figure 1.5 Connective tissue.

for metabolic exchange of nutrients and waste products between tissues to form organs. The different types of connective tissue vary according to their density, cell components, and specialisms.

The basic structure of connective tissue is a ground extracellular matrix, which contains cells and protein fibres (Figure 1.5). Connective tissues need a good blood supply due to the exchange of nutrients and waste products that occur within them.

Structure of connective tissue

As already mentioned, the basic structure of connective tissue is an extracellular matrix containing protein fibres and cells.

Ground/extracellular matrix

The ground matrix is a thick, clear, and colourless fluid that fills up the space between the cells and the protein fibres. It acts as a sieve for molecules that can travel between the blood and the cells, therefore aiding the exchange of nutrients, oxygen, and waste products.

There are three protein fibres that could be present in the ground matrix:

- *Collagen* – produced by fibroblasts. Not very elastic but has great tensile strength and flexibility. Tendons by which muscles are attached to the bones are composed of collagen fibres.
- *Elastic* – It is found where the tissue is regularly required to stretch and bend. Can be found in ligaments which hold the bones of the skeleton together, the walls of large blood vessels, and in the skin.
- *Reticular* – It is found where greater support is needed, such as in the walls of blood vessels, smooth muscle cells, and nerve fibres.

There are two types of cells (split into subtypes) that can be present in the ground matrix:

- *Fixed/resident* cells – permanent residents of connective tissue.
- *Fibroblasts* – most common type of connective tissue cell.
- *Adipose* – present in smaller numbers except in adipose tissue.
- *Transient/Wandering* cells – can move through extracellular space.
- *Macrophages* – phagocytic cells that remove dead cells and tissue.
- *Mast cells* – containing secretory granules in their cytoplasm that release their contents when the cell is damaged.
- *Plasma cells* – antibody-producing cells derived from lymphocytes that are present in small numbers.
- *Leucocytes* – present in small numbers for a short time. Their quantity is higher if the animal has an infection.

Types of connective tissue

The proportion, density, and type of protein fibres and cells contained in the ground matrix determine the type of connective tissue.

Loose connective tissue fills layers between the epithelial tissue of other organs almost like a packing material. As the name suggests, the protein fibres are arranged loosely within this type of tissue. It is quite fragile and not very resistant to stress. There are three types of loose connective tissue:

- *Areolar tissue* – there is a high distribution of this type of tissue across the body, and it is predominantly comprised of collagen fibres and fibroblasts with equal amounts of ground matrix, fibres, and cells. Can be found in subcutaneous and dermal layers of skin, in mucous membranes, and around blood vessels.
- *Adipose tissue* – comprised of many adipocytes that store lipid droplets. It is a source of stem cells for repair of cells and tissues. White adipose tissue is predominant and found across the body and is a site of storage for fat droplets. Brown adipose tissue is so called as it is darker in colour and is more energy dense. It is spread between mitochondria and releases heat to maintain body temperature. There is a high proportion of brown adipose tissue in newborn animals (neonates) as they are not yet able to maintain their own body temperature.
- *Reticular tissue* – contains a greater proportion of reticular fibres throughout. Reticular tissue can be found in places such as the liver, spleen, lymph nodes, and bone marrow.

Dense connective tissue provides tough support in the skin. It contains a greater number of protein fibres that are thicker and more densely packed than in loose connective tissue. It is found where strength is required in the tissues but little flexibility such as in tendons, ligaments, large blood vessels, and the lungs. There are three types of dense connective tissue:

- *Dense regular* – provides strength and strong attachments, e.g. tendons and ligaments.
- *Dense irregular* – provides resistance against stress, e.g. dermal layer of the skills and surrounding capsules of body organs.
- *Elastic* – contains a high number of elastic fibres which provide stretch and expansion as needed, e.g. in lungs and large blood vessels.

Specialised connective tissue – There are several specialised connective tissue types in the body:

- *Bone* – a connective tissue made up of cells called osteocytes, osteoblasts, and osteoclasts embedded in an extracellular matrix that becomes calcified for strength. Bone can either be compact or spongy. Compact bone is the strongest. Spongy bone has spaces in its structure that are filled with red bone marrow, which is responsible for producing and destroying blood cells.
- *Cartilage* – a strong and resilient supportive tissue that has some degree of flexibility. It has no direct blood or nerve supply; nutrients are obtained from surrounding capillaries through diffusion. The only cells in cartilage tissue are *chondrocytes*. There are three types of cartilage:
  - *Hyaline cartilage*
  - *Elastic cartilage*
  - *Fibrocartilage*
- *Blood* – Blood is a fluid connective tissue that contains a range of cells and an extracellular material called *plasma*. Blood cells are formed from stem cells in bone marrow. Plasma makes up approximately 55% of the total volume of blood. The primary function of blood is to transfer nutrients and respiratory gases (oxygen and carbon dioxide) to and from the right locations. Blood is classified as a connective tissue because it connects all the cells in the body together.
- *Fibrous connective tissue* – It is like dense connective tissue. It is involved in the repair of damaged tissues, and it is often called scar tissue but can also be found in the covering of organs such as the kidney and the brain, as well as in ligaments.
- *Lymphoid tissue* – It is a specialised form of reticular connective tissue. It makes up the lymphatic system and is therefore found in bone marrow, the thymus, spleen, and lymph nodes.

Blood

Blood is a highly specialised connective tissue consisting of different types of cells held in an aqueous fluid called *plasma* (Figure 1.6). Plasma makes up 55% of total blood volume, and the cellular components therefore make up 45%. The main blood cells are:

- Red blood cells (*erythrocytes*)
- White blood cells (*leucocytes*)
- Platelets (*thrombocytes*)

It is important to note that the proportions of cells in blood can vary according to the physiological state of the body. For example, an animal with an infection will have a higher proportion of white blood cells and an animal with a wound will have a higher proportion of platelets in the injured area. Some illnesses are caused by a change in blood cells in the body. For example, *anaemia* is a lack of healthy red blood cells in the body.

Blood performs a wide range of functions, but its key role is as a transportation system. Living animals continuously take in valuable substances such as respiratory gases (oxygen) and nutrients,

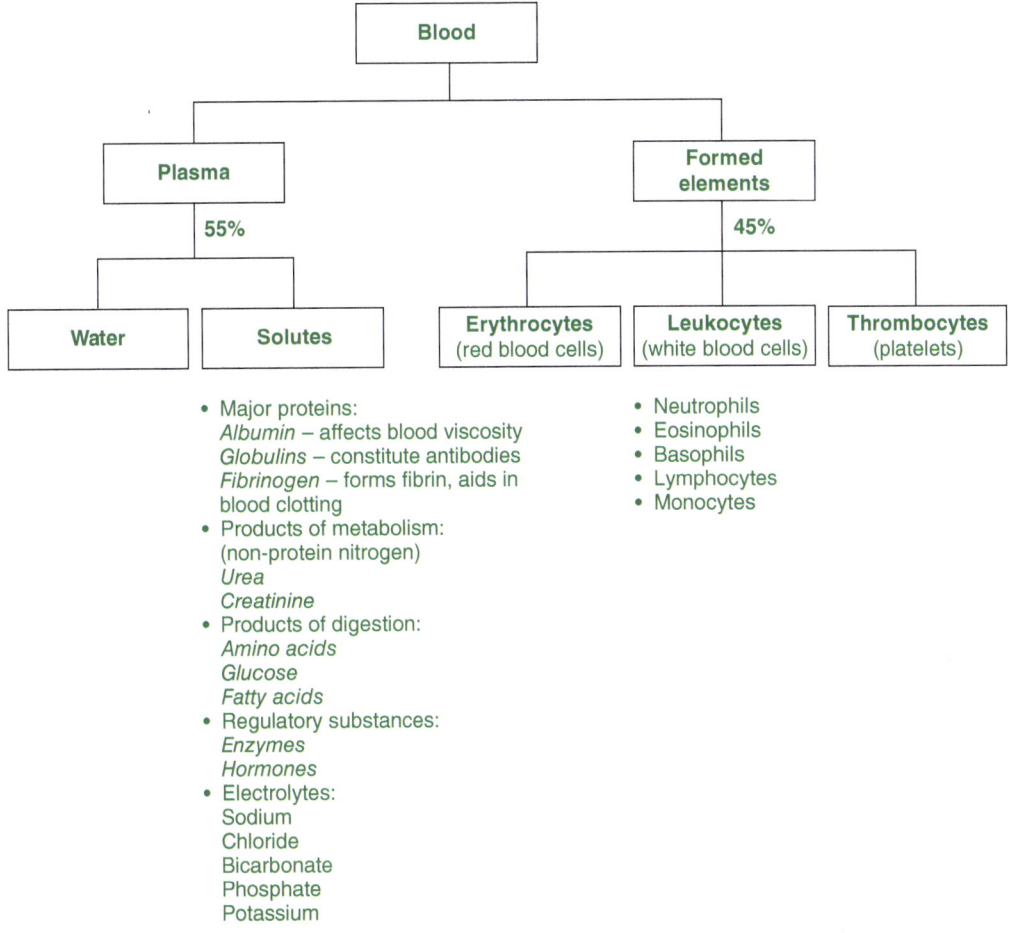

Figure 1.6 Components of blood.

which need to be distributed throughout their bodies. They produce an endless stream of waste materials, such as carbon dioxide, which must be removed from their bodies before they reach harmful levels. These distribution and waste removal processes are performed by blood.

Composition of blood

Plasma makes up about 55% of blood. Cells and other components make up the remaining 45%. The amount of blood in an animal is known as *total blood volume*. The amount varies according to the size of the animal and its physiological state. Blood volume can be affected by metabolic conditions, illnesses, cardiac function, sex (usually higher in males than females), and weight. Blood sample analysis gives a good indicator of what is happening in the body at any one time.

To analyse a blood sample, it is mixed with an *anticoagulant* (stops clotting) and placed into a *centrifuge*, which spins at high speed. This centrifugal force causes the components within the blood to separate out into layers. The plasma is at the top of the tube, followed by the platelets, and then the white blood cells with the red blood cells at the bottom (Figure 1.7). The white blood cells and platelets may be referred to in combination as the *buffy coat*.

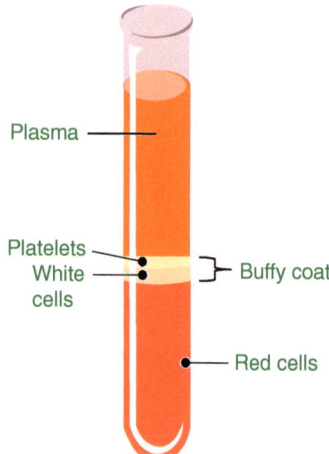

Figure 1.7 Blood separated into layers.

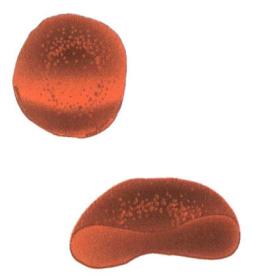

Figure 1.8 Cross-section of a red blood cell showing its biconcave shape.

Components of blood

Plasma – It is approximately 92% water and contains a variety of dissolved substances such as plasma proteins (6–7%) and salts/glucose (1%), which are transported from one part of the body to another. For example, nutrients from food breakdown (glucose, lipids, and amino acids) are taken from the small intestine to the liver where they are metabolised. The resulting waste product of urea is transported from the liver to the kidneys to be excreted. Another example is when hormones are transported from their various production sites in endocrine glands to their target organ location. There is a continuous exchange taking place in the body between blood and cells.

Three key plasma proteins carried in blood are called *albumin, globulin,* and *fibrinogen*. Fibrinogen plays an important role in the process of blood clotting. When fibrinogen has been used up by clot formation at the site of injury, then the fluid part of blood seen is called *serum*. Serum is simply plasma with fibrinogen removed.

Plasma	Serum
Fibrinogen (protein for clotting) plus water, protein, glucose, lipids, amino acids, salts, enzymes, hormones, and waste products	Contains water, protein, glucose, lipids, amino acids, salts, enzymes, hormones, and waste products but no proteins for clotting (these have been used up)

About 92% of blood is made of water, and the water can be forced into the tissues where it is then called *tissue fluid* because of its location. Both plasma and tissue fluid are the environments that keep body cells alive.

Imagine it as a fish tank where the plasma/tissue fluid is the water, and the cells are the fish that get their nutrients and oxygen from that water and subsequently excrete their waste products into the same water, which is then filtered to remove them. The filters in the body are the kidneys, which are discussed in Chapter 3.

Red blood cells (erythrocytes)

Red blood cells (RBC) are produced from stem cells in red bone marrow. Their main function is to carry oxygen from the respiratory organs to the tissues. To do this effectively, their structure is adapted, and they have no nucleus. Due to this, red blood cells are biconcave discs in shape with a surrounding thin elastic membrane (Figure 1.8). RBC are filled with the red pigment *haemoglobin*. Haemoglobin combines with oxygen to form the molecule *oxyhaemoglobin* and carries the oxygen to the tissues. Haemoglobin also combines with carbon dioxide to carry this waste product away from the tissues. The quantities of red blood cells present are what give blood its red colour. When combined with oxygen, it is a brighter red but duller without. The lifespan of a red blood cell is approximately 120 days in the body.

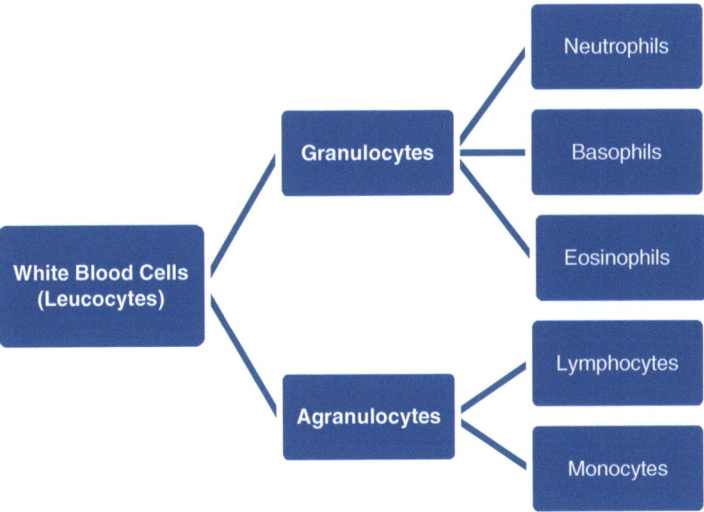

Figure 1.9   Categorisation of white blood cells.

White blood cells (leucocytes)
White blood cells (WBC) exist in lower quantities in the blood (approximately 1% of total blood volume), and their key role is to protect the body from infection and disease, as well as aiding repair from injury. All white blood cells have a nucleus. WBC are produced in the bone marrow and are categorized into two key groups (Figure 1.9).

Functions of WBC
The term *phagocyte* or *phagocytic* means 'cell eater'. Phagocytic cells eat/engulf and destroy other cells that can be harmful to the body, e.g. pathogens, toxic materials. WBC are transported via the blood stream where they push through the walls of capillaries into the tissue spaces. Phagocytic WBC will gather areas where there are injury and damage to the body to destroy bacteria, viruses, and other harmful materials. They are one of the first lines of defence the body has in fighting infection.

Granulocytes
- Have granules in their cytoplasm that contain enzymes to protect from pathogens.
- The proportion present in the blood increases during times of infection as they are the first line of defence.

Neutrophils
Neutrophil

- Make up 40–60% of WBC
- Lifespan of 12–20 days
- *Phagocytic* cells that remove and destroy pathogens

Basophils

Basophil
(granules are blue)

- Make up 1–3% of WBC
- Life span of 1–2 days
- Fight parasite infection
- Prevent blood clotting as they contain *heparin*
- Respond to allergic reactions

Eosinophils

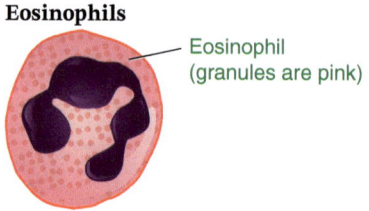

Eosinophil (granules are pink)

- Make up 1–4% of WBC
- Lifespan of 5–6 days
- Eliminate parasites
- Respond to histamine released during allergic reactions
- Help dissolve blood clots as contain *plasminogen*
- Sustain an inflammatory response

Agranulocytes

Have no granules in their cytoplasm

Integral part of the animal's immune system

Lymphocytes

Lymphocyte

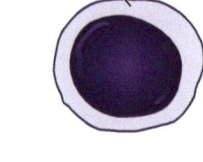

- 18–40% of WBC
- Lifespan of a few weeks to years
- Large nucleus
- Recognise and respond to foreign *antigens*
- 3 main types – T Cells, B cells, and NK cells (natural killer cells)

Monocytes

Monocyte

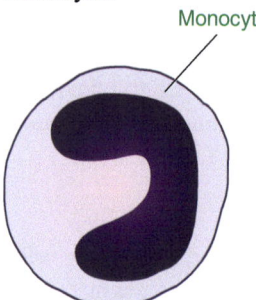

- 2–10% of WBC
- Lifespan 2–3 days
- Largest of the WBC
- Mature into macrophages and dendritic cells
- Part of the innate and adaptive immune system

Bone and Cartilage

There are two kinds of specialised skeletal connective tissue: bone and cartilage.

Bone

Bone is a connective tissue made up of cells called osteocytes, osteoblasts, and osteoclasts that are embedded in an extracellular matrix that becomes calcified for strength.

Bone can either be compact or spongy. Compact bone is the strongest. Spongy bone has spaces in its structure that are filled with red bone marrow, which is responsible for producing and destroying blood cells.

Cartilage

Cartilage is a dense, clear, blue/white material found mainly in skeletal joints that provides support for the body. Cartilage can be elastic or rigid. Cartilage has no blood vessels or nerve supply but is covered by a membrane called the *perichondrium* from which it receives its blood supply. The cells of cartilage are called *chondroblasts*.

There are three types of cartilage that have been previously identified:

- *Hyaline cartilage* – It contains many collagen fibres and is found in mobile articular joints, ribs, and the C-shaped rings of cartilage that keep the trachea open for air passage into the lungs. Hyaline cartilage also forms the embryonic skeleton until it is replaced by bone.
- *Elastic cartilage* – This has a high number of elastic fibres and is found where flexibility is needed in the structure, e.g. the ear pinna, the external ear canal, the epiglottis, and larynx and the upper respiratory tract.
- *Fibrocartilage* – It is found where strength is required for support in the body such as the inter-vertebral discs, the hip joints, and tendons. Its collagen fibres tend to be thicker than those of hyaline cartilage. The knee joint contains thick pads of fibrocartilage called menisci.

Muscle tissue

Muscle cells are usually long, thin cells known as *myocytes*. Individual myocytes combine to form bunches of cells called *muscle fibres*. Groups of muscle fibres are joined together by connective tissue to form muscles. The structure of the muscle fibres gives muscles the ability to contract as the cells are excitable and elastic in their nature. These characteristics enable movement of the skeleton and the function of organs and systems within the body.

The cell membrane of muscle cells is called the *sarcolemma* and as with all other cell membranes, it is selectively permeable and controls the movement of substances in and out of the cell. The cytoplasm of muscle cells may be referred to as *sarcoplasm*.

There are three main types of muscle tissue:

- *Skeletal* (also called voluntary and striated) (Figure 1.10)
- *Smooth* (also called involuntary, non-striated, and visceral) (Figure 1.11)
- *Cardiac* (Figure 1.12)

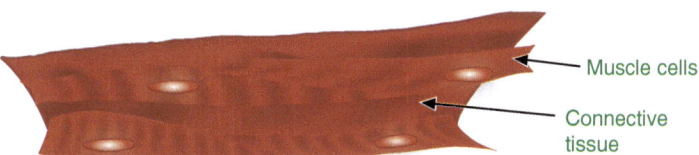

Figure 1.10   Skeletal (striated) muscle fibre.

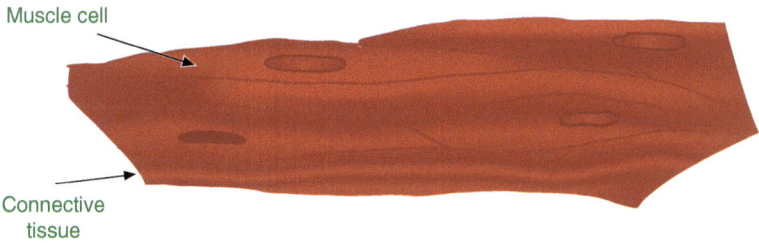

Figure 1.11   Smooth (non-striated) muscle fibre.

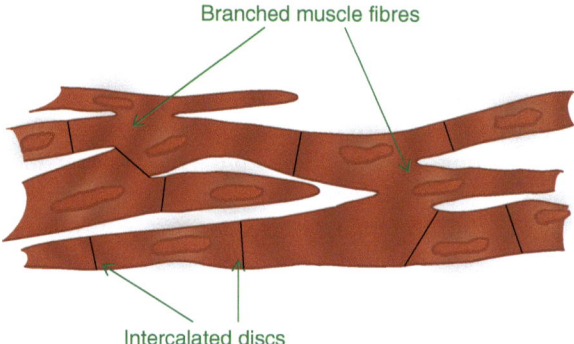

Figure 1.12   Cardiac muscle fibre.

Skeletal muscle tissue

Skeletal muscle tissue is found in the muscles attached to the skeleton by tendons. The cells are cylindrical and vary from 1 mm to 5 cm in length. Skeletal muscles are also called *voluntary muscle* as most of the time, they move due to thought processes of the animal. As well as enabling movement in an animal, skeletal muscles also support body posture and contribute towards the regulation of body temperature.

Skeletal muscles are constructed from parallel muscle fibres being held together in small bundles by connective tissue. These are collected into larger groups, which ultimately form the muscle and are surrounded by more connective tissue called the *muscle sheath*. When muscles are close to one another, the muscle sheaths may thicken to form *intermuscular septa*.

Skeletal muscle appears striped when viewed under the microscope. These stripes are known as striations leading to skeletal muscle tissue being called *striated* muscle. The striped appearance is due to the arrangement of two proteins called *actin* and *myosin*, which form muscle units called *sarcomeres*. These sarcomere units are repeated throughout the muscle fibre. Actin and myosin are the key proteins referred to in the most widely accepted theory of muscle contraction called the *sliding filament theory*. This theory states that a muscle contracts due to the thinner actin filaments sliding over the thicker myosin filaments within muscle cells to cause contraction.

Skeletal muscle cells are cylindrical in shape and have more than one nucleus (multi-nucleated). These cells contain many mitochondria due to their role in energy production. Their endoplasmic reticulum is more specialised *(sarcoplasmic reticulum)* as it stores and releases calcium ions that are needed for muscle contraction to take place.

While skeletal muscle can be quickly stimulated to respond, and can contract rapidly, it becomes tired easily (fatigued). Muscle fibres may be categorised as fast twitch and slow twitch fibres. Twitch refers to the process of contraction. Slow twitch fibres move more slowly but do not tire as easily, whereas fast twitch fibres help fast movement over a shorter time frame but are easily fatigued.

Tendons

At either end of a muscle, the muscle sheath continues into the connective tissue of the structure to which the muscle is attached, i.e. bone. In most cases for skeletal muscles, the connective tissue leaves the muscle as a fibrous band called a *tendon*. Tendons connect muscle to bone and do not stretch very easily. They help with supporting the body structure. Tendons have little blood supply and so, if damaged, they heal very slowly.

Examples of tendons:

- *Achilles tendon* – connects the calf muscle to the heel bone to enable walking
- *Superficial flexor tendon* – helps transfer energy from the upper leg to the lower leg through flexion of the joint in animals

In some areas of the body, fibrous sheets called *aponeurosis* connect muscles to bones and contribute to the body's strength and stability. Aponeuroses are also responsible for absorbing energy when the body moves in stabilising posture. Examples of aponeurosis are as follows:

- *Epicranial aponeurosis* – found in the skull. Works with the skin and other connective tissue to support the muscles of the skull that control facial expression
- *Plantar aponeurosis* – found in the foot. Works to support the foot when running and walking

Ligaments

Ligaments hold bones together across a joint to give it more protection and stability. They stop bones from over-twisting or moving too far apart.

Examples of ligaments:

- *Anterior cruciate ligament* – found around the *stifle* (knee) joint. The common site of injury causing lameness in dogs.
- *Nuchal ligament* – found in the neck from the skull to the vertebral joints at the base of the neck. The nuchal ligament helps to support the weight of the head in species such as cows, horses, and dogs.

Smooth Muscle

Smooth muscle cells are spindle shaped and usually no longer than 0.5 mm in length. When viewed under the microscope, they look smooth (not striated) and contain a single nucleus (Figure 1.11). Smooth muscle cells contain fewer mitochondria than skeletal muscle cells as they do not produce rapid bursts of energy, but they appear to contain more Golgi bodies and endoplasmic reticulum. Within smooth muscle, there are layers known as circular muscle and longitudinal muscle, and these layers work together to move objects through the relevant tract, e.g. digestive, reproductive.

Smooth muscle is specialised for continuous low-force contractions that are applied over a greater section of muscle tissue. Smooth muscle may also be called *involuntary* muscle as their movement is involuntary, i.e. the animal does not need to think about moving them. For example, smooth muscle is found in the intestinal walls of the digestive tract, where it contracts in a continuous rhythm, to move food through the tract by *peristalsis*. Peristalsis occurs when the circular muscle layer contracts and the longitudinal muscle relaxes behind the food bolus to move it along. The longitudinal muscles contract and the circular muscles relax at the other side of the bolus to enable it to move further down the digestive tract.

Smooth muscle can be found in the respiratory tract, the urinary and the reproductive systems, where they are responsible for changing the size of blood vessels and organs. They form a supportive lining and can also be called visceral muscles due to this.

Cardiac Muscle

Cardiac muscle is only found in the heart. Cardiac muscle helps to pump blood through the body to ensure that nutrients and oxygen are delivered to all cells, tissues, and organs.

Cardiac muscle produces continuous forceful contractions that use a lot of energy. For continuous contraction to take place, the muscle fibres are branched and have specialised junctions with the surrounding fibres. These specialised junctions are called *intercalated discs*, and they allow rapid electrical signalling between the cells to enable rapid contraction of nearby tissue. Cardiac myocytes are elongated and striated in appearance with only one nucleus per cell unlike skeletal muscle (Figure 1.12). They contain many mitochondria for a constant energy supply. They are held together by very small amounts of connective tissue.

Nervous Tissue

The function of nervous tissue is to receive, transmit, and coordinate electrical messages from one part of the body to another to effect a change. Nervous tissue is therefore complex. Individual nerve cells can transmit and sometimes store information because of this complexity.

Nerve cells are called *neurones* (Figure 1.13). Neurones connect and communicate to form pathways so that the body can respond to information received from stimuli. Neurones vary in size and shape depending on where they are in the nervous system. However, all neurones have the same basic structure:

- A large *cell body (soma)* containing the nucleus surrounded by cytoplasm, with two types of processes extending from the cell body: a single axon and one or more dendrites. The cell body maintains the nerve cell and is involved in its growth and development.
- *Dendrites* are processes like tree branches that receive electrical impulses from specialised *sense receptors* (information) and convert them into electrical impulses to transfer the information into the cell body.
- *Axons* extend from the cell body as a tube-like structure of variable length, carrying the electrical signal away to the next nerve cell at their *terminal ending*. The point at which the axon leaves the cell body is called the *axon hillock*.

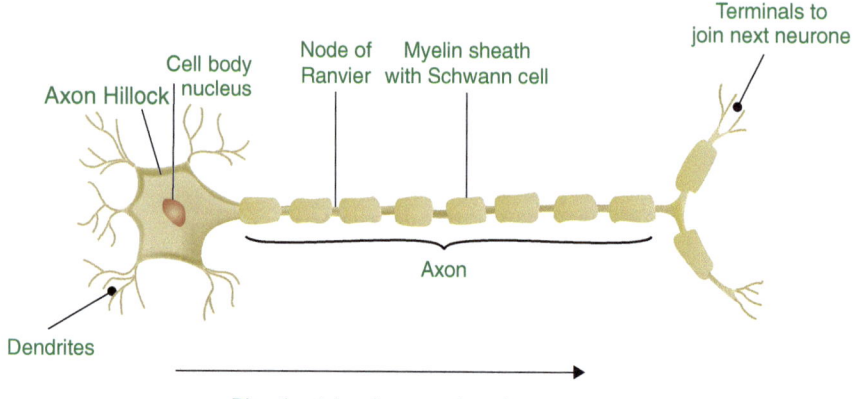

Figure 1.13   A neurone.

- The primary function of the axon is to transmit electrical signals at the *axon terminal* to other neurones, muscles and glands or form junctions (*synapses*) with adjoining neurones from which they receive electrical stimuli, which are passed to the cells beyond.

Additional structures

- Along the axon, most neurones have a protective layer called the *myelin sheath*, which aids in speeding up the transmission of the electrical impulses. The myelin sheath is formed by structures called *glial cells*. The myelin sheath is comprised of individual segments called *Schwann cells*. In between the Schwann cells are gaps called nodes of Ranvier. The structures aid transmission of the electrical impulse through a process called *saltatory conduction*.

While the basic structure is the same, neurones can be classified into three types:

1. **Sensory neurones**
   Receive information from the *external environment* via specialised tissues called sensory receptors and transmit electrical impulses to the central nervous system (CNS) for processing. Because they transmit information towards the CNS, sensory neurones are also called *afferent* neurones. Sensory neurones detect external stimuli such as touch, taste, smell, pain, and temperature.
2. **Motor neurones**
   Receive information from the CNS and transmit electrical impulses to voluntary (skeletal) and involuntary (cardiac and smooth) muscles. Because they transmit information away from the CNS, sensory neurones are also called e*fferent* neurones.
3. **Interneurones**
   Interneurones are the connecting cells between the sensory neurones and the motor neurones. There may be several interneurones involved in the transfer of electrical impulses from stimuli receipt to muscle movement. They are the most abundant type of nerve cells, and they are only found in the CNS.

The point at which neurones meet each other to transfer information is called a *synapse* or synaptic gap. The neurone that is sending the signal is called the *presynaptic neurone* and the neurone receiving the signal is called the *post-synaptic neurone*. Transmission across the synapse may be electrical or chemical. Chemical transmission is via chemicals called *neurotransmitters*.

Summary of Tissues

There are many different tissue types within the body with their own specialised function reflected in the diversity of cells that the tissues contain. The four main tissue types are as follows:

- Epithelial
- Connective
- Muscle
- Nervous

All tissue types work together to form organ systems that integrate and collaborate to enable functioning of the animal body and respond to its external environment.

2

Movement of Materials Within the Body

Learning goals

In this chapter, the learning goals are:

- To identify active and passive transport processes in the body
- To describe the following transport processes in the body:
  - Diffusion
  - Osmosis
  - Endocytosis
  - Active transport
- To identify the structure and function of the lymphatic system

Animal cells have a cell membrane, which is *semi-permeable* (or selectively permeable). This means that the membrane controls the substances that can move in and out of the cell. The exchange of substances in and out of the cell occurs via one of several transport processes. Transport process can be categorised as being *active* or *passive*. The difference is that active transport processes require energy to happen, whereas passive transport processes do not need energy to occur.

Passive transport processes:

1. Diffusion
   a. Simple
   b. Facilitated
2. Osmosis

Active transport processes:

3. Active transport
4. Endocytosis

Diffusion

Diffusion is the process of the movement of molecules from a region of high concentration to a region of lower concentration.

No energy is needed for the process of diffusion to successfully take place.

Animal Biology and Care, Fourth Edition. Emily Jewell.
© 2026 John Wiley & Sons Ltd. Published 2026 by John Wiley & Sons Ltd.
Companion Website: https://www.wiley.com/go/animal/biology4e/jewell

Diffusion continues until the molecules are evenly distributed throughout the area. This process is very important in the movement of molecules and salts (electrolytes or ions) in and out of cells.

Example: Respiratory gas exchange in cells

All cells need oxygen to live. Oxygen is continually being used in cell respiration processes that take place in the mitochondria. Oxygen is brought to cells via blood. The concentration of oxygen inside the cell is lower than in the blood and surrounding tissue. Oxygen molecules will diffuse from the blood into the cell, therefore supplying the oxygen that the cell needs.

With carbon dioxide, the reverse is true: its concentration is highest inside the cells, where it is continually being formed. This results in carbon dioxide molecules diffusing out of the cells into the blood and surrounding tissues.

Osmosis

Osmosis is the movement of water from an area of high-water molecule concentration to an area of low-water molecule concentration through a semi-permeable membrane (Figure 2.1).

Water exists in *solutions*. Solutions are made up of two parts – the *solvent* and the *solute*. When the solute dissolves in the solvent, a solution is formed. An example of a solution is salt water. The salt is the solute, and the water is the solvent. The cytoplasm of cells is a solution with solutes such as amino acids, glucose, and *electrolytes* dissolved in it.

The proportions of solvent and solute present in a solution determine how concentrated the solution is:

- A solution that has a high concentration of water molecules is a *dilute* (weak) solution, i.e. high solvent, low solute.
- A solution with a low concentration of water molecules is a *concentrated* (strong) solution, i.e. low solvent, high solute.

Osmosis continues until the concentration of water is the same on both sides of the semi-permeable membrane, i.e. solution concentration is equal.

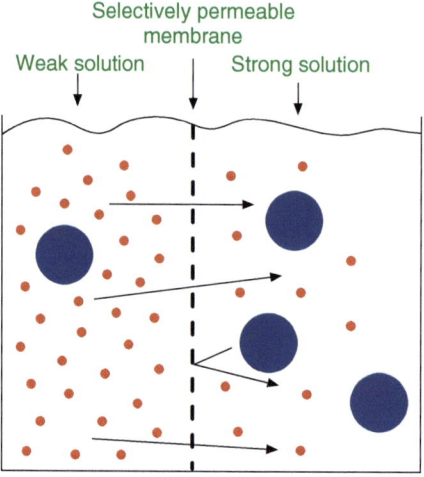

Figure 2.1 Osmosis.

Solutions surrounding cells in the body can exist as three different types:

- *Isotonic* – Same concentration of solutes both inside and outside of the cell, and therefore, there is no overall movement of water (solvent). The amount of water going in and out of the cell is equal.
- *Hypotonic* – The solute concentration (dissolved substances) inside of the cell is higher than on the outside of the cell. More water (solvent) moves into the cell than leaves it to balance out the solute concentration.
- *Hypertonic* – The solute concentration (dissolved substances) inside the cell is lower than on the outside of the cell. More water (solvent) moves out of the cell than into it to balance the solute concentration.

The ideal environment for a cell is in an *isotonic solution*. Isotonic solutions are often used in treating sick animals as they are easily absorbed and replace glucose, amino acids, and electrolytes quickly, preventing further complications.

A cell can tolerate small changes in solution concentration, but if there are great changes to the solution surrounding a cell, then the impact can be profound.

For example, if the cell is hypotonic and takes in too much water, the cell can burst (lyse).

If the cell is hypertonic and too much water leaves the cell, then it can shrivel and die – a prime example of this is when slugs or snails encounter salt on the ground. Water leaves their cells, and the slug/snail shrivels up and dies.

Water concentration is particularly important in aquatic environments.

Saltwater is hypertonic to the fish that live in it (more salt in the surrounding water than in the fish). Water, therefore, leaves the fish to help balance the surrounding environment. Due to this, saltwater fish (marine) need to take in a lot of water to prevent dehydrating.

Freshwater is hypotonic to the fish that live in it (more salt in their body than in the surrounding water). Water, therefore, moves into their body to balance, and therefore, freshwater fish excrete a lot of water from their system.

This is a simple representation and more complex physiological processes and adaptations come into consideration, but if a fish is put into an environment that has a different salt concentration than they need, then water may rapidly enter or leave their bodies causing their death.

In veterinary practice, fluid therapy may be used when treating sick patients. The type of fluid chosen for administration is based upon its sodium (Na) concentration and how equal it is to that of a red blood cell. An isotonic fluid has the same concentration of sodium (saline) as a red blood cell (0.9%). A hypotonic fluid contains less than 0.5% saline, and a hypertonic fluid contains much more (approximately, 7% saline). Fluid therapy is a complex veterinary process and must not be undertaken without a full understanding.

Osmotic pressure

Osmotic pressure is the amount of pressure needed to prevent the movement of water (the solvent) through the semi-permeable membrane. Osmotic pressure is important in patients undergoing kidney dialysis.

Endocytosis

Some molecules are unable to cross the cell membrane via diffusion or osmosis due to their size, and therefore, a different process of transport is needed. For molecules that need to be transported into the cell, *endocytosis* is the process of actively transporting molecules into the cell by engulfing it with the cell membrane. The process of transporting molecules out of the cell is called *exocytosis*.

Note: endo = into, exo = out of

Two types of endocytosis are as follows:

- Phagocytosis
- Pinocytosis

Phagocytosis

Phagocytosis = cell eating

When a molecule or pathogen (solid particle) needs to be consumed by the cell (phagocytosed), the membrane of the cell begins to fold inwards. As this occurs, projections from the cell membrane fold around the molecule/pathogen enclosing it. This structure is now known as a *phagosome*, and it is transported towards the centre of the cell where it is broken down by *enzymes* within the cell. Any useful products are used by the cell, and any unused products are expelled from the cell via exocytosis.

Phagocytosis is a common operation of white blood cells, which take up and destroy bacteria and other particles that could be harmful to the body (Figure 2.2).

Pinocytosis

Pinocytosis = cell drinking

Pinocytosis is a very similar process to phagocytosis with the difference being that the cell takes in fluids within the phagosome rather than solid molecules. Examples of pinocytosis include the absorption of nutrients by microvilli in the intestines and secondly, the reabsorption of nutrients in the kidneys, where the nutrients are separated from urine before excretion.

Active Transport

The previous transport processes described are passive and rely on the natural physical processes where molecules or salts move from a region of high concentration to low concentration, i.e. they move with the concentration gradient.

In some biological situations, however, the reverse happens: molecules or salts move from a region of low concentration to a region of higher concentration, i.e. they move against the concentration

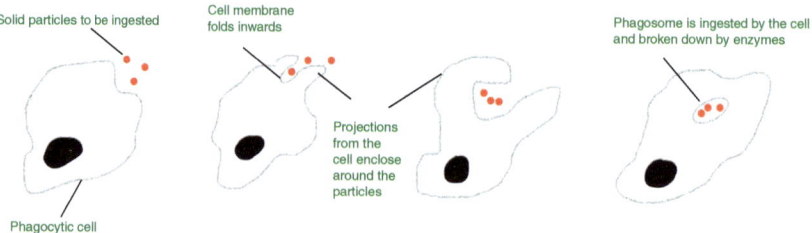

Figure 2.2 Phagocytosis.

gradient. This process is known as *active transport* and needs energy to occur, and therefore, active transport only takes place in organisms that produce energy via respiration processes that take place in the mitochondria. This energy source is known as adenosine triphosphate (ATP).

Examples of where active transport occurs in the body are as follows:

- The movement of Ca^{2+} ions out of cardiac muscle cells
- Transport of glucose molecules across cell membranes

Summary of Transport Processes

There are passive and active transport processes within the body.

- *Diffusion* – a passive transport process where molecules work with the concentration gradient until the concentrations become equal.
- *Osmosis* – a passive transport process where water moves with the concentration gradient until the concentration of solutions becomes equal.
- *Endocytosis* – an active transport process where particles or fluids are taken into the cell through the cell membrane changing shape to enclose the particles/fluids.
- *Active transport* – an active transport process where molecules work against the concentration gradient until the concentration becomes equal. Active transport needs respiratory energy to occur in the form of ATP.

Body Fluid

Body fluid is not just made up of water. It is a fluid containing dissolved essential salts called electrolytes or ions. They are called electrolytes because they carry one or more electrical charges. Those that are positively charged are called cations, i.e. sodium and potassium. Those that are negatively charged are called anions, i.e. chloride and bicarbonate.

The role of electrolytes is to:

- Help control the osmotic pressure
- Assist the pH and buffer mechanisms
- Support the enzyme systems

About 60% of the body consists of fluids, and body fluid can be divided into two main areas:

- Intracellular fluid – 40%
- Extracellular fluid – 20%

Extracellular fluid is further divided into:

- Tissue fluid (interstitial), which bathes the tissues and cells.
- Plasma, which is the water part of blood, is needed to transport the cells, nutrients, gases, hormones, and waste products.

Acids and bases in the body

The acidity of a solution is expressed as its pH (per hydrogen). A pH of 7.0 represents neutral. A solution with a pH of less than 7.0 is acidic, and the lower the figure, the higher the acidity (the greater the hydrogen ion concentration). A solution whose pH is greater than 7.0 is basic or alkaline, and the higher the figure, the more basic is the solution.

The cells of the body function within a normal range of 7.35–7.45 pH. This normal range must be maintained by the body systems at all times for the correct internal environment.

Tissue fluid and the lymphatic system

Each tissue and organ in the body contains a dense network of capillaries (blood vessels that are one cell thick). These are called the capillary beds. Tissue fluid is forced under pressure through the capillary walls. This process tends to occur at the artery end of the capillary bed, since blood pressure is greatest at this point.

When tissue fluid is being forced out of the capillaries, the capillary wall acts as a filter holding back the red blood cells, most of the white cells, and large protein molecules.

Substances that pass through the capillary wall include the following:

- Water
- Oxygen
- Glucose
- Fatty acids
- Amino acids
- Vitamins and minerals
- Hormones and enzymes

Tissue fluid flows out of the capillaries and moves between body cells, which absorb oxygen, nutrients, and other requirements from it while releasing carbon dioxide and other waste products into it.

The Lymphatic System

The lymphatic system consists of a system of open-ended tubes within the capillary bed areas, as numerous as the blood capillaries. The lymphatic system transports a fluid around the body. This fluid is called *lymph*.

Lymph is tissue fluid that is not absorbed back into the bloodstream after carrying required substances to the cells. This tissue fluid drains into the open-ended tubes of the lymph system known as *lymph vessels*. The structure of these vessels is similar to that of veins, in that they have a valve system to make sure fluid only flows in one direction. The movement of lymph in these vessels is achieved by the movement of surrounding tissues, which squeeze or 'milk' the fluid in the lymph vessels.

At intervals in the lymphatic system, there are *lymph nodes* (Figure 2.3), some of which are located near the surface of the skin (Figure 2.4). These structures contain a system of narrow channels through which the lymph fluid will drain and be filtered. This filtering is assisted by phagocytic white blood cells, therefore filtering harmful substances out of the lymph, making the fluid safe enough to return to the main blood circulation.

Where this fluid returns into the bloodstream, *lymph ducts* can be found. From the right side of the head, neck, and right forelimb, lymph drains via the right lymphatic duct. From the rest of the

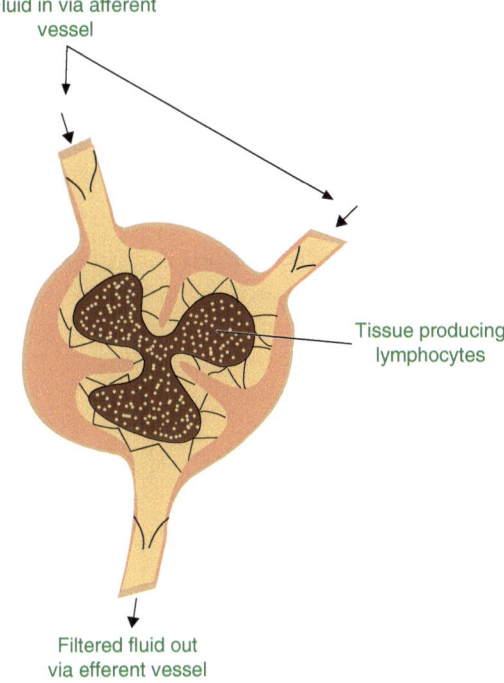

Figure 2.3 Lymph node.

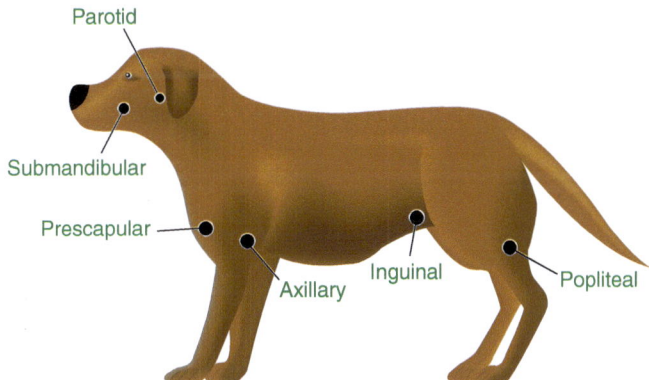

Figure 2.4 Surface nodes.

body, lymph drains via a collecting area called the *cisterna chyli* into the thoracic duct in the thorax or chest. This fluid will contain:

- Fats from the digestive system
- Water
- Electrolytes
- White blood cells
- Antibodies

Functions of the lymphatic system

The lymphatic system has several functions in the body:

- Return excess tissue fluid to the blood.
- Add lymphocytes (white blood cells) to the blood for the immune protection of the body.
- Absorb fats in the lacteals of the villi in the small intestine and carry them to the bloodstream.
- Filter out bacteria and other harmful substances via the nodes.

The lymphatic system is complementary to the blood and circulation system. Between them, they move fluid and other substances through the tissue spaces and help to keep the internal environment of the body within normal limits for healthy functioning (Figures 2.5 and 2.6).

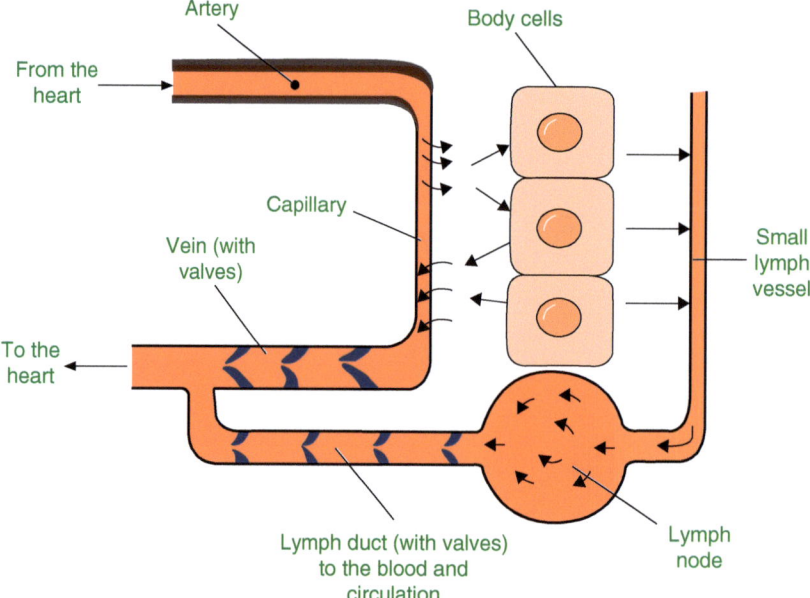

Figure 2.5   Fluid movement from blood to lymph and back to blood.

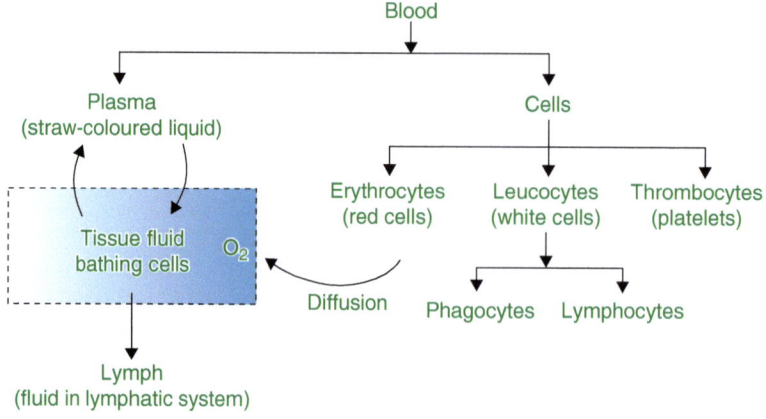

Figure 2.6   Constituents of blood and their functions.

Summary of Movement of Materials

Materials in the body are in constant movement, and this may be via active or passive transport processes.

The key movement processes to be aware of are as follows:

- Diffusion
- Osmosis
- Endocytosis and
- Active transport

The lymphatic system works to maintain the fluid balance in the animal's body and keep it at the right levels for homeostasis to be achieved.

3

Body Systems and Functions

Learning goals

In this chapter, the learning goals are:

- To identify the anatomy and functions of the following systems:
  - Circulatory system
  - Respiratory system
  - Digestive system
  - Urinary system
  - Nervous system
    - ○ Central nervous system
    - ○ Peripheral nervous system
  - Endocrine system
  - Sensory organs
  - Integumentary system
  - Skeletal system
  - Reproductive system
- To define the term homeostasis and explain its importance in the body

The Circulatory System

The circulatory system is a major system of the animal body. It is made up of:

- A pump – the *heart.*
- A circuit of tubes which leave the pump, permeate the body, and return to the pump – these tubes are the *arteries, veins*, and *capillaries.*

For body cells to survive, they need a supply of oxygen and nutrients that is quickly replenished. Waste substances need to be removed swiftly to avoid a toxic build-up in the body. For both of these processes to be achieved, the body needs an active supply and removal system. This is provided by the circulatory system, which is powered by the heart.

The circulatory system connects with all tissues and body cells and transports:

- *Nutrients* – sugars, lipids, amino acids, vitamins, minerals, and salt.
- *Oxygen* and other respiratory gases.

Animal Biology and Care, Fourth Edition. Emily Jewell.
© 2026 John Wiley & Sons Ltd. Published 2026 by John Wiley & Sons Ltd.
Companion Website: https://www.wiley.com/go/animal/biology4e/jewell

- *Hormones* – chemical messages controlling the metabolism, development, and operation of the body.
- *White blood cells* – which provide a defence system for the protection of the body.

It also:

- *Provides a clotting mechanism* – to prevent loss of blood from minor damage to blood vessels.
- *Carries heat* – to and from the cells and tissues depending on their requirements.
- *Removes waste products* – such as carbon dioxide and other nitrogenous waste like urea and creatinine.
- *Carries water* – to replenish the tissues and transport materials in circulation.

Blood vessels

There are several types of blood vessels in the body (Figure 3.1), going from the large vessels of the aorta and vena cava through arterioles, capillaries, and venules.

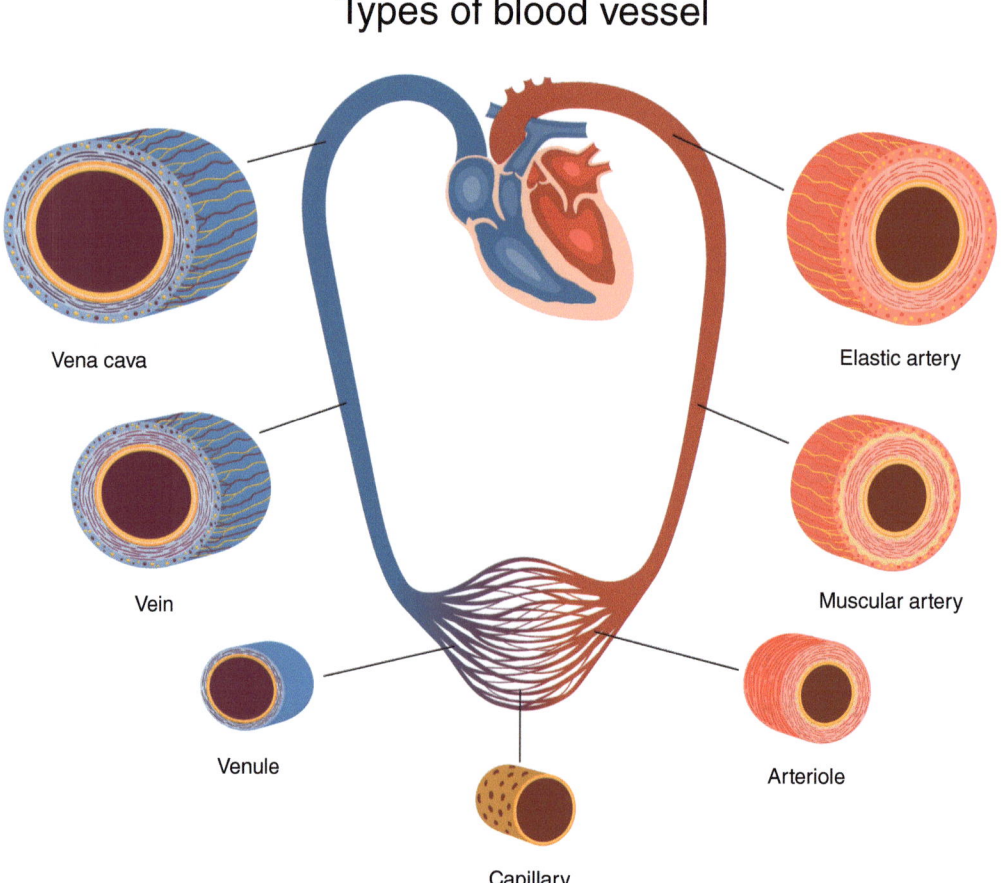

Figure 3.1 Types of blood vessel in the body.

Arteries

- Carry blood away from the heart.
- Carry oxygenated blood (except for the pulmonary artery that carries deoxygenated blood to the lungs).
- Have thick muscular walls to assist with the movement of blood.
- Carry blood under high pressure due to heart muscle contractions.
- Have a narrow *lumen* (the centre channel of the vessel).
- Connective tissue provides strength to the vessel.

Veins

- Carry blood towards the heart.
- Carry deoxygenated blood (except the pulmonary vein from the lungs to the heart).
- Have thin walls (less muscular than arteries).
- Blood moved under low pressure and by the action of surrounding tissues.
- Have a valve system to prevent backflow of the blood (Figure 3.2).
- Have a wide lumen.
- Less connective tissue involved.

Capillaries

- Carry blood from the smaller artery branches to veins.
- Blood movement is slower to allow maximum diffusion of substances across the capillary.
- Only one cell thick.
- Connects all cells and tissues in networks called capillary beds.
- Narrow, may only be wide enough for one blood cell at a time to pass through.

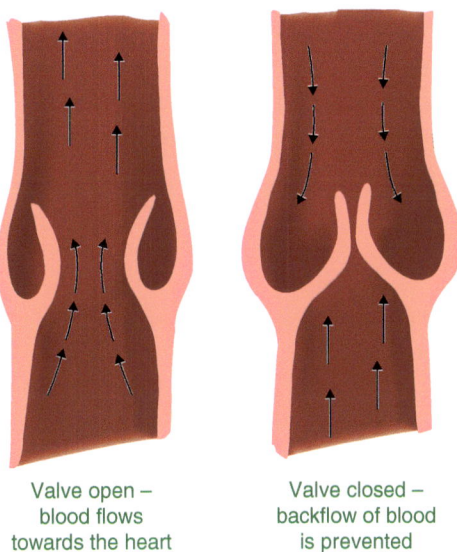

Valve open –
blood flows
towards the heart

Valve closed –
backflow of blood
is prevented

Figure 3.2 Valve system in the veins to prevent backflow of the blood.

Blood vessels have the capability of expanding and contracting according to the requirements of the body. The technical terms associated with this are:

- *Vasodilation*
- *Vasoconstriction*

Blood vessel location names

The more significant larger blood vessels in the body have names. For example, the main artery leaving the left side of the heart is called the *aorta*. Whenever the aorta divides to supply an organ, it takes a *location name* to describe where the blood vessel is in the body. An example of this would be the aortic division to supply the kidney with blood, called the *renal artery*. When blood leaves the kidney, the vessel is called the *renal vein*, and this will rejoin the main collecting vein of the body called the *vena cava*.

Consider where the following blood vessels may be found in the body:

• Cardiac artery	• Hepatic vein
• Pulmonary artery	• Femoral vein
• Carotid artery	• Cephalic vein
• Coronary artery	• Tibial vein

The Mammalian Heart

The heart (Figure 3.3) lies between the two sides of the chest *(thorax)*. It is surrounded by the lungs and held in place by a structure called the *mediastinum*. The heart is comprised of cardiac muscle, which is a specialised type of muscle that differs from other types of muscles in three ways:

1. It is comprised of branching muscle fibres connected to each other in a network. This enables contractions to begin at one point in the heart and spread outwards in all directions.
2. Cardiac muscle contracts and relaxes rhythmically in 'beats'. The rhythm is generated within the muscle itself and not by impulses from the nervous system.
3. Cardiac muscle does not get tired, despite continuous and rapid contractions over many years.

The mammalian heart consists of two pumps fused together, each of which has two chambers:

- Right atrium and right ventricle
- Left atrium and left ventricle

The right side of the heart is less muscular than the left side. The right side is responsible for pumping deoxygenated blood received from the body to the lungs for reoxygenation. The left side of the heart is very muscular and is responsible for pumping oxygenated blood received from the lungs to the body (Figure 3.4). The blood pumped from the left side of the heart is under considerably high pressure and this ensures:

- Fast supply of materials to the cells and tissues
- Pushing of fluid from the circulation into the tissues

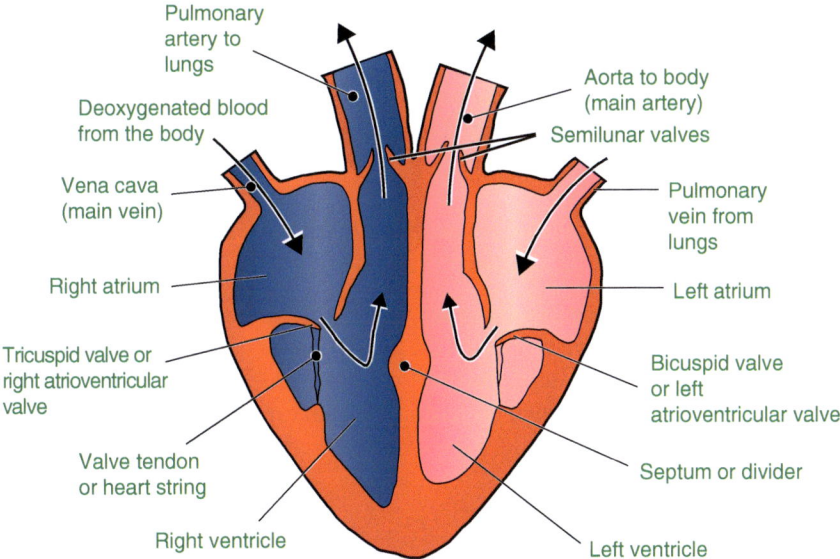

Figure 3.3 The mammalian heart – arrows indicate the direction of blood flow.

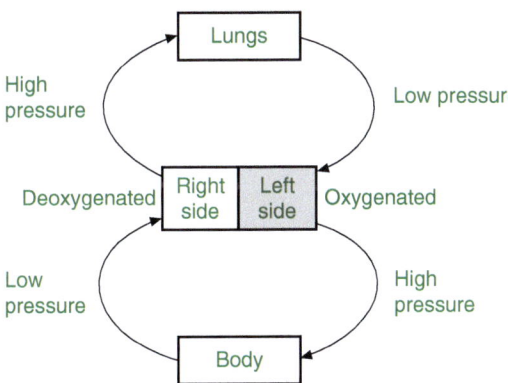

Figure 3.4 The heart pumping system.

The heart is surrounded by a thick fibrous sac called the *pericardium*.

1. Blood enters the heart from the body (systemic circulation) via the great veins (the vena cava, caudal, and cranial vessels).
2. The *right atrium* contracts to fill the *right ventricle*. When the right ventricle contracts, it pushes blood out into the *pulmonary artery* where it is carried to the lungs (deoxygenated blood).
3. After oxygenation of the blood in the lungs, the blood returns via the *pulmonary veins* to the *left atrium*.
4. The left atrium then contracts to pump blood into the *left ventricle*. The left ventricle is the most muscular chamber of the heart and can pump blood around the rest of the body via the *aorta*.

To stop blood flowing backwards (in the wrong direction), there are *valves* located in the heart. On the *right* side of the heart, there are the:

- *Right atrioventricular valve*, also called the tricuspid valve.
- *Semilunar valve*, also called the pulmonary semilunar valve.

And on the *left* side of the heart, there are the:

- *Left atrioventricular valve*, also called the bicuspid or mitral valve.
- *Semilunar valve*, also called aortic semilunar valve.

At the base of the aorta, just above the semilunar valves, are the entrances to the left and right *coronary arteries*, which supply the *myocardium* (the heart muscles). If these vessels become narrowed, due to fatty deposits or cholesterol, this will reduce the blood flow to the heart muscle, causing a lack of oxygen *(ischaemia)* when exercising. This, in turn, could lead to a heart attack, also called a *coronary attack*.

Heartbeat

Most muscles contract once they are stimulated by nerve impulses. Cardiac muscle, however, does not require these nerve impulses. Cardiac muscle beats rhythmically due to signals within its own structure. It has special fibres embedded in the wall of the right atrium called the sinoatrial node (*SA node*) or, more commonly, the *pacemaker* (Figure 3.5). This area also responds to chemicals such as adrenaline to increase the heart rate in situations of flight, fight or fear.

The electrical message from the pacemaker passes to the right and left atrium, causing them to contract in unison. The impulse then arrives at the *atrioventricular (AV) node*, before passing along

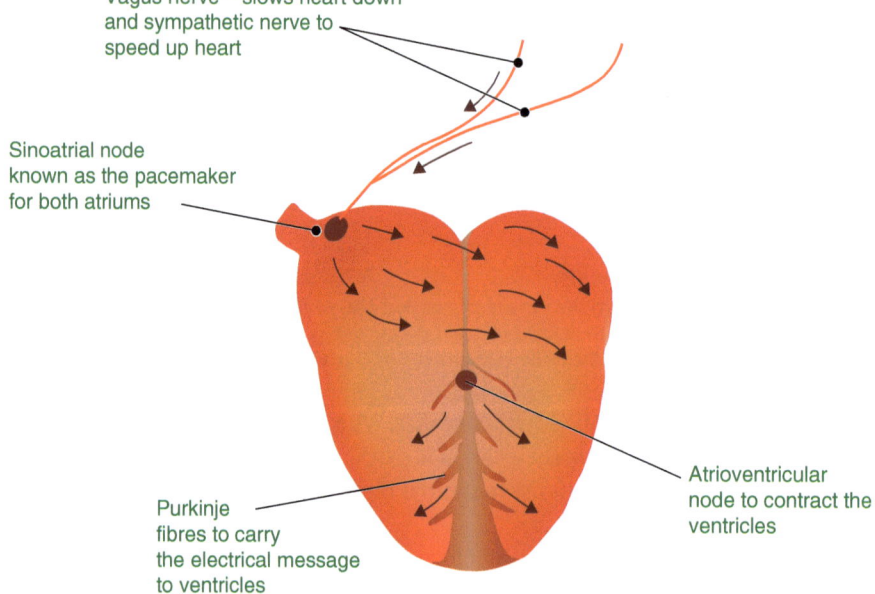

Figure 3.5 Electrical activity during the contraction of the heart (pumping). The rhythm for this is provided by the pacemaker.

Table 3.1 Comparison of heart rate between species.

Heart rate comparison (beats/minute)

Organism	Average rate	Normal range
Human	70	58–104
Cat	120	110–140
Cow	65	60–70
Dog	115	100–130
Ferret	200	180–250
Guinea pig	280	260–400
Hamster	450	300–600
Horse	44	23–70
Rabbit	205	123–304
Rat	328	261–600

Source: Cardiovascular System: The Heart and Vessels of Mammals, Birds, Fish and Amphibians, 2025 / https://www.petcoach.co/article/cardiovascular-system-the-heart-and-vessels-of-mammals-bird/, last accessed on 31 March 2025.

special conducting tissue pathways called the *bundles of His*. These fibres lead to smaller bundles of conducting tissues called *Purkinje fibres*, which cause contraction of the ventricles.

If the pacemaker region of the heart is malfunctioning, the heart rate may fall and not increase with exercise. An animal with this condition will have a slow heart rate with poor exercise tolerance and may faint. Heart rates vary between species (Table 3.1).

Heart sounds

There are two sounds heard when listening to a heart:

- *Lub* and *Dub*

The first sound, *Lub*, is produced by the closure of the right and left atrioventricular valves, as the ventricles begin to contract.

When the valves at the base of the aorta and pulmonary artery (semilunar valves) snap shut at the end of the ventricle contraction, then the second sound, *Dub*, is produced.

If blood within the chest is flowing unevenly or turbulently, a murmur may be detected. This sounds like *Lub–woosh*. The heart and flow of circulation can be seen in Figure 3.6.

Heart structure of non-mammalian species

Avian species have a heart with four chambers like mammals. Their hearts tend to be proportionally larger than that of a mammal, due to the energy demands and oxygen requirements of flight. The heart of a bird also tends to pump more blood than that of a mammal of a similar size.

Reptilian species (except for crocodile species) have a heart with three chambers. The atria are separate, but the ventricles are only partially separated, which means that oxygenated and

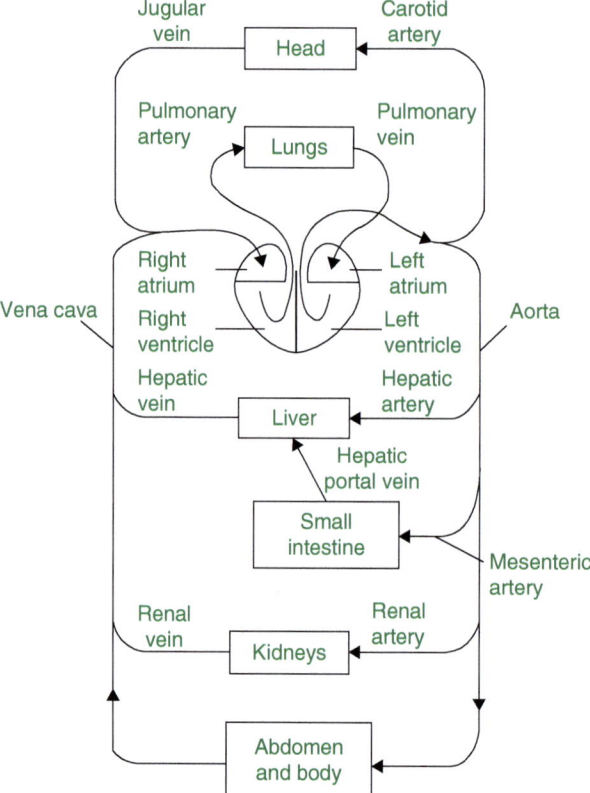

Figure 3.6 Heart and circulation flow.

deoxygenated blood mix in the heart. Reptile hearts also possess two aortas. Reptiles can exist with a three-chambered heart that is less muscular than a mammalian heart due to being *ectothermic* animals. It is important to note that heart structure can vary between reptile species, and this is an ongoing area of scientific investigation.

Amphibian species also have a heart with three chambers (Figure 3.7). Heart rate in amphibians and reptiles is affected by environmental temperature.

Fish have a heart with two chambers – one atrium and one ventricle, which are separated by a simple valve. Blood is pumped from the ventricle to the gills, where the blood is oxygenated (Figure 3.8). The blood is then transported to the remainder of the body before returning to the atrium. Heart rate in fish is affected by water temperature.

Summary of the Circulatory System

This essential system consists of:

- The heart (cardiac muscle which is self-innervating).
- Different types of blood vessels that travel from the pump, through the body and return to the pump.
- Blood vessels that take blood from the heart are called arteries.
- Blood vessels that return blood to the heart are called veins.
- Capillaries are a network of vessels reaching all cells of the body.

The circulatory system works to:

- Transport respiratory gases, hormones, nutrients, and water around the body.
- Maintain heat in the body.
- Respond to other body systems according to the animal's activity levels.

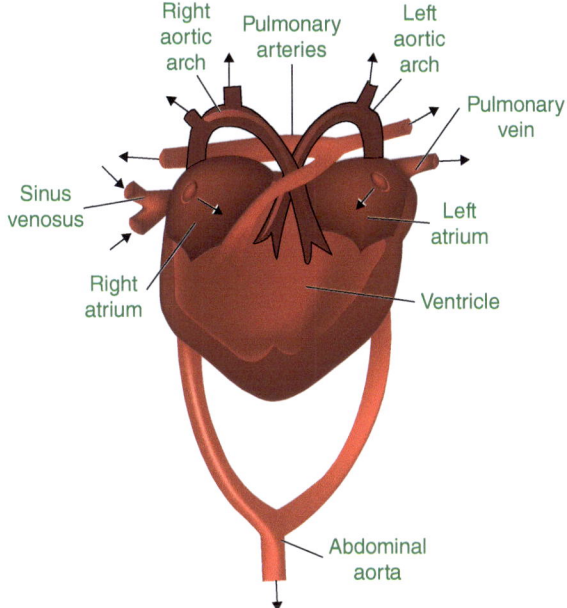

Figure 3.7 Amphibian heart. *Source*: Adapted from http://www.peteducation.com/article.
cfm?c=16+2160&aid=2951, accessed 13 March 2014. Reproduced with permission of Foster and Smith, Inc.

This link has been updated to: https://www.petcoach.co/article/cardiovascular-system-the-heart-and-vessels-of -
mammals-bird/, accessed 30 October 2024.

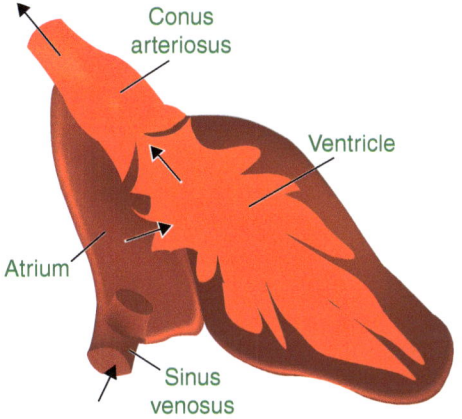

Figure 3.8 Fish heart. *Source*: Adapted from http://www.peteducation.com/article.
cfm?c=16+2160&aid=2951, accessed 13 March 2014. Reproduced with permission of Foster and Smith, Inc.

This link has been updated to: https://www.petcoach.co/article/cardiovascular-system-the-heart-and-vessels-of -
mammals-bird/, accessed 30 October 2024.

Anatomy of heart in vertebrates

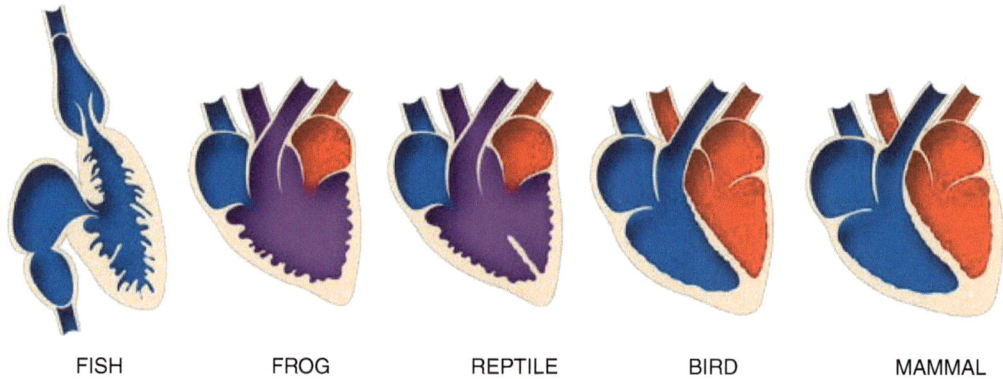

FISH   FROG   REPTILE   BIRD   MAMMAL

Figure 3.9   Comparative image of vertebrate hearts. *Source*: Adobe Stock photo #543457187.
https://stock.adobe.com/uk/images/comparative-anatomy-of-heart-in-vertebrates-
diagram/543457187?prev_url=detail - accessed 30th October 2024

The Respiratory System

The respiratory system is the term given to the organs of the body that allow *gaseous exchange* to occur between a living organism and its environment. In animals, this usually involves taking oxygen into the body and releasing carbon dioxide as a waste product. The process of gaseous exchange in an animal occurs in the *alveoli*.

Structures through which the oxygen and carbon dioxide must pass in a mammal are:

- *External nares* – nose
- *Turbinate bones* – scroll-shaped tubes with epithelial lining in nasal chambers
- *Nasopharynx* – back of the throat
- *Larynx* – voice box
- *Trachea* – open tube for passage of gases only
- *Bronchus* – branching of the trachea to the two sides of the chest (thorax)
- *Bronchioles* – further branching, getting smaller in diameter
- *Alveoli* – air sacs
- Blood capillaries of the pulmonary system
- Tissue cells around the body

Characteristics of respiratory surfaces

A respiratory surface is one where *gaseous exchange* occurs. They enable oxygen and carbon dioxide to be exchanged rapidly between an organism and the air surrounding it. Respiratory surfaces must have certain features for gaseous exchange to be effective and efficient:

- A *large surface area* to ensure maximum contact with the inhaled air. A mammal's respiratory surface consists of millions of tiny bubble-like air sacs called *alveoli*.
- All respiratory surfaces are *moist*. This is necessary because oxygen and carbon dioxide can only diffuse in solution across a respiratory surface (alveoli to blood vessel).

- A respiratory surface is very *thin* – only one cell thick for diffusion to take place.
- The inner layer of the respiratory surface is *in contact with a network of capillary blood vessels* to allow gas exchange to take place between the blood and gases.
- In many species of animals, a respiratory surface is usually *well ventilated*, in that it receives a steady flow of air. Breathing movements increase the rate of gas exchange by continually removing carbon dioxide and renewing supplies of oxygen to the tissue cells.

The role of breathing and the circulatory system

The respiratory and circulatory systems determine how much oxygen and carbon dioxide are present in the body at any given moment. They work together to ensure that a balance is maintained of both gases within the body. If the amount of oxygen in the blood is low and carbon dioxide high, the body responds by increasing:

- The rate and depth of breathing – *ventilation rate.*
- The rate at which the heart beats – *cardiac frequency.*
- The diameter of the arterioles serving those structures that are short of oxygen – *vasodilation.*

The respiratory organs of mammals

Most of the respiratory organs of animals are contained within the head and thoracic cavity – also known as thorax or chest:

- *Nasal passages* (found in the head)
- *Pharynx* and *larynx*
- *Trachea*
- *Lungs*
- Major blood vessels (indicated by the term *pulmonary*)
- Lymph ducts
- Major nerves

The walls of the thorax are strengthened by the *ribs* (skeletal system), and caudally (towards the tail), there is a sheet of muscle called the *diaphragm*.

The upper respiratory tract

A system of passageways leads from the mouth and nostrils into the lungs and are referred to as the upper respiratory tract (Figure 3.10).

The nasal passages

The nasal passages are where air enters the body and is warmed to body temperature. The membranes covering the nasal passages also contain the organs responsible for the sense of smell. The walls and base of the nasal passages are lined with a carpet of microscopic hair-like structures called *cilia*. The cilia extend down the trachea to create a surface of moving hairs beating in an upward manner. They help to expel *mucus*, which contains dust and micro-organisms which are trapped in this thickened liquid. The *turbinate bones* give structure to the nasal passages.

Air is drawn out of the nasal passages into the *pharynx* at the back of the mouth. From here, air is drawn into the *trachea* via the *larynx* and past the *vocal cords* to activate the voice of the animal.

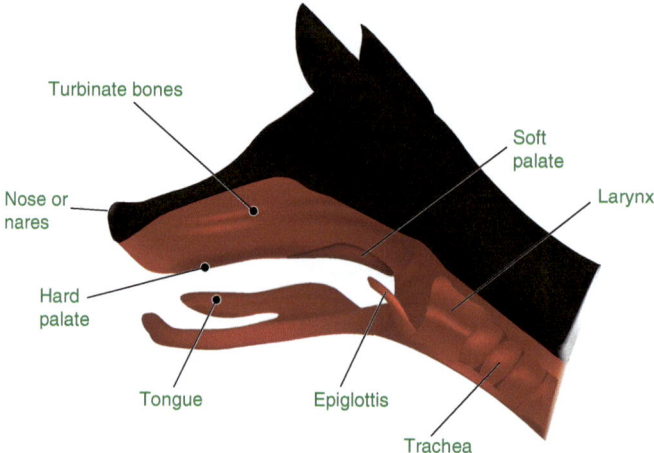

Figure 3.10 Upper respiratory tract.

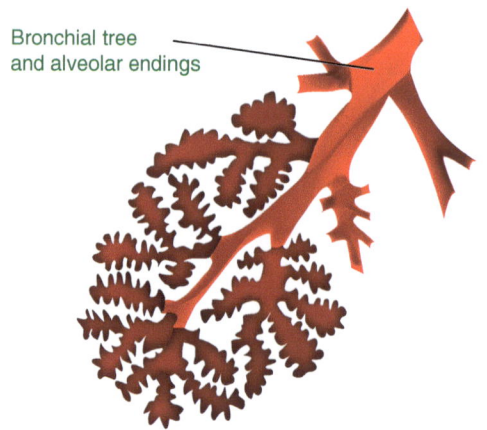

Figure 3.11 Lung tissue.

The bronchial tree

The trachea delivers the air breathed into the body to the lungs. On reaching the lungs, the trachea branches to supply the lung tissue on both sides of the thorax. Each initial division feeding from the trachea into the lungs is known as a *bronchus* (collectively known as the *bronchi*) (Figure 3.11). The bronchi will further divide many times to form a mass of fine branches called the *bronchioles* and so form a *bronchial tree*. Inflammation of the bronchi is known as *bronchitis*, and inflammation of the bronchioles is known as *bronchiolitis*.

The alveolar ducts

At the end of the bronchioles are structures called *air sacs* or *alveoli* (Figure 3.12) where the process of gaseous exchange occurs. The alveoli are the respiratory surface of the lungs and give lung tissue its spongy appearance. The outer surface of the alveoli is covered by a dense network of capillary blood vessels. All these capillaries originate from the *pulmonary artery* (deoxygenated blood) and drain into the *pulmonary vein* (oxygenated blood) to return to the left side of the heart, for pumping around the body.

Gas exchange in the lungs

Blood entering the lungs is deoxygenated because it has already travelled around the body, and the *haemoglobin* (red pigment) in its red cells has given up all its oxygen to the body tissues.

The internal diameter of the lung capillaries is smaller than the diameter of the red cells which pass through them. The red cells are squeezed out of shape as they are forced through the lungs by blood pressure and the speed at which they move is considerably reduced by the resulting friction. This increases the rate of oxygen absorption in two ways:

1. As the red cells squeeze through the narrow capillaries, they expose more surface area to the capillary walls, through which oxygen is diffusing and absorbed.
2. Their slow rate of progress increases the time available for oxygen to diffuse into the vessels and combine with haemoglobin.

The continuous removal of oxygen as fast as it diffuses into the lung capillaries and the continuous arrival of oxygen in the alveoli owing to breathing movements mean that there is always a higher concentration of oxygen molecules in the alveoli than in the blood. As a result of this, carbon dioxide is exchanged (Figure 3.13).

Breathing: ventilation of the lungs

The *pleural cavity* in the thorax is completely airtight and contains a partial vacuum. Its internal pressure is always less than the atmospheric pressure outside the body. The lungs are open to the atmosphere through the trachea, and therefore, there is always a higher

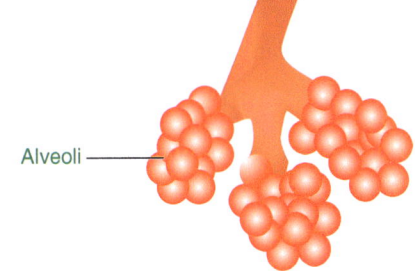

Alveoli

Figure 3.12 Alveoli.

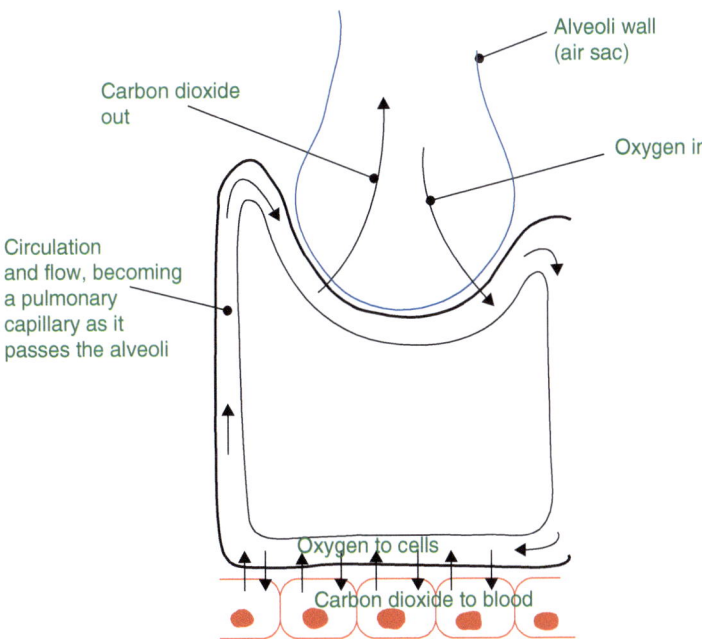

Carbon dioxide out

Alveoli wall (air sac)

Oxygen in

Circulation and flow, becoming a pulmonary capillary as it passes the alveoli

Oxygen to cells

Carbon dioxide to blood

Figure 3.13 Gas exchange between the alveoli and the blood and between the blood and body cells.

pressure in the lungs than in the thorax or pleural cavity which surrounds them. This pressure difference is extremely important for two reasons:

1. The higher pressure in the lungs in relation to the *pleural cavity* around them stretches the thin elastic alveoli walls so that the lungs almost fill the thorax on *inspiration.*
2. Since this pressure difference is maintained during breathing movements, when the thoracic cavity increases in size (inspiration), the lungs inflate to fill the extra space available.

At normal atmospheric pressure, this process could not happen; hence, there is a need for negative pressure in the thorax.

The muscles that bring about these volume changes are as follows:

- The *diaphragm* – a dome-shaped sheet of muscle, which separates the thorax from the abdomen.
- The *intercostal muscles* – both internal and external, which cross the gap between each rib and pull the ribs outwards on inspiration (Figure 3.14).

Diaphragm

Immediately before inspiration, the diaphragm is dome shaped and its muscle relaxed. Inspiration takes place when the diaphragm muscle contracts, making the muscle sheet a flatter shape.

Ribs

At the same time, contraction occurs in the external intercostal muscles between each rib. This increases the size of the rib cage, leading to an increase in lung volume:

- *Inspiration* – the movement of the diaphragm and external intercostal muscles, causing the ribs to move visibly outwards.
- *Expiration* – or breathing out is when the diaphragm and external intercostal muscles relax. This reduces the size of the thorax and the ribs move inwards to the resting position.

Air can be forced out of the lungs by contraction of the internal intercostal muscles, but expiration tends to be passive, simply allowing these structures to fall back into the resting position.

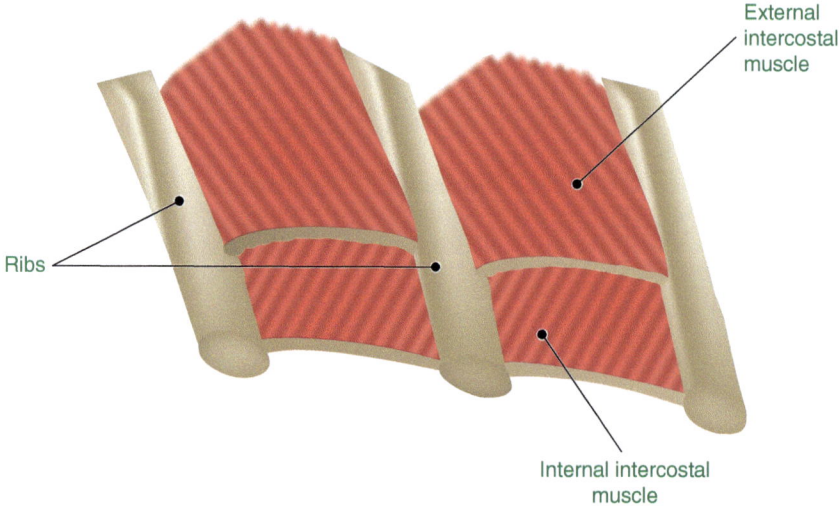

External intercostal muscle

Ribs

Internal intercostal muscle

Figure 3.14 Intercostal muscles and ribs for breathing.

Respiration

The word 'respiration' is derived from the Latin *respirare* which means 'to breathe'. At first, this term referred to the breathing movements which cause air to be drawn into and pushed out of the lungs, hence where the respiratory system obtained its name from. Now, when defined with strict accuracy, the term respiration refers to an entirely different process.

The modern definition of respiration

Respiration is the processes which lead to, and include, the chemical breakdown of materials to provide energy for life. These processes occur inside the living cells of every type of organism and cause the release of energy from food, which is essential for life.

Cells cannot use energy as soon as it is released from respiration. This energy is first used to build up a temporary energy store, which takes the form of a chemical called *adenosine triphosphate* (ATP) for short. Think of ATP as 'packets' of power used to transfer energy from the chemical reactions which release it to the body processes which use it. Respiration fills these ATP packets with energy, and they are 'emptied' when energy is needed anywhere in the body.

There are four main advantages to the ATP energy transfer system:

1. ATP takes up some energy, which would otherwise be lost as heat during the breakdown of glucose by respiratory enzymes.
2. Energy is released from ATP the instant it is required without cells having to go through the many different reactions of respiration, allowing for sudden bursts of energy.
3. ATP delivers energy in precise amounts.
4. Energy can be delivered from ATP to other chemicals without energy loss, for example, from sources of sugars, fats, or proteins.

The release of energy at the cellular level is known as the *Krebs cycle*, which takes place in mitochondria.

Respiratory system in birds

Respiration in birds is much different than in mammals, mainly because the respiratory system in birds has additional structures (Figure 3.15):

- An organ known as the *syrinx* replaces the voice box. Birds do have a larynx, but it is not used for making sounds.
- As well as lungs, birds have additional unique structures called *air sacs*. There can be seven or nine air sacs, depending on the species of bird. The air sacs are located throughout the body cavity of the bird. The cervical air sacs are not present in some species.
- The air sacs of birds replace the diaphragm. Pressure changes in the air sacs cause air to flow through the respiratory system of the bird. Muscular contractions in the chest area cause the *sternum* to be pushed out, and so air enters the respiratory system. Further muscle contraction causes air to be exhaled from the bird. It is therefore important not to hold a bird too tightly during handling; otherwise, its respiratory system could be affected.
- Gas exchange occurs in the *air capillaries* rather than in alveoli.
- A bird's respiratory system is more efficient than a mammalian one as more oxygen is released and exchanged with each breath, which is beneficial to sustain flight.

Respiratory system in reptiles

The structure of the respiratory system in reptiles is like that of mammals, but the mechanics of the process vary between different reptile groups. Some groups have a diaphragm; some groups don't.

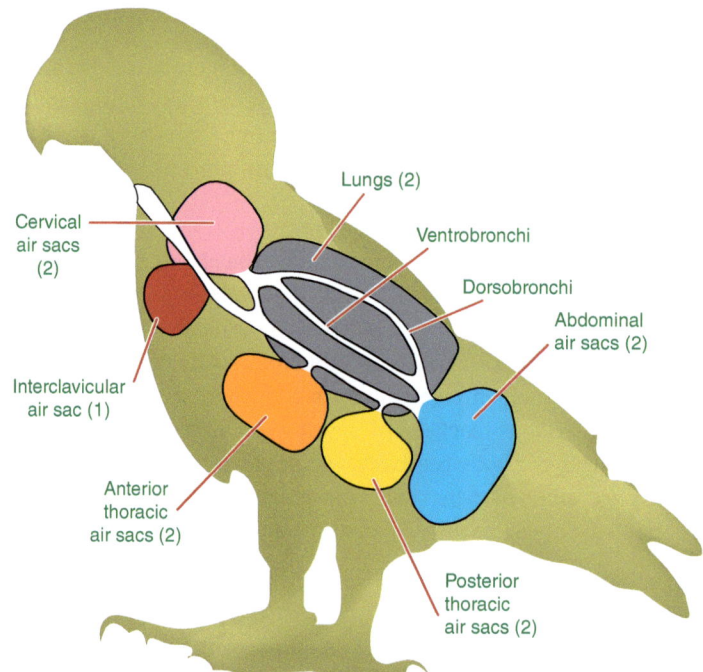

Figure 3.15 Respiratory system of a bird. *Source*: Adapted from PetCoach, 2025, http://www.peteducation.com/article.cfm?c=15+1829&aid=2721, accessed 13 March 2014.

This link has been updated to: https://www.petcoach.co/article/respiratory-system-of-birds-anatomy-and-function/, accessed 30 October 2024.

Some draw air into their body through the movement of their limbs, but others have additional processes to aid breathing. Some hold their breath while locomotion occurs, but others do not. Further research is occurring in this area of study.

Respiratory system in amphibians

Gaseous exchange can occur in amphibians in three different ways:

- Through the lungs
- Through the gills
- Through the skin

Structurally, most amphibians do not have a diaphragm. Gas exchange does not occur through alveoli as amphibian lungs are like the air sacs of birds. Amphibians do not have a regular respiratory rate; they tend to breathe as and when they need more oxygen (Figure 3.16).

Amphibian skin allows water through as it is very thin. Just as water can be absorbed through the skin, so can oxygen. During their larval stages, amphibians acquire oxygen through their gills.

Respiratory system in fish

Respiration in fish is achieved via their *gills*. Gills contain *gill filaments* to increase the surface area for gas exchange (Figure 3.17). A good capillary supply serves the gills and allows the efficient absorption of oxygen into the bloodstream. The gills are kept moist (as needed in a respiratory surface) by the water that surrounds the fish.

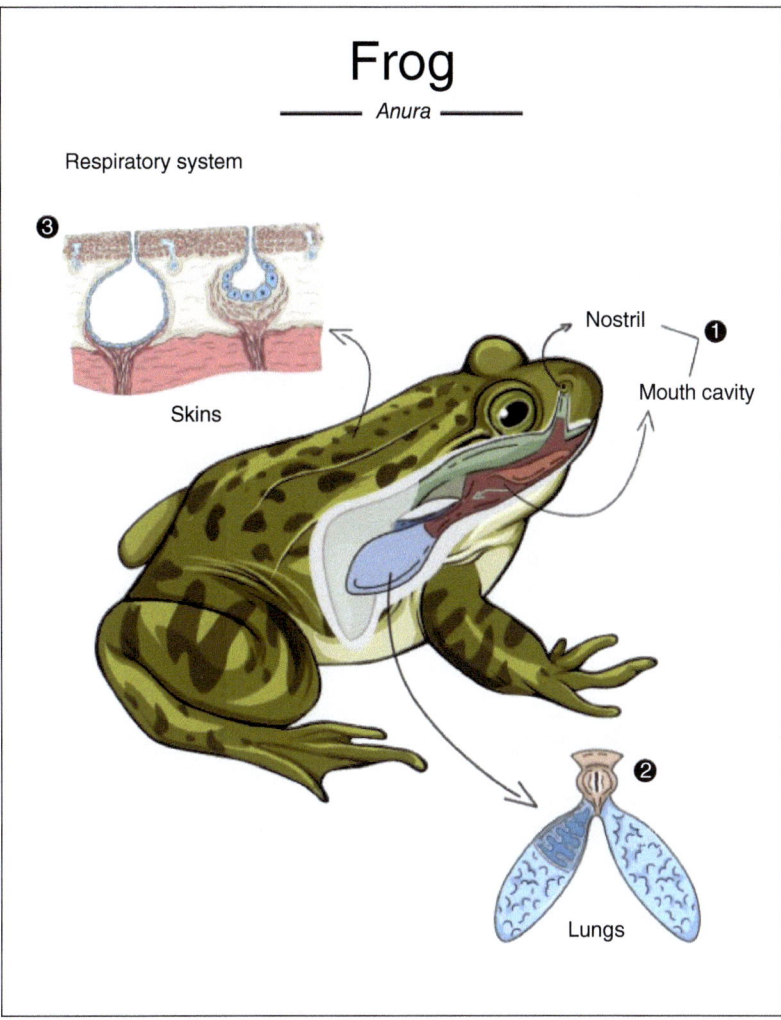

Figure 3.16   Respiratory system of an amphibian.

Bony fish possess an additional structure known as the *operculum*, which protects the gills. As water is taken into the mouth of the fish, the fish moves its mouth to pump water through the gills, and therefore, the oxygen that is dissolved in the water is absorbed across the gills into the bloodstream of the fish.

Carbon dioxide is also released through the gills.

Summary of the respiratory system

This essential system consists of:

- The nasal passages.
- The trachea, bronchi, and bronchial tree that end in the alveoli.
- Associated muscles that assist with the breathing process.

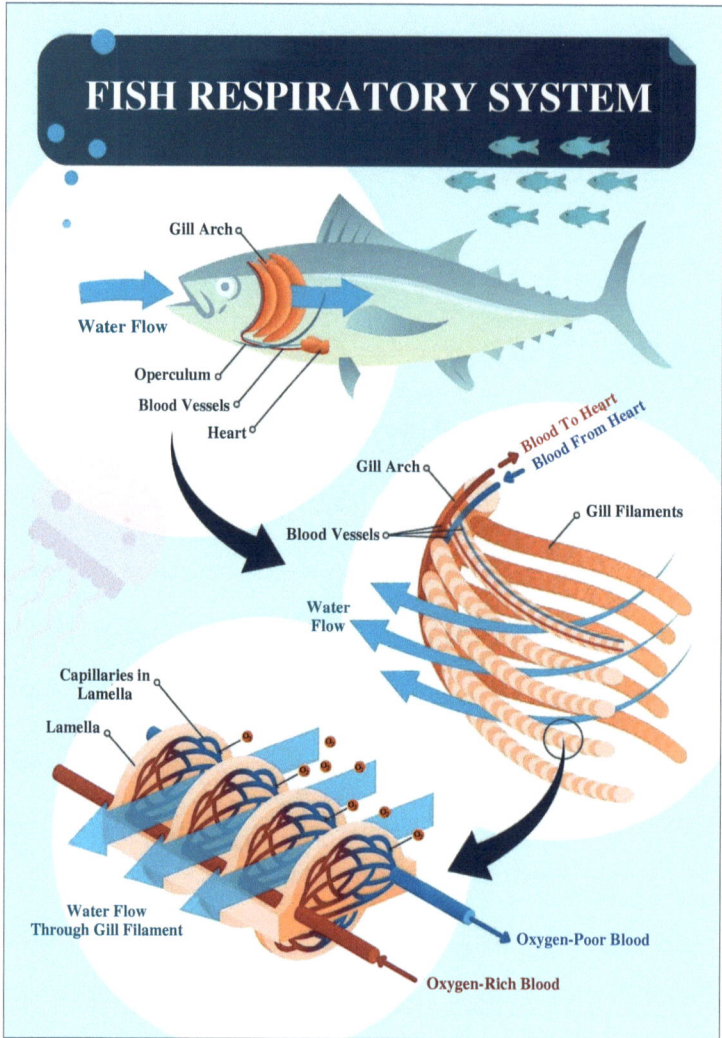

Figure 3.17 Respiratory system of fish.

The respiratory system works to:

- Transport respiratory gases around the body.
- Respond to other body systems according to the animal's activity levels – for example, breather faster when undertaking exercise in response to the muscle requirements for more oxygen.

The word *pulmonary* is linked to the respiratory system.

The Digestive System

Animals can make full use of the food they eat once it has passed through its digestive system (Figure 3.18). The digestive system may also be called the alimentary canal. The digestive system is basically a continuous tube that starts at the mouth and ends at the anus of the species with the different regions

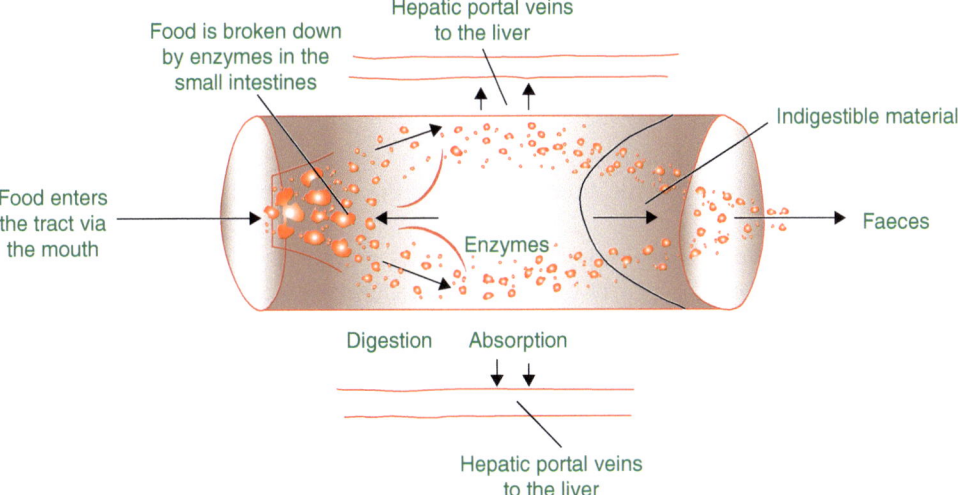

Figure 3.18 Digestive tract process.

along its length performing different functions. Food is carried through the tube and the nutrients are extracted and absorbed leaving the waste products to be excreted from the body. Nutrient extraction and absorption are enhanced via the presence of digestive enzymes and the presence of naturally occurring bacterial species often referred 'gut flora'. Smooth muscle assists with the movement of food along the tube in a peristaltic action as mentioned in Chapter 1. Technically, digestion occurs outside of the cells of the body and its end products are absorbed into the cells for use. Imagine the body as a donut with the centre hole being the digestive tract and the external perimeter being the skin of the animal.

At the start of the digestive system, whole food is reduced into smaller pieces through a chewing/tearing/crushing process (*mastication*) so that they can be easily swallowed. Digestive enzymes released into the mouth via *saliva* aid the process of digestion at this point.

These smaller pieces of food are swallowed from the mouth into the *oesophagus* where they travel towards the stomach to continue the digestive process. The swallowed food is now called a *food bolus*. The oesophagus does not secrete any digestive enzymes, only mucus to lubricate the movement of the food bolus down the tract.

Having entered the stomach, the bolus is mixed with hydrochloric acid and more digestive enzymes (*chemical digestion*). The stomach also contracts and squeezes its contents to help with breakdown of the bolus (*mechanical digestion*). By the time the bolus exits the stomach, the components exist as a partially digested liquid called *chyme*, which then progresses into the small intestine. Please note that some species have more than one stomach compartment, e.g. camelids and ruminants.

Further digestion continues in the *small intestine* (comprised of three parts: the *duodenum*, the *jejunum*, and the *ileum*) where the soluble nutrients pass through the walls of the intestine into the bloodstream. This process is called *absorption*. The presence of *villi* in the small intestine increases the surface area available for the absorption of nutrients.

Blood transports the digested, soluble food to all parts of the body requiring the nutrients. The nutrients enter the cells and are metabolised into useful products. This process is called *assimilation*.

Any solid substances in food that cannot be digested, such as fibre, progress through into the *large intestine*, where water is absorbed from them and the resulting waste is expelled from the body as *faecal matter* or *faeces*.

The control of digestion of food is both voluntary and involuntary:

- Voluntary
    - **i.** *Ingestion* – placing in mouth
    - **ii.** Chewing (*mastication*)
    - **iii.** Swallowing (*deglutition*)
    - **iv.** Control of anal sphincter – the muscle controlling the opening and closing of the anus
- Involuntary
    - **v.** *Opening and closing of sphincters in the digestive system*
    - **vi.** Peristaltic movement (a ripple or wave of muscle) squeezing the food through the gut
    - **vii.** Release of digestive enzymes

Digestion of food

Digestive processes exist because most foods that animals eat cannot be used in their original form for two main reasons:

1. Most foods are insoluble and so cannot pass through semi-permeable cell membranes into cells.
2. Most foods are chemically different, and therefore, they must be broken down (chemically and physically) and processed by the body before the end products can be metabolised by cells.

Digestive enzymes

All enzymes, whether digestive or belonging to another body system, are *catalysts*. They speed up chemical reactions, which would otherwise happen very slowly. Digestive enzymes are just one example of the many types of enzymes that exist in living animals. The reactions which these enzymes speed up involves the splitting of complicated molecules into simpler ones (Table 3.2).

Enzymes combine briefly with food molecules that undergo a rapid chemical change to split the molecules apart into chemically simpler substances. These substances separate from the enzyme, leaving it immediately available for another identical reaction. Enzymes are not used up in the reactions which they control but are used countless times in rapid succession. The efficiency of the enzymes can be affected by the body's internal environment and is temperature sensitive.

Table 3.2 Enzymes of the digestive tract.

Secretion	Source	Site of action	Enzyme	Acting on
Saliva	Salivary gland	Mouth	Water and mucus	All foods
Gastric juice	Stomach	Stomach	Gastrin, pepsin	Protein
Bile	Liver	Duodenum (SI)	Bile salt	Fats
Pancreatic juice	Pancreas	Duodenum[a] (SI)	Amylase	Starch
			Trypsin	Protein
			Lipase	Fats
Intestinal juice	Intestine wall	Small intestine	Amylase	Starch

[a]The cells in the duodenum release the hormone enterokinase, which activates the pancreatic enzymes only when they reach the small intestine. Otherwise, the pancreas would be damaged/digested by these enzymes.

Comparative digestive anatomy

Anatomically, different species of mammals are grouped according to their digestive anatomy (Figures 3.19 and 3.20):

- Ruminants/polygastric animals (cattle, sheep, camelids).
- Monogastric/simple-stomached animals (e.g. dog, cat, pigs, ferrets, and humans).
- Avian (all birds).
- Hindgut fermenters (e.g. horses and rabbits).

Other groupings also exist that refer to the type of food eaten:

- *Carnivores* – meat eating
- *Omnivores* – eat both meat and plant matter
- *Herbivores* – plant eating
- *Granivores* – grain eating
- *Piscivore* – fish eating
- *Frugivore* – fruit eating

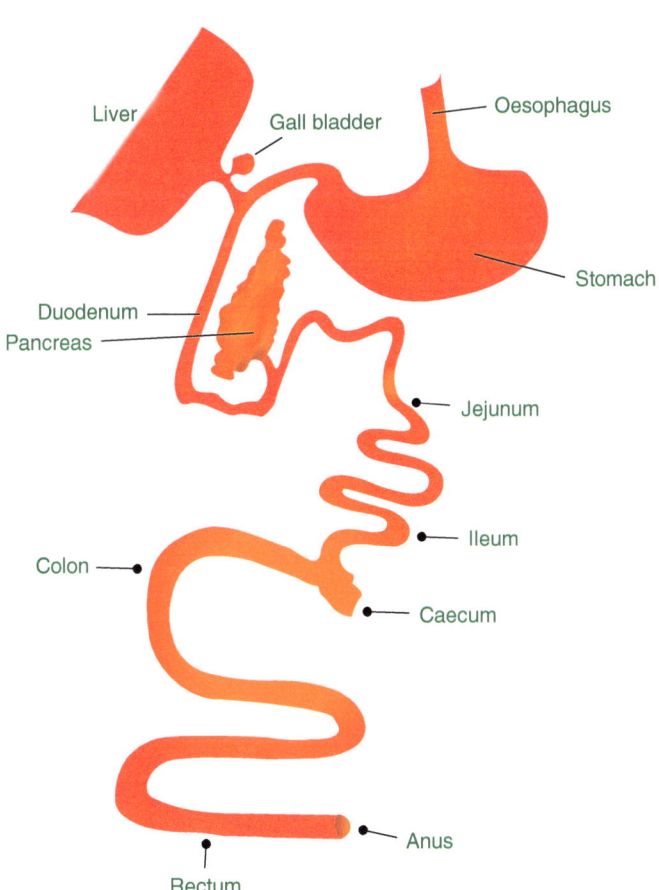

Figure 3.19   Monogastric digestive anatomy, e.g. dog, cat, pig, and human.

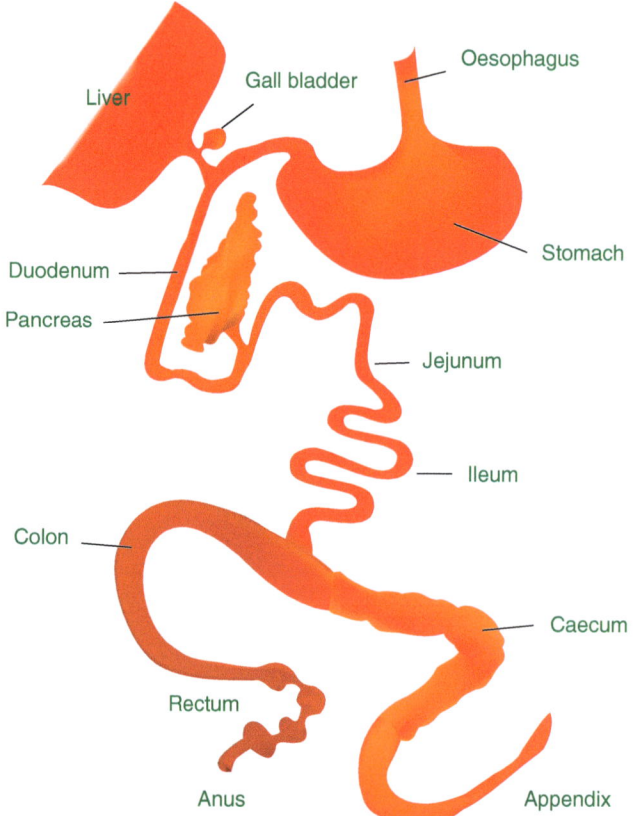

Figure 3.20 Rabbit digestive tract showing enlarged caecum and appendix. New food is mixed with soft caecal pellets, which are eaten by the rabbit from its own anus (*coprophagia*).

Monogastric digestive tract

The key parts of the monogastric digestive tract are:

- Mouth
- Pharynx
- Oesophagus
- Stomach
- Small intestines
- Duodenum
- Jejunum
- Ileum
- Large intestines
- Caecum
- Ascending colon
- Transverse colon
- Descending colon
- Rectum
- Anal canal

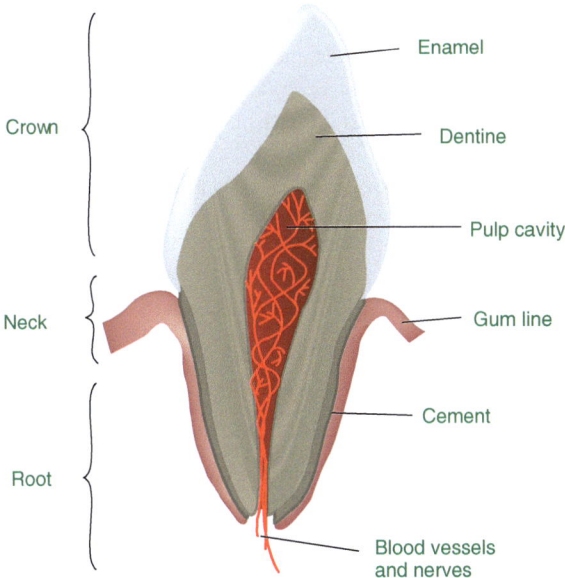

Figure 3.21 Structure of the basic tooth.

The mouth

The mouth is also called the *oral or buccal cavity* and contains the tongue, teeth, and salivary glands. The teeth are responsible for grinding, crushing, or tearing up the food, and with the aid of the tongue and saliva, the food is mixed into a *food bolus*. Saliva is supplied from four glands located around the face. Saliva is usually present in the mouth, but its flow is increased by the sight and smell of food. This effect is known as a *gustatory response*. Saliva is made of water with about 1% of it being mucus, electrolytes (salts), and enzymes. The mucus acts as a lubricant and helps in the swallowing of the food bolus.

The *tongue* helps to move the bolus. The tongue is a mass of striated muscle fibres. It is a sensitive structure with some taste buds on its surface. In animals such as cats, the tongue has the additional function of helping to groom the fur and keep the coat in good condition.

Common to the digestive and respiratory systems is the *pharynx* area. There are lymphoid areas in the mucous membrane of this area called *tonsils*.

Dentition

Dentition of an animal reflects its prevalent diet, but the basic tooth structure is the same (Figure 3.21), even if the overall shape differs. The layout of the teeth in an animal's mouth is known as its *dentition*, and the types of teeth present can be represented by a *dental formula*.

Types of teeth

There are several different types of teeth in the animal mouth, each with a different purpose:

Incisors	Chisel-shaped teeth found at the front of the mouth	Cutting, biting, gnawing, tearing
Canines	Long, pointed teeth found behind the incisors. Also called fangs.	Tearing and ripping

(Continued)

(Continued)

Premolars	Teeth found between the canines and molars.	Chewing and grinding food
Molars	Large, flat teeth found at the back of the mouth.	Chewing & grinding food
Carnassials	Found in carnivore species at the side of the mouth as adapted premolar/molar teeth.	Shear food from bone

Dental formula

The dental formula is used to indicate the different types of teeth in the mouth and the number that should be present at a certain stage of life in a species.

Dog	Deciduous or milk teeth $-I\frac{3}{3}C\frac{1}{1}PM\frac{3}{3}=$ Total 28
	Permanent or adult teeth $-I\frac{3}{3}C\frac{1}{1}PM\frac{4}{4}M\frac{2}{3}=$ Total 42
Cat	Deciduous $-I\frac{3}{3}C\frac{1}{1}PM\frac{3}{2}=$ Total 26
	Permanent $-I\frac{3}{3}C\frac{1}{1}PM\frac{3}{2}M\frac{1}{1}=$ Total 30
Rabbit	Open rooted $-I\frac{2}{1}C\frac{0}{0}PM\frac{3}{2}M\frac{3}{3}=$ Total 14

Figure 3.22 shows the variation in skulls and dentition of different species.

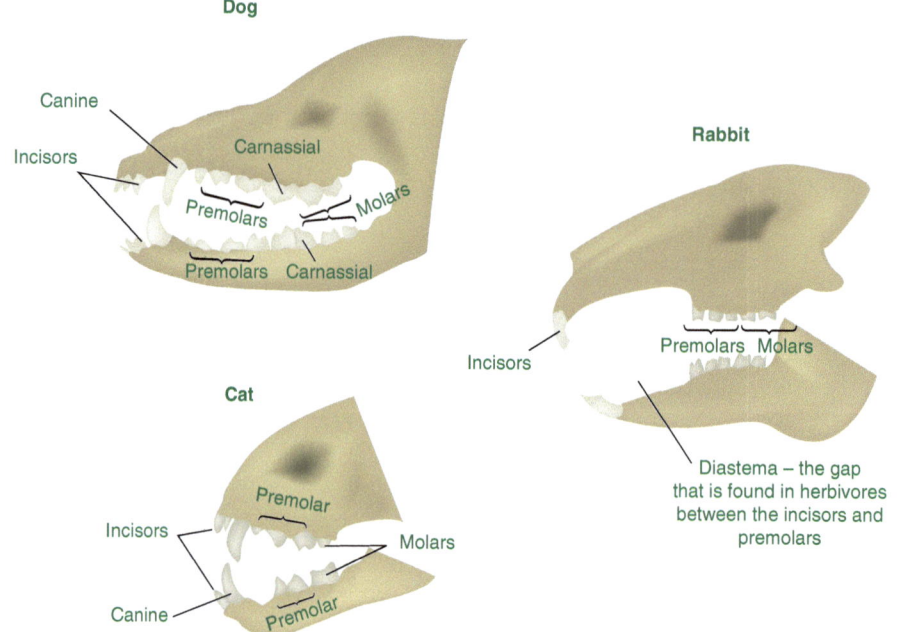

Figure 3.22 Dentition variation in animals.

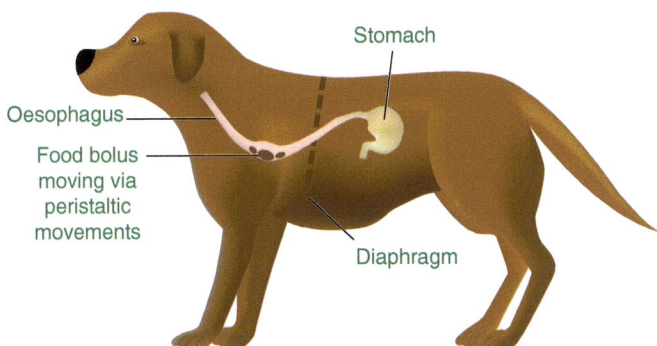

Figure 3.23 Oesophagus and stomach showing food being moved by peristalsis.

The oesophagus

The food bolus is moved into the oesophagus by the pharyngeal muscles. The swallowing process is now complete. No digestive enzymes are secreted here, but oesophageal cells produce mucus to lubricate the process of peristalsis, the wave-like contraction and relaxation that propels the food along the tract (Figure 3.23). These contractions are stimulated by the presence of food.

The stomach

The oesophagus meets the stomach at a ring of muscle called the *cardiac sphincter*. The stomach can adapt its size according to the quantity of food eaten as it fulfils its role as a temporary storage reservoir. Some chemical digestion occurs in the stomach due to the presence of gastric juices comprised of enzymes and hydrochloric acid. Mechanical digestion occurs in the stomach through churning and contraction of the smooth muscle in the stomach walls. The partially digested substance that leaves the stomach is known as *chyme* and it moves through the *pyloric sphincter* into the first part of the small intestine called the duodenum.

The small intestines

The small intestines are narrow tubes (hence their name) located between the stomach and the large intestine. The small intestines are frequently long in length. Chemical digestion via enzymes is completed in the small intestines.

Chyme is mixed with more enzymes in the *duodenum*. Some of these enzymes will originate from the duodenum and others from the *pancreas* (its exocrine function). The *liver* also secretes a digestive fluid into the duodenum via the *gall bladder*; this fluid is ducted into the small intestine to reduce the size of fatty acid molecules and is called *bile*. The alkaline bile helps by emulsifying fats and neutralising the acidic stomach fluids.

The *jejunum* is the second section of the small intestines, and it continues the mixing and exposing of the chyme to the fluids that reduce it sufficiently for absorption.

The third section of the small intestines is the *ileum*, where the digestive processes are completed. Following travel through the small intestines:

- Proteins are converted to amino acids.
- Fats are converted to fatty acids + glycerol.
- Carbohydrates are converted to simple sugars.

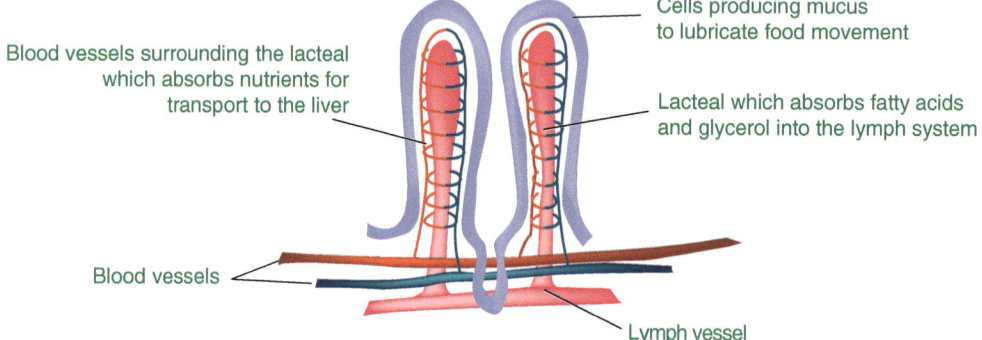

Cells producing mucus to lubricate food movement

Blood vessels surrounding the lacteal which absorbs nutrients for transport to the liver

Lacteal which absorbs fatty acids and glycerol into the lymph system

Blood vessels

Lymph vessel

Figure 3.24   The villi.

Digestion and absorption are improved by the increased surface area in the small intestine, which is due to:

- The length of the small intestines.
- The presence of folds of tissue, increasing the surface area.
- The presence and arrangement of finger-like projections called villi.
- The great number of villi on the surface of the small intestine, particularly in the final area, the ileum, for maximum absorption of nutrients.

Absorption. This takes place via the villi (Figure 3.24). They contain smooth muscle, which allows them to contract and expand. This action brings them into contact with the newly digested food. Simple sugars (mainly glucose) and amino acids are absorbed by a combination of diffusion and active transport across the epithelial lining of the villi into the waiting capillaries beneath. These capillaries drain into the hepatic portal vein, which leads to the liver.

Fat is dealt with differently. The fatty acids and glycerol are absorbed into the columnar epithelial cells lining the villi and are pushed into the lymph vessels of the villi as a white emulsion of tiny globules of fat. These globules give the lymph vessels a milky appearance, and therefore, they are known as *lacteals*. The lymph system finally opens into the veins in the thorax and empties via the thoracic *duct* into the vena cava near the heart.

Mineral salts, vitamins, and water are also absorbed in the small intestine.

The caecum
The first part of the large intestines is called the *caecum*. It is a blind-ended sac, which has no function in carnivores but is enlarged in herbivores as a site of bacterial breakdown of vegetable food matter.

The large intestines
The large intestine is also called the *colon*, and this section of intestines is a wider tube structure and contains no villi. Food materials that are of no nutritious value or cannot be broken down to an absorbable size pass from the small to the large intestine through the *ileo-caecal valve*. The large intestine in carnivores is relatively short in length, and its main purpose is to absorb salts and water. The walls of the large intestine are much folded for this purpose. By the time the digested materials reach the *rectum*, the indigestible food is in a semisolid condition and ready to be excreted through the anus as *faeces*.

The colon is divided into three sections:

- Ascending
- Transverse
- Descending

The colon terminates in the rectal area, where waste products are held before excretion.

The large intestine is lined with a mucous-secreting surface as this assists in the movement of materials by a lubricating action. The mucus prevents the total drying out of the faeces, which might then damage the lining on excretion.

The last part of the digestive tract is closed by sphincter muscles and is known as the anal canal, over which the animal has control via skeletal muscle (voluntary control). Defaecation involves relaxation of the anal sphincter, but diarrhoea or illness may override this control. Diarrhoea is defined as the frequent evacuation of watery faeces. If defaecation is delayed too long, constipation may result.

Digestion and absorption of the main food constituents:

- *Proteins* – come from muscle meat, egg, or vegetable proteins like soya bean. These are broken down in the stomach and small intestines to become *amino acids* and absorbed into the bloodstream for transport to the *liver*, where they are processed.
- *Carbohydrates* – They are found as cereals like biscuit, potatoes, or pasta. They are broken down into *simple sugars* (e.g. *glucose*) and absorbed into the bloodstream for transport to the liver, where they may be stored as *glycogen*. When required by the body for energy, glycogen can be turned back into glucose.
- *Fats* – They are found as animal fat or vegetable oils and are broken down into *fatty acids and glycerol* by bile and enzymes in the small intestines. Most will enter the lacteals in the villi to travel via the lymph system, finally reaching the bloodstream for use or storage.
- The process and products of digestion are shown in Figure 3.25.

The liver

The liver is the largest organ of the body, situated immediately caudal to the diaphragm in the abdomen. About 75% of the liver's blood supply comes from the *hepatic portal system* of vessels (Figure 3.26). This ensures that the products of digestion are absorbed into the bloodstream and travel to the liver for processing, before being used or stored in the body. The remaining 25% of blood to the liver arrives via the *hepatic artery*.

The liver itself is a very complex chemical factory, which generates materials for use within the body from the products of digestion, which come directly to it from the gut. The specialised epithelial cells that make up the liver are called *hepatocytes*.

Functions of the liver

It is thought that the liver performs over 500 functions. The main functions are as follows:

- Regulation of sugar which has four possible fates:
  - used as an energy source (Krebs cycle)
  - stored as glycogen in the liver
  - converted to fat and stored around the body
  - passed directly into the circulation
- Regulation of lipids (fats)
- Regulation of amino acids and proteins

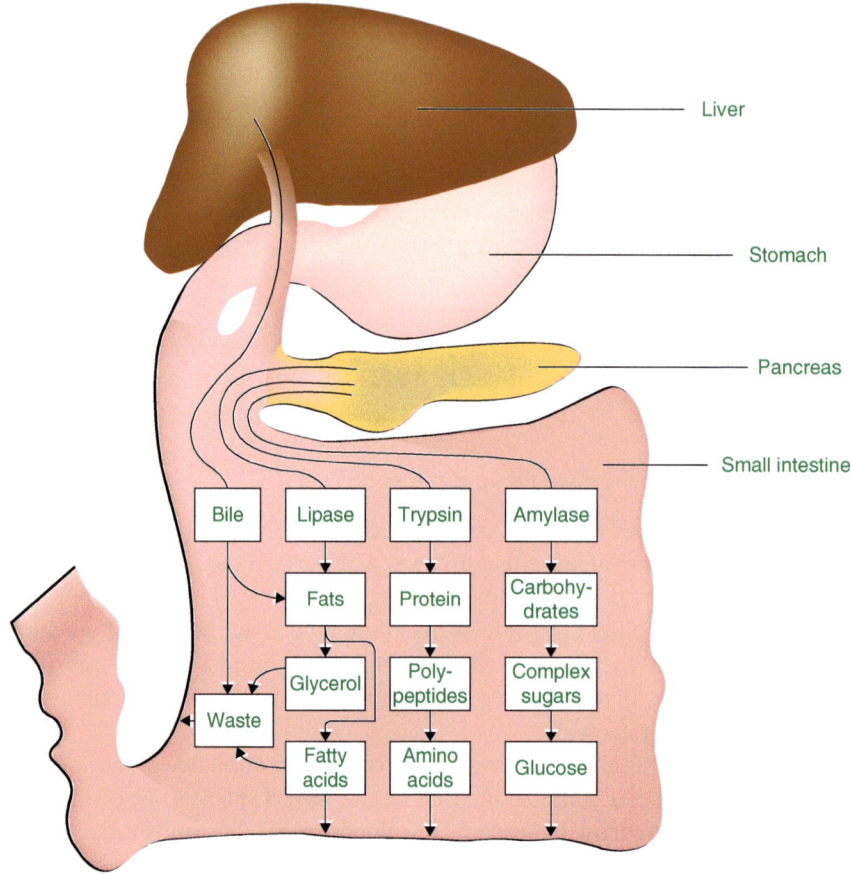

Figure 3.25 The process and products of digestion.

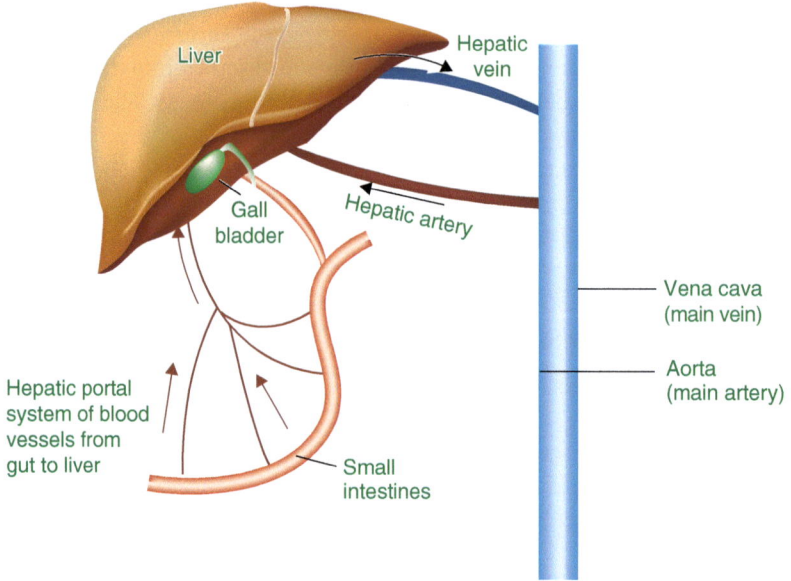

Figure 3.26 Blood supply to the liver.

- Heat production
- Bile production
- Formation of cholesterol
- Elimination of sex hormones
- Storage and filtration of blood
- Elimination of haemoglobin from exhausted red blood cells
- Formation of urea to be passed on to the kidneys for removal from the body
- Creation of plasma proteins (synthesis)
- Storage of vitamins A, D, and B12 and minerals like iron and copper

The pancreas

The *pancreas* is a large grey-pink gland, which lies in the abdomen close to the stomach and the duodenal section of the small intestine. It is made up of two parts which are joined together, giving the pancreas its boomerang shape.

There are two types of tissue present within the gland, and these have very different functions:

- *Exocrine tissue* – produces digestive enzymes
- *Endocrine tissue* – produces hormones like insulin to help in controlling sugar in the body.

Summary of the digestive system

This essential system consists of the following:

- A tube extending from the mouth to the anus with specific regions for different digestive processes.
- Specialised cells that work to carry out specific processes involved in digestion.

The digestive system works to:

- Breakdown food that is ingested by the animal by mechanical and chemical processes.
- Extract, absorb, and metabolise the nutrients of the food ingested.

The urinary system

The urinary system has several functions, but its main one is to remove and excrete waste liquid products from the body. Wastes are toxic if allowed to accumulate, so this removal of harmful materials, which are the end products of metabolism, is essential and continuous.

The mammalian urinary system consists of:

- two kidneys (left and right)
- two ureters (left and right)
- one bladder
- one urethra

Functions of the urinary system include:

- expulsion or conservation of body water
- excretion of unwanted substances or those in excess to requirements
- storage of products before their removal from the body
- as an endocrine organ producing hormones

The kidneys

The kidneys of small mammals are bean shaped, single lobed and situated one on each side of the abdomen (Figure 3.27). Each contains specialised cells, which filter out potentially toxic materials

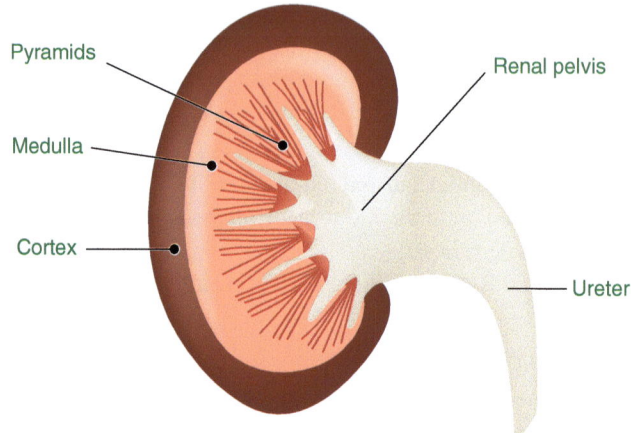

Figure 3.27 The simple mammalian kidney.

from the body and conserve those which the body needs. These cells are called the *nephrons*, from which we get the term *nephritis*, meaning inflammation of the kidney nephron cells.

The blood supply to the kidneys is via the *renal artery* directly from the aorta and drains away from the kidney via the *renal vein* directly into the vena cava.

Larger mammals may have more than one lobe as part of their kidney structure.

The nephron

This is the unique specialised cell of the urinary system. The structure is seen in Figure 3.28. Parts of the nephron include:

- *Glomerulus* – a network or knot of artery from branches of the renal artery in the cortex section of the kidney.
- *Bowman's capsule* – the cup-shaped part of the nephron at the start of the tubule. The glomerulus fits into the Bowman's capsule, initiating the blood filtration and the removal of urea and other nitrogenous wastes.
- *Proximal tubule* – the start of the long tube through which the filtered substances will pass.
- *Loop of Henle and distal tubule* – this is where, on instruction from hormones, the nephron conserves water, salts, and sugars or, if the body has an excess, it is instructed to add the excess to the forming urine for removal from the body.

The distal tubule joins a collecting duct, which directs the urine to the pelvis region of the kidney, where all nephrons drain, and then along the ureter to the bladder for temporary storage. When the bladder is full, the animal receives this information from the brain and relaxes the sphincter muscle from the bladder to the urethra and the outside (Figure 3.29). The act of passing urine is called *micturition*.

It is important to note that mammals excrete nitrogen in the form of the chemical *urea*, which is highly soluble and when water is added, then urine is formed. Reptiles and birds excrete nitrogen in the form of *uric acid* which is less soluble than urea. For uric acid to be excreted, protein is required, and so diagnostic testing will indicate the presence of protein. In mammals, very little protein should be detectable in urine.

Kidney structure in birds and reptiles is like that of mammals but does have some differences. Reptile kidneys follow a specific organisation of nephrons in their kidneys. There are also differences in the proportional lengths of the proximal and distal tubules.

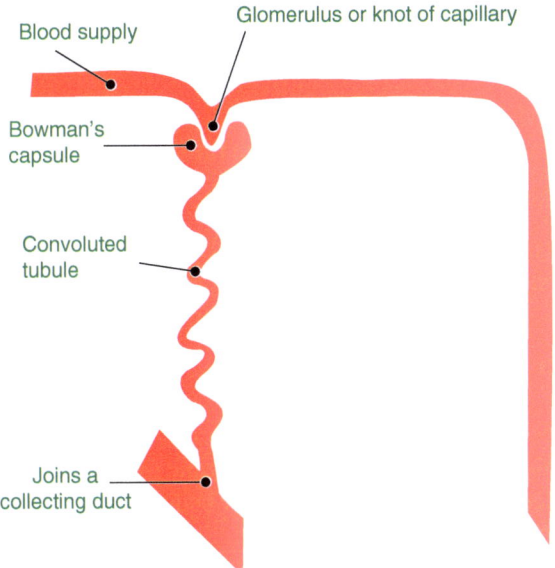

Figure 3.28 The nephron.

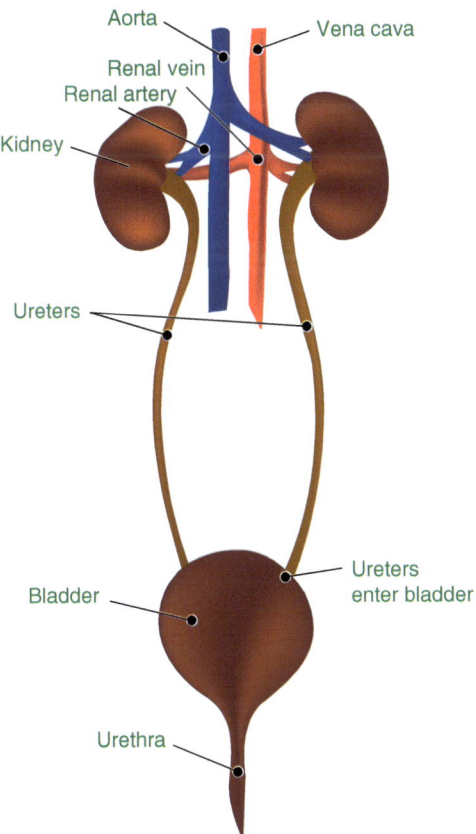

Figure 3.29 The urinary system.

Summary of the urinary system

This essential system consists of:

- Structures to filter blood and create urine.
- Structures to store the urine prior to expulsion from the body.

The urinary system works to:

- Remove toxic products from the body continuously to avoid build up in the body.
- Balance the water levels in the body through urine dilution or concentration.

The Nervous System

The nervous system provides the quickest means of communication within the body. Information is received both from outside the animal (the environment) and from inside the animal's body. The response to information received must be coordinated for body systems to unite in their response and produce the desired effect.

Messages to the body are carried in two ways:

- *Electrical* – These are impulses that travel along the nerves and give fast response to a situation or stimulus (*nervous system*). The electrical messages stimulate movement of muscles.
- *Chemical* – These are hormones which, once released into the bloodstream, will travel more slowly to their target organ. The body response is seen after a period of time (*endocrine system*).

Body coordination by nervous system tissue is conducted by nerve cells called *neurones* (Figure 3.30), together with various forms of supporting tissue in which they are embedded. These cells are the basic functional unit of the nervous system and are found in bundles called *nerves*.

There are three main types of neurones:

1. *Sensory* – those attached to the sense organs, (i.e. eyes, ears, tongue, nose, and skin). These carry information about the animal's external environment to the brain.
2. *Interneurone* (relay) – carry information or messages between sensory neurones and motor neurones.

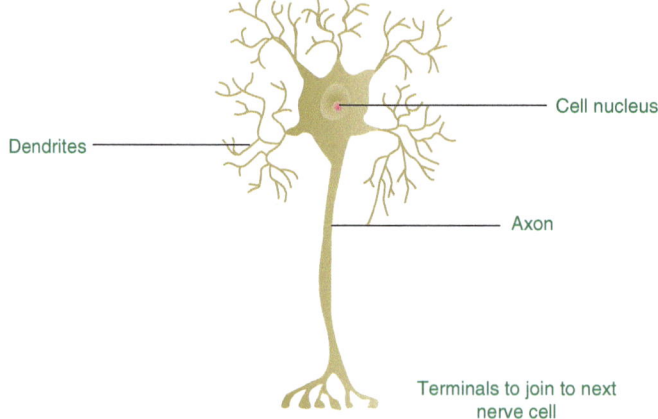

Figure 3.30   Nerve cell – a basic neurone.

3. *Motor* – these link from interneurones to muscle or gland cells to deliver messages from the central nervous system (brain and spinal cord) to initiate an action. This may be the release of more hormones or the movement of a muscle.

All neurones work together to form a *neural network* that links the cell branches to keep the information and action by the brain and spinal cord networked like a computer.

The shape of the nerve cell will vary to suit the tissue into which it links, but the basic components remain the same:

- a cell body containing the nucleus.
- cell processes which lead to and from the cell body (Figure 3.31).
- the axon – which carries the impulses away from the cell body.
- the dendrite – which carries impulses towards the cell body.

The cell membrane of a neurone is electrically charged by the action of ions (salts or electrolytes), such as potassium (K^+) or sodium (Na^{2+}). The voltage carried is small, but once discharged along the length of neurone, it allows the system to act as a high-speed electrical signalling system. After the signal, the membrane is recharged and returns to a resting position, awaiting the next signal.

The junction between two or more neurones is called a *synapse* (Figure 3.32). Electrical impulses cannot pass across this gap, so communication is dependent upon a chemical substance known as a

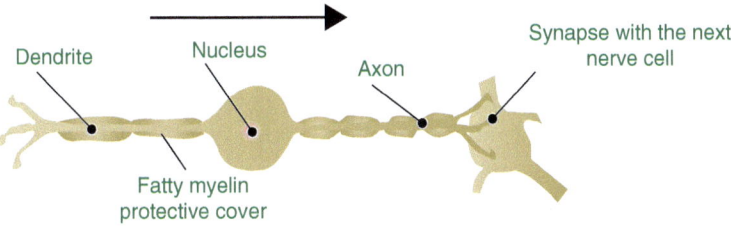

Figure 3.31 Nerve cell and direction of electrical impulse.

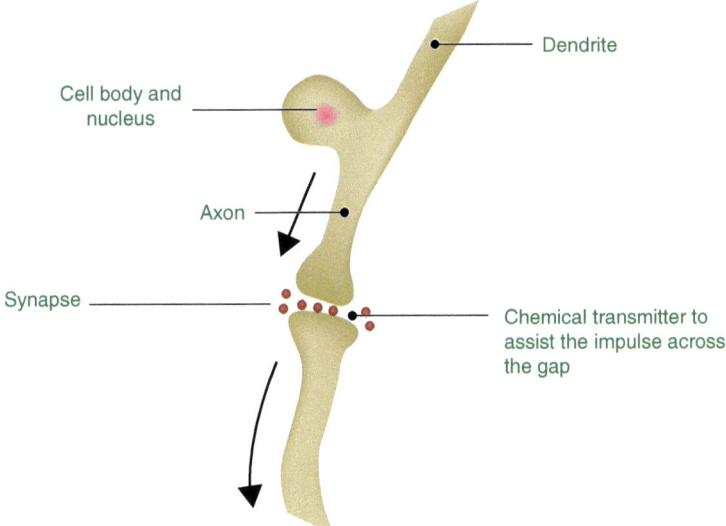

Figure 3.32 A synapse – the junction between two or more neurones.

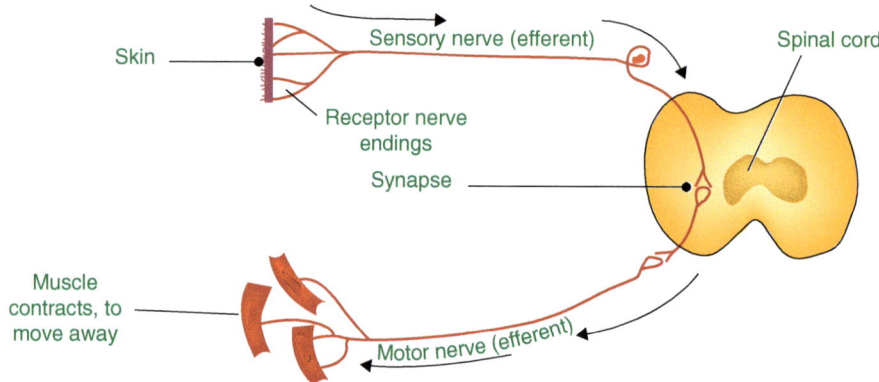

Figure 3.33   Reflex arc.

neurotransmitter. This substance will connect two neurones for less than 1 ms, allowing the impulse to progress. The chemical is then destroyed by another substance and recreated again before each future impulse.

Reflex action or arc

A reflex action is an automatic and very rapid response to a potentially harmful stimulus, which is usually external to the body. It is a survival response (Figure 3.33).

The structural basis of the reflex action is the *reflex arc*, which represents the series of units of nerve tissue through which impulses must pass in order to bring about a *reflex response*. The sensory tissues receiving the information are called *receptors* and may be scattered sensory cells in the skin or special sense receptors like the eye or ear. Their stimulation results in impulses being generated in sensory (*afferent*) neurones located in the peripheral nerves (on or near the body surface). These afferent neurones take the impulse to the central nervous system (only to the spinal cord) where a connection nerve in the cord connects to a motor (*efferent*) neurone. This will take the impulse or message to an *effector* tissue like a gland or to a muscle for the desired effect – survival.

A common example used is touching a hot surface, when the reflex arc ensures that the animal suffers minimal harm as the paw is speedily withdrawn from the danger.

Central nervous system

The central nervous system consists of the *brain* and the *spinal cord*.

The brain

The function of the brain is to coordinate the body's activities. It receives all sensory information and processes it for:

- Immediate use in a reflex action/arc.
- Later use – storing it in memory, passing orders via neurones and hormones, and constantly monitoring the internal body systems for any change.

The brain is divided into three parts (Figure 3.34):

- *Forebrain* – *cerebrum*, divided into two areas called the cerebral hemispheres (including the *hypothalamus*) and involved with voluntary movement and the senses.

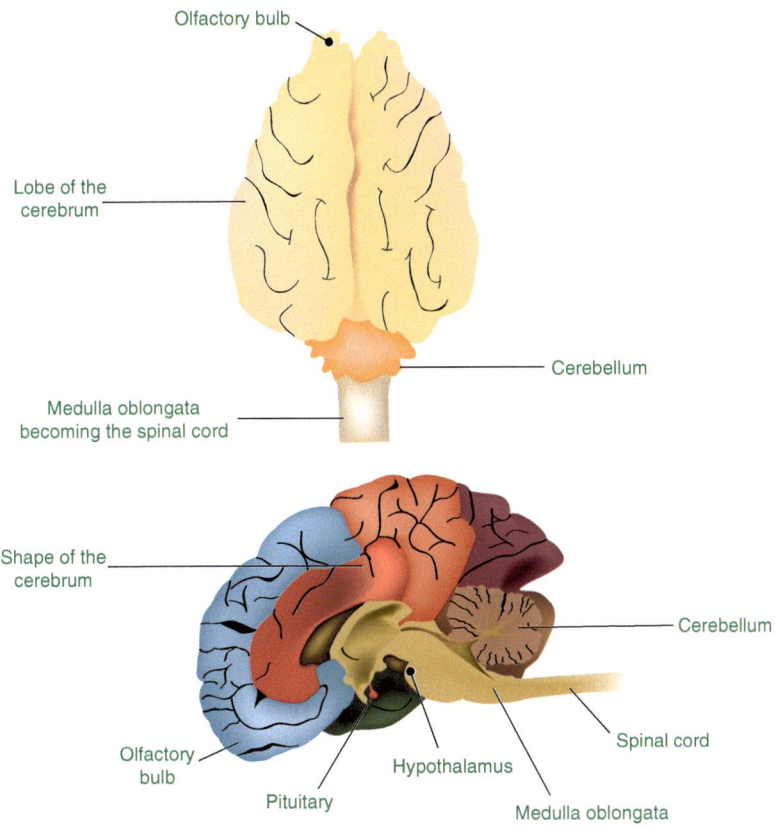

Olfactory bulb

Lobe of the
cerebrum

Cerebellum

Medulla oblongata
becoming the spinal cord

Shape of the
cerebrum

Cerebellum

Olfactory
bulb

Spinal cord

Hypothalamus

Pituitary

Medulla oblongata

Figure 3.34   Parts of the brain, from two views.

- *Midbrain* – involved with sight, hearing, muscle control, and body position.
- *Hindbrain* – the *cerebellum*, the *pons*, and the *medulla oblongata*. It is involved with complicated movements of the body, control of circulation and respiration, and awareness of surroundings.

The spinal cord

The cord extends from the base of the skull to the lumbar/sacral region of the spine, over the pelvis. It is a continuation of the hindbrain and medulla oblongata. The cord is protected by the *vertebrae* and the *meninges*. A spinal canal runs through each vertebra and houses the spinal cord.

The spinal cord divides into many branching spinal nerves. This continues first inside the vertebrae and then on the outside of the coccygeal vertebrae as the *cauda equina* (resembling a horse's tail), to supply motor and sensory nerves to the tip of the animal's tail.

Protection of the brain and spinal cord

- *Bones* – skull and vertebrae (bones of the spine).
- *Meninges* – three protective membranes covering the brain and spinal cord, which in turn are separated by the cerebrospinal fluid (CSF).
- *Dura mater* – the tough outer membrane, in contact with the bone of the skull and the vertebrae.
- *Arachnoid mater* – a fine network of collagen and elastic fibres, underneath the dura mater.

- *Pia mater* – the membrane in contact with the surface of the brain and spinal cord tissue.
- *Blood–brain barrier* – a mechanism located in a continuous layer of endothelial cells, which allows only useful substances to enter the brain.

Peripheral nervous system

The *peripheral nervous system* receives the information from the animal's surrounding environment and transfers it to the central nervous system where a response is coordinated.

The peripheral nervous system is comprised of the *voluntary* and *involuntary* nervous systems.

Voluntary nervous system
- Paired spinal nerves containing both sensory and motor fibres, forming a mixed spinal nerve.
- Twelve cranial nerves. These are mixed nerves and can contain motor and sensory, voluntary, and autonomic fibres (Table 3.3).

Involuntary or autonomic nervous system
- *Sympathetic* nervous system
- *Parasympathetic* nervous system

The involuntary or autonomic nervous system is not under conscious control and is involved with the regulation of body functions. It is divided into two parts, distinguished by their function and by the chemical transmitters (neurotransmitters) used at the synapse between nerve cells (Table 3.4).

Table 3.3 The 12 cranial nerves.

Number	Name	Type	Function
I	Olfactory	Sensory	Smell
II	Optic	Sensory	Vision, pupil light response
III	Oculomotor	Motor	Eye movement, pupil constriction
IV	Trochlear	Motor	Eye movement
V	Trigeminal	Mixed	Mastication, touch, and pain receptors
VI	Abducens	Motor	Eye movement
VII	Facial	Mixed	Salivation, facial expression, taste
VIII	Auditory/ vestibulocochlear	Sensory	Hearing, balance
IX	Glossopharyngeal	Mixed	Taste, laryngeal muscles
X	Vagus	Mixed	Vocalisation, swallowing Decrease in heart rate Abdominal organs
XI	Accessory	Motor	Head movement
XII	Hypoglossal	Motor	Tongue movement

Table 3.4 Function of neurotransmitters.

Sympathetic system	Parasympathetic system
• Chemical – adrenaline	• Chemical – cholinesterase
• Prepares body for fight, fright, and flight	• Stimulates salivation
• Inhibits salivation	• Assists in day-to-day function of the body
• Increases heart rate	• Decreases heart rate to normal
• Increases respiratory rate	• Decreases respiratory rate

Summary of the nervous system

This essential system:

- Consists of various types of neurones that are found in the central and peripheral nervous systems.
- Transmits electrical impulses around the body to cause a specific effect.

The nervous system works to:

- Respond to stimuli to keep the animal alive and safe within its environment.

The Endocrine System

The endocrine system is a system of *ductless glands*, which are sites for *hormone* production (Figure 3.35). Hormones are the chemical messengers of the body. They are discharged directly into the circulating bloodstream for transportation to the target organ or tissue.

The word 'endocrine' means 'internal secretion', and the organs of this system are therefore glands of internal secretion. Although endocrine glands are sited all over the body, they influence one another and, through their interactions, are integrated into a highly coordinated system.

The messages from the hormones:

- Have long-lasting effects on their targets (hours to days).
- Aid in the constant adjustment of the internal body environment.
- Arrive at their target via circulating blood.

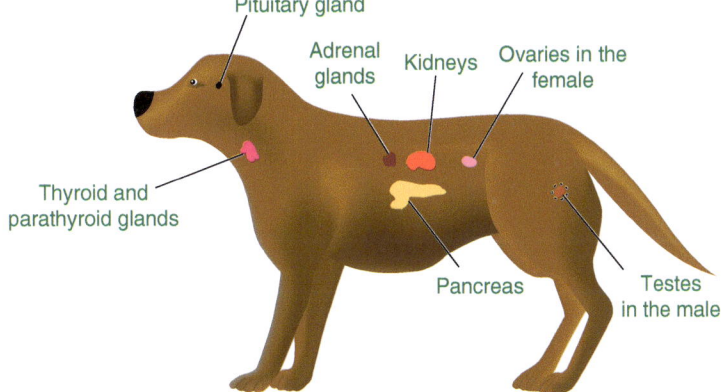

Figure 3.35 Endocrine glands in the dog.

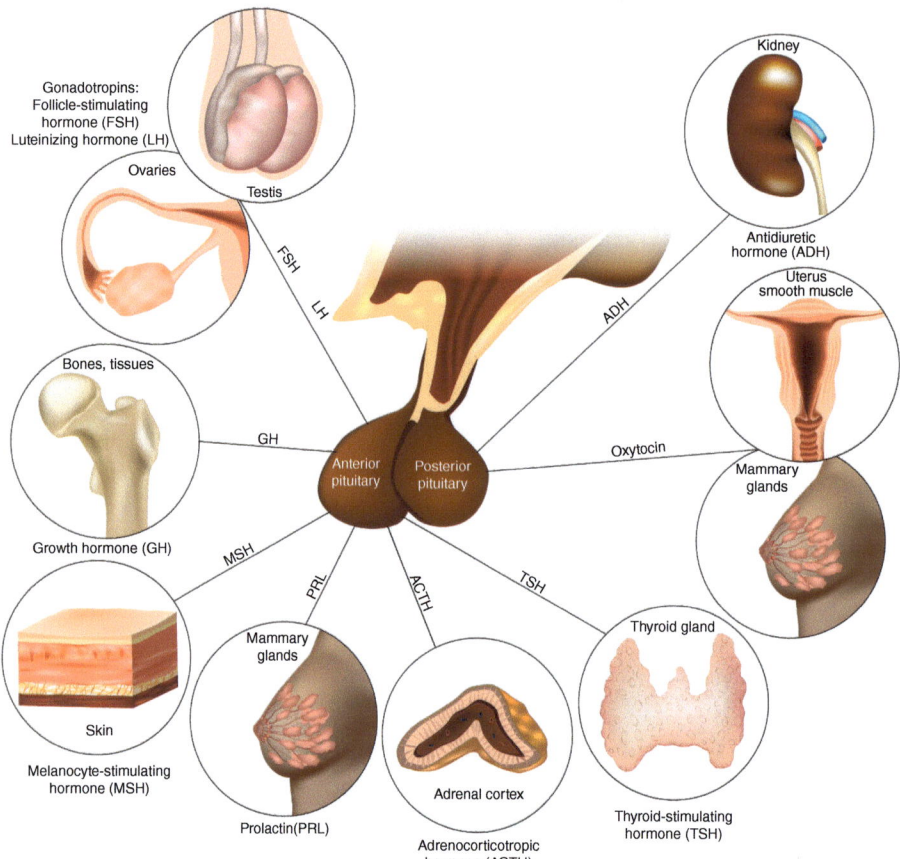

Figure 3.36   Effects of the pituitary gland.

The nervous and endocrine systems are linked. The *pituitary gland* controls the functions of all the other glands in the endocrine system and is found in the brain close to the *hypothalamus*.

Endocrine glands

Pituitary gland

The pituitary gland controls all other endocrine glands and so may also be referred to as the master gland. Situated at the base of the brain near the hypothalamus, the pituitary gland also has an influence on body growth and maintenance of the internal body environment (Figure 3.36). It is divided into two parts:

- The *anterior* pituitary
- The *posterior* pituitary

The *anterior pituitary* produces:

- Thyrotropic or *thyroid-stimulating hormone* (TSH) for production of thyroid hormone.
- *Adrenocorticotropic hormone* (ACTH) for control of adrenal glands and release of corticosteroids.
- *Growth hormone* (GH) or somatotropin, which promotes the body's growth.

- *Gonadotropins*, which influence the ovaries and testes:

    a. *Follicle-stimulating hormone* (FSH) promotes the ripening of the eggs in the ovaries and the secretion of oestrogen in the female. In the male, FSH assists the development of the sperm cells.
    b. *Luteinising hormone* (LH) stimulates ovulation and the secretion of *oestrogen* and *progesterone* in the female. In the male, it stimulates the development and release of *testosterone*.
    c. *Prolactin* or lactogenic hormone develops mammary tissues during pregnancy for milk production.

The *posterior pituitary* produces:

- *Antidiuretic hormone* (ADH) or vasopressin, which prevents excessive loss of water from the body via the kidneys.
- *Oxytocin*, which stimulates the release of milk and uterine contractions during *parturition* (birth) and *lactation*.

Thyroid gland

The thyroid gland regulates growth, body development, and metabolism. It is located below the larynx near the trachea. It produces and secretes the *thyroid hormone T4*, which regulates metabolism, growth, and development.

Parathyroid glands

The parathyroid glands are situated near the thyroid gland. It produces *parathyroid hormone (PTH)*, which regulates the calcium and phosphorus levels in the blood and bones.

Adrenal gland

The adrenal gland regulates the growth of bones, muscle development, and secondary sex characteristics. These two small glands are located near the kidneys. The glands are divided into:

- *Adrenal Cortex* – produces steroids which are concerned with the regulation of sodium and potassium and water (fluid) balance in the body. An example of a hormone produced here is *aldosterone*. Corticosteroids produced assist in the metabolism of nutrients, antibody formation and dealing with stress. Also produced here are androgen hormones responsible for the male and female sex characteristics.
- *Adrenal Medulla* – secretes adrenaline and noradrenaline, which prepare the body for fight or flight in stressful situations. Dopamine is also secreted in small amounts.

The pancreas

The pancreas regulates the use and storage of glucose in the body and is considered a part of the digestive system. It lies close to the stomach in a loop of the small intestine (duodenum). It produces insulin for the use and storage of simple sugars from the breakdown of carbohydrates in the diet.

Pineal gland

This is a small oval gland situated attached to the base of the posterior pituitary gland near the base of the brain (Figure 3.37). The pineal gland is responsible for controlling the body's circadian rhythms. It secretes melatonin and plays a part in the control of breeding cycles in animals that are seasonal breeders such as sheep and ferrets by inhibiting gonad function. The pineal gland also contributes to the production of serotonin. In reptiles and amphibians, research has shown that the pineal gland acts a photoreceptor, along with contributing to temperature control and

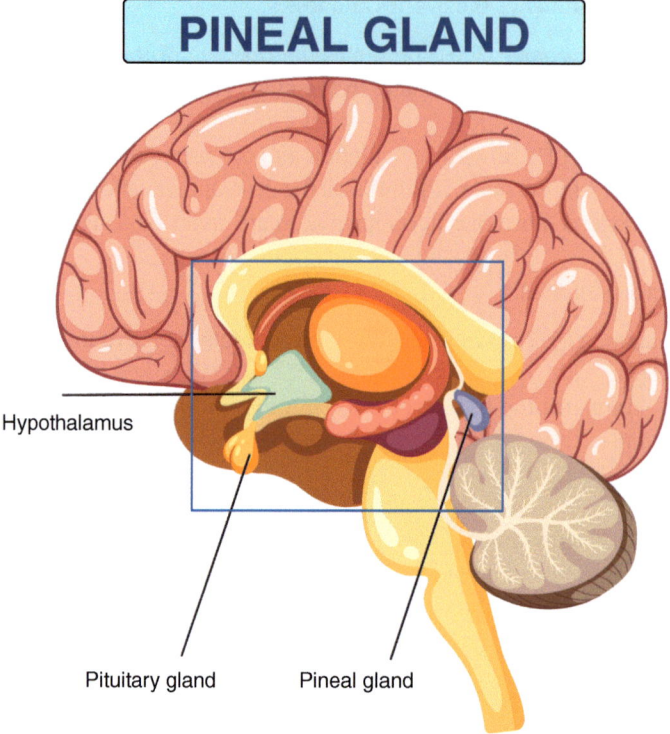

PINEAL GLAND

Hypothalamus

Pituitary gland   Pineal gland

Figure 3.37   Pineal gland.

breeding cycles. The pineal gland is involved in the processes of hibernation, estivation, navigation, and migration and is therefore thought to be sensitive to the earth's magnetic fields. Research is ongoing in this area.

Gonads

Female *(ovaries)* and male *(testes)* gonads produce hormones for the functioning of the reproductive systems of each sex:

- *Ovaries* – produce some of the oestrogen hormone responsible for the secondary sex characteristics and oestrous cycles. They also produce progesterone for the preparation and maintenance of the uterus in gestation (pregnancy).
- *Testes* – produce testosterone, responsible for male secondary sex characteristics.

The following organs are not endocrine glands but do produce hormones:

- Kidney – produces the hormone *erythropoietin*, which stimulates the production of red cells in active bone marrow sites.
- Stomach – produces *ghrelin* and at high levels indicates hunger – appetite stimulator.
- Adipose tissue – produces *leptin*, which at high levels tells the body to stop eating – appetite suppressor.
- Intestines – produce hormones to promote the production of digestive enzyme compounds from organs such as the pancreas. Regulatory enzymes are also produced that control appetite such as *gastrin, secretin*, and *gastric inhibitory peptide* (GIP).

Summary of the endocrine system

This essential system consists of:

- A network of ductless glands and organs that produce chemical messages called hormones to regulate the body.
- Controlled by the pituitary gland and hypothalamus

The endocrine system works to:

- Secrete hormones to travel to target organs for specific effects.
- Regulate growth, metabolism, temperature, and reproductive processes in the body.

The Sense Organs

Sense organs collect information from the surrounding environment, both internal and external. Each piece of information received is known as a *stimulus*. The stimuli are interpreted by the brain once it receives the information via the nerves. Sense organs collect information from inside and outside the body:

Inside the body

- Temperature monitored by the hypothalamus of the brain.
- Regulation of breathing by measuring the carbon dioxide levels.
- Tension of muscles or tendons, which prevents over-exercise and damage.

Outside the body

- Light, dark, shape, or colour becomes sight.
- Sound and changes in body position become hearing and balance.
- Airborne chemicals become smells.
- Ingested chemicals become tastes.
- Touch, heat, and cold pass survival information to the brain.

The eye

The eye is the organ of vision (Figure 3.38). The eye resembles a camera in at least three ways:

1. Both focus light. In the eye, this is due to the transparent *cornea* and *lens*. These act like the glass lens of the camera in forming the image.
2. This image falls on a layer of receptors called the *retina*, which, like the film in a camera, is sensitive to light.
3. Eyes and cameras have a mechanism called an *iris* diaphragm, which is an opaque disc with a hole at the centre. This increases or decreases in size to control light entering the eye.

   The *retina* transforms light into a stream of nerve impulses, which pass down the *optic nerve* to the brain to form a picture. The frequency and pattern of these impulses vary according to patches of colour, light, and shade, which make up the retinal image. The visual area of the brain interprets these impulses to form moving impressions.

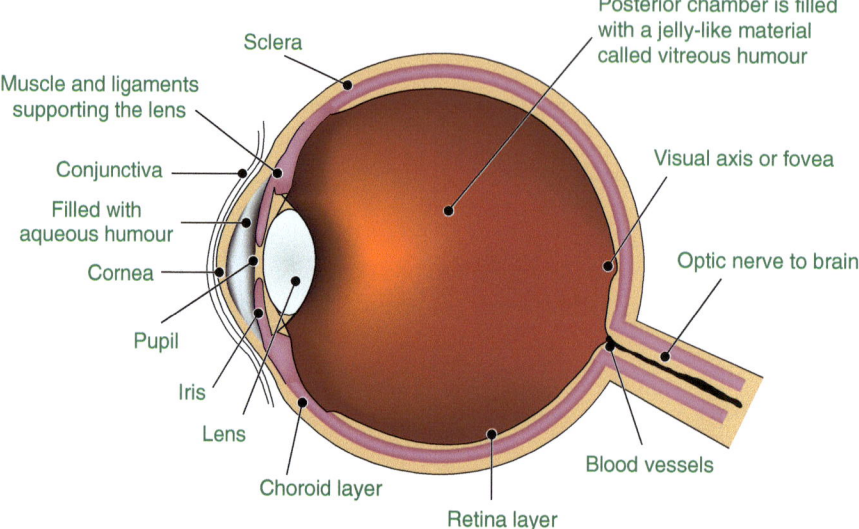

Figure 3.38   The eye.

Protection of the eyes

There are several features that aid in the protection of eyes:

- Cavities in the skull called the *orbits* protect the eyeball with a bone and cartilage ring.
- The transparent, self-repairing skin on the eye called the *conjunctiva*.
- *Tears* keep the eyes moist; a stream of liquid from the *tear glands* is wiped across the eye by blinking and prevents the tissues from becoming too dry.
- The *blink reflex* to guard against dust and other objects which might enter the eye socket.
- The *eyelashes* to guard against dust and other objects, which might enter the eye socket (Note: eyelashes are not present in all species).

Structures of the eye

- The eye receives oxygen via the blood vessels, which enter with the *optic nerve*, at the back of the eye. These vessels spread out through the *choroid layer* and over the surface of the *retina*.
- The *cornea* and *lens* obtain oxygen and food by diffusion from vessels in the liquid in the front chamber of the eye – *the aqueous humour*.
- *Vitreous humour* is a jelly in the back cavity of the eye, which helps to maintain the shape of the eye.
- The *iris* is the coloured part of the eye and has a round hole in its centre called the *pupil*. The iris consists of muscles which radiate out and contract to enlarge the size of the pupil and circular muscles, which make it smaller in size. The iris regulates the amount of light reaching the retina.
- The *lens* consists of layers of transparent material arranged like the skin of an onion, which are enclosed in an elastic outer membrane. These are held in place by *suspensory ligaments*, which in turn are attached to a ring of muscle called the *ciliary muscle*.
- The retina is covered with light-sensitive receptors called *rods and cones* (due to their shape). These are buried under nerve fibres and a layer of blood capillaries, which conduct

the impulses to the brain. These layers are absent from the area where the clearest image is formed, the *fovea*. This area is directly opposite the lens and is the most sensitive part of the eye for colour vision.

- The retina contains an area called the *blind spot* (Figure 3.39). It consists of blood vessels and nerve fibres leading to the optic nerve. Due to these tissues, this area is completely insensitive to light.

Figure 3.39 Detecting the eye's blind spot.

1. Hold this page with the cross and spot at arm's length.
2. Close the left eye and stare at the cross with the right eye. Note that the black circle is still visible.
3. Bring the page slowly towards the face. At a certain point, the circle will disappear.
4. This happens when its image falls on the blind spot.

The ear

The anatomy of the ear is shown in Figure 3.40. The functions of the ear are:

- Hearing
- Detecting change in body position
- Balance

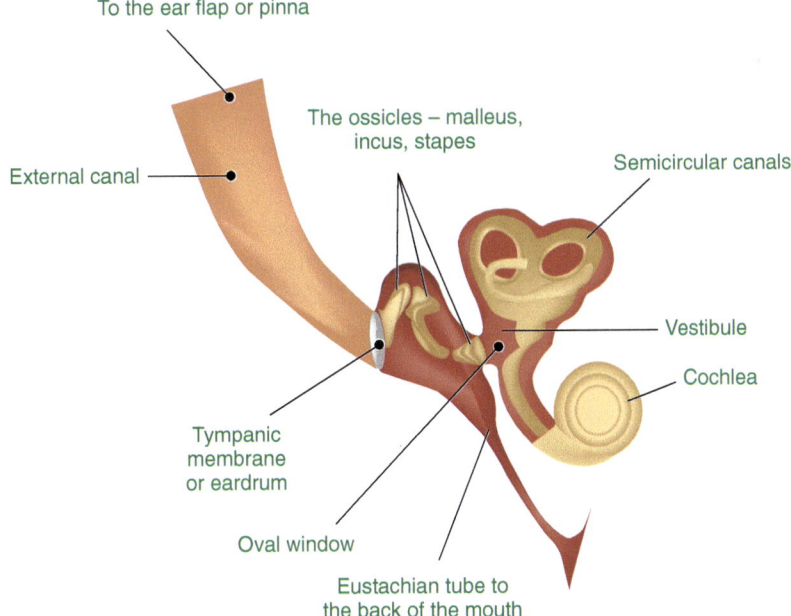

Figure 3.40 Anatomy of the ear.

The ear is divided into three sections:

1. *Outer* – for sound gathering.
2. *Middle* – transmits vibrations to the oval window of the inner ear.
3. *Inner* – receives the sound waves and passes them to the nerve that connects to the brain for conversion into hearing.

Outer ear

This is made up of the ear flap or *pinna* and the *ear canal*. The shape of the canal varies between species and breeds, but the function is the same and that is to collect sound waves and direct them into the canal, which is lined with modified sebaceous glands. These glands produce *wax*, as a protective layer. The canal leads to the eardrum or *tympanic membrane*.

Middle ear

This lies beyond the eardrum in the *tympanic cavity*, which is made of bone, on the ventral surface of the skull. The cavity contains three small bones called *ossicles*:

i. *Malleus* – known as the hammer (contacts the eardrum)
ii. *Incus* – known as the anvil
iii. *Stapes* – known as the stirrup (contacts the oval window)

The vibrations of the eardrum (tympanic membrane) are transmitted by these small bones to the *oval window*, which is the junction between the middle and inner ear.

The link between the middle ear and the throat/pharynx is the *auditory tube* (*Eustachian tube*). This tube allows air pressure to be equalised on either side of the eardrum.

Inner ear

This is protected by the *temporal bone* of the skull. The sound vibrations are converted into nervous impulses here and the inner ear is also involved in maintaining balance.

This area consists of a closed system of delicate tubes, called the *membranous labyrinth*, which contains a fluid called *endolymph*. The labyrinth is itself bathed in a separate fluid, the perilymph.

The labyrinth is made up of:

- The *vestibule* – a sac-like structure.
- The *semicircular canals* – these are three loops at right angles to each other. They respond to the movement of the endolymph, the angle of the head and changes in body position.
- The *cochlea* – a snail-shaped structure responsible for converting sound waves into nerve impulses which are converted in the brain to hearing.

The labyrinth is also known as the *vestibular system* (Figure 3.41).

Other senses

Smell or *olfaction* is important for the selection of food and scenting other animals. Olfactory membranes can also receive stimuli from the mouth; as a result, taste is sometimes actually smell. For some species, the smell is the major sense through which they detect changes in their environment, e.g. star-nosed mole.

Jacobson's organ or the *vomeronasal* organ (Figure 3.42). It is specifically involved in the location of an animal on heat (in oestrus) for reproductive purposes. The intake of air to analyse for pheromones

Vestibular system

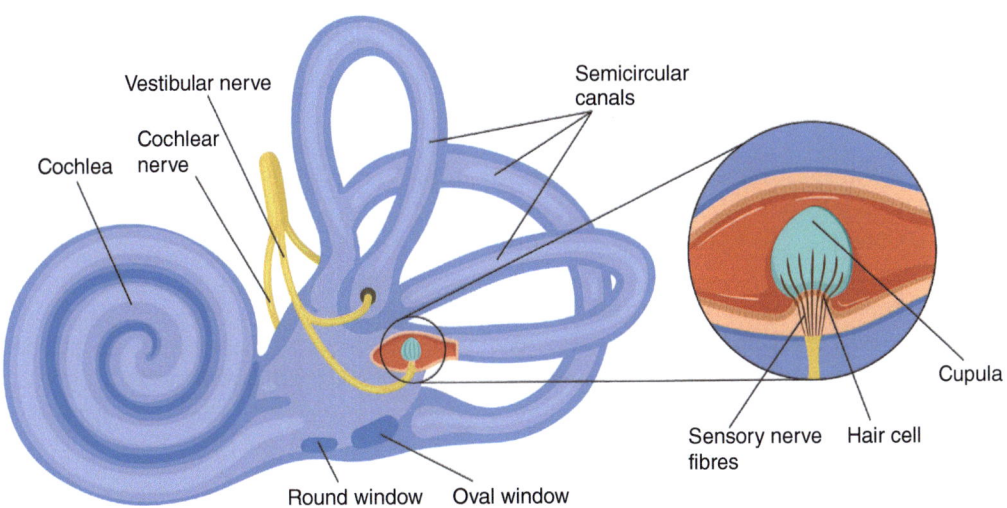

Figure 3.41   The vestibular system.

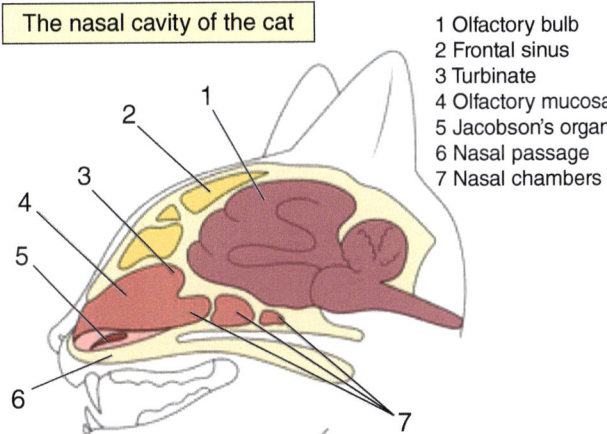

The nasal cavity of the cat

1 Olfactory bulb
2 Frontal sinus
3 Turbinate
4 Olfactory mucosa
5 Jacobson's organ
6 Nasal passage
7 Nasal chambers

Figure 3.42   Jacobson's organ in the cat.

in mammals can often be characterised by a specific behaviour known as the *Flehmen response* where the animal curls its top lip and exposes its top teeth/gums for a few seconds to allow the air to travel up the duct that connects the mouth to the vomeronasal organ. The Flehmen response can be seen in a range of animal including cats (wild and domestic), sheep, horses, and goats.

Snakes and lizards possess a vomeronasal organ and gather scent information when they flick their tongues in and out.

Taste or *gustation* arises from taste cells contained in the mucous membranes of the mouth and on the base of the tongue. Taste and smell will stimulate salivation and the digestive tract in readiness for food to be swallowed.

The Integumentary System

The skin is also known as the *integument* and is the outer protective layer of the body. The anatomy of the skin is shown in Figure 3.43.

Functions of the skin

- *Protection* from the external environment and the controlled internal environment of the body, actively preventing:
  - **i.** water loss
  - **ii.** absorption of toxic or harmful substances
  - **iii.** entry of disease-producing micro-organisms (pathogens)
- *Production* of vitamin D, which is required for the absorption of calcium from the intestines.
- *Sense organ* with receptor nerves throughout the skin's surface that respond to:
  - **i.** touch
  - **ii.** temperature
  - **iii.** pressure
  - **iv.** pain
- *Storage* of fat as adipose tissue. This is an energy store of the body and acts as an insulation layer to help maintain body temperature in cold weather.
- *Temperature control*
  - **a.** For heat loss:
    - **i.** *vasodilation* of surface blood vessels (widening of the vessel wall)
    - **ii.** sweating

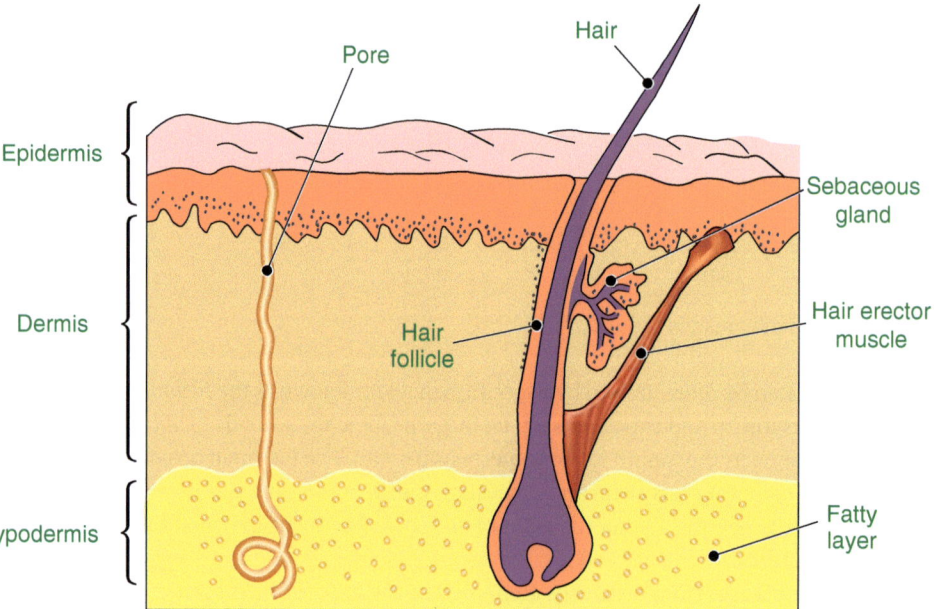

Figure 3.43   The skin.

   b. For heat gain:
       i. *vasoconstriction* of blood vessels (narrowing of the vessel wall)
      ii. erection of surface hair/coat/feathers to trap a layer of air for insulation
    iii. a fat layer under the skin (*subcutaneous* layer)
- *Scent gland* for communication with other animals for reproductive purposes (production of pheromones) or territorial purposes (use of the anal glands on either side of the anus).

Structure of the skin

- *Epidermis* – is the outer layer, which is hard and dry and contains no blood vessels. This layer continually loses dead cells.
- *Dermis* – is the layer below the epidermis and is a type of connective tissue containing nerves, blood vessels, glands, and hair roots.
- *Hypodermis* – is the innermost layer of the skin.

Hair

This covers most of a mammal's surface area. It is made of *keratin* (a protein made by the body) and pigments for colour. It grows from the *hair follicle*, and attached to the deepest section of the hair is the smooth (involuntary) muscle called the *erector pili muscle*, which is responsible for moving the hair upright.

   In other species, hair may be replaced with feathers or scales.

Sweat glands

Sweat or *sebaceous* glands produce *sebum*, which contains pheromones. Other very specialised glands in the skin include mammary glands for milk production and anal glands for scenting territory.

Summary of the Sense Organs

This essential system consists of:

- A range of organs that detect external stimuli to enable an animal to respond appropriately.
- The five key sense organs are: eyes, ears, nose, tongue, and skin.

The sense organs work to:

- Provide an animal with information about its external environment. Sense organs are continually detecting stimuli that is received in the central nervous system, which then coordinates a response.

The Skeleton

The anatomy of the skeleton is shown in Figure 3.44a. Figures 3.44b, c shows the differences between dog and cat skeletons.

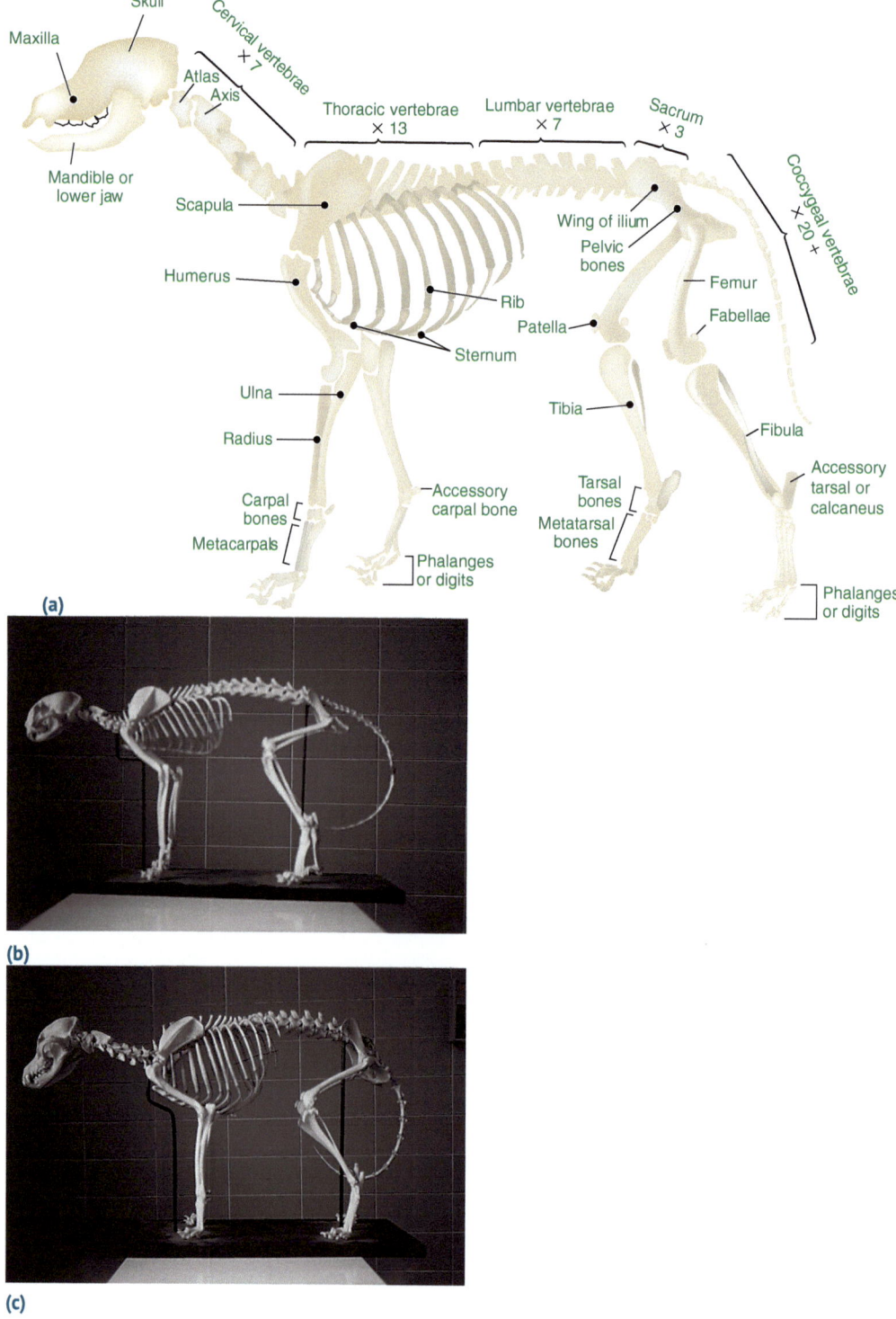

(a)

(b)

(c)

Figure 3.44   (a) Anatomy of the skeleton, (b) skeleton of cat, and (c) skeleton of dog.

The skeleton is divided into three parts:

1. *Axial* – skull, vertebral column (spine), ribs, and sternum.
2. *Appendicular* – the fore- and hindlimbs.
3. *Splanchnic* – bones that develop in tissues, such as the *os penis* and *fabellae*.

Bone structure

Bone is hard and to some extent also flexible (Figure 3.45). The cells in bone are arranged as cylinders and in layers to give bone its strength. They also produce minerals like calcium and phosphorus, which provide bone's rigid nature. The structure of bones allows for maximum resistance to mechanical stresses, while maintaining the least mass.

Bone is made of two types of cells:

- *Osteoblasts* are responsible for the secretion of material which, when mineralised, will become bone. Osteoblasts become trapped in the forming bone and are then called *osteocytes*.
- *Osteoclasts* are responsible for reabsorbing materials and therefore for the remodelling of bone.

In the general structure of long bones, there are two types of bone materials:

- *Compact bone*, which will form the dense walls of the bone shaft.
- *Cancellous or spongy bone*, which is found in the central medullary cavity. As the name suggests, this bone consists of a network and spaces all linked to each other.

The *medullary cavity* of most bones contains active or red marrow, which is responsible for the production of platelets, red and white blood cells. The yellow, rather fatty-looking, material sometimes found in the medullary cavities is the inactive bone marrow.

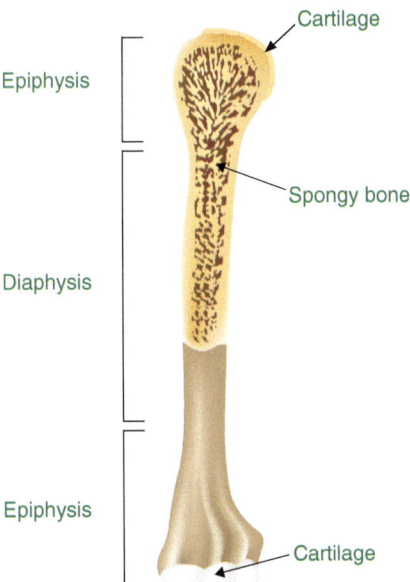

Epiphysis

Cartilage

Spongy bone

Diaphysis

Epiphysis

Cartilage

Figure 3.45   Bone structure.

The outer surface of bone is covered with a layer of dense fibrous connective tissue called the *periosteum* into which are inserted muscles, tendons, and ligaments for attachment. The inner surface of bone is covered by a delicate connective tissue layer, called the *endosteum*. Both these layers contain cells, which assist in the remodelling and repair of bone if it becomes damaged.

The function of bone and the skeletal system is to:

- Support the body
- Provide levers for movement
- Protect organs
- Maintain mineral levels in the body
- Produce blood cells (both red and white)

Please note that in birds, there are adaptations in the bone to enable the species to fly. Bones in birds have more of a honeycomb structure and lack bone marrow. These two features enable the bones to be light but strong and therefore suitable for flight.

Joints

Joints are the articular surfaces of the ends of bones, always protected by a layer of *cartilage* (hyaline). The study of joints is termed *arthrology*. When joints become inflamed, this is termed *arthritis*.

Joints are places where different bones come into anatomical contact with each other:

- *Synarthroses* – are joints which are immovable, e.g. joints of the skull.
- *Diarthroses* – are joints where movement of adjacent bones can occur, and these are usually related to the limbs, e.g. synovial joints.
- *Amphiarthroses* – are joints which share some of the characteristics of the synarthroses and diarthroses but have limited movement, e.g. between the vertebrae of the spine.

Joints can be described as:

- *Fibrous* – no movement at all, also called suture joints, such as the bones of the skull.
- *Cartilaginous* – some movement to these. Examples are found where there are right and left sides, e.g. the lower jaw (mandibles) and in the pelvis.
- *Synovial* (Figure 3.46) – plenty of movement to these joints. They also have other features:
    - i. cartilage surfaces at bone ends
    - ii. joint membrane or capsule
    - iii. joint fluid for lubrication (synovial fluid)

Synovial joints may be called *simple joints* if they contain two articular surfaces, e.g. the two bones which make up the shoulder joint. *Compound joints* have more than two articular surfaces, as in the elbow where three bones come together to form the joint.

The following simple and compound joints are generally recognised:

- i. Ball and socket (femur/acetabulum) (Figure 3.47)
- ii. Hinge (humerus/radius and ulna) (Figure 3.48)
- iii. Pivot (radius/ulna or atlas/axis) (Figure 3.49)
- iv. Saddle (between phalanges of toes) (Figure 3.50)
- v. Plane or gliding (between carpals/tarsals) (Figure 3.50)
- vi. Condylar (stifle or knee)

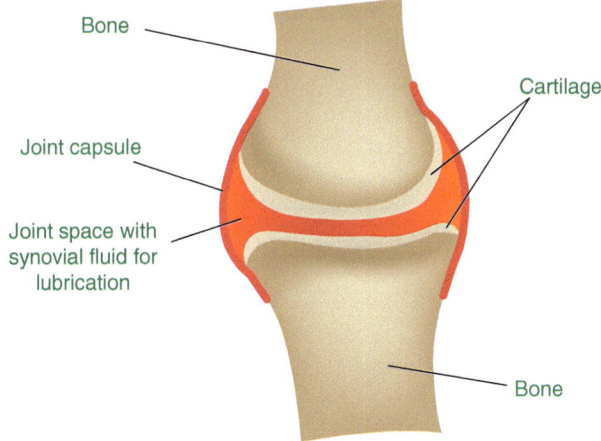

Figure 3.46 Simple synovial joint.

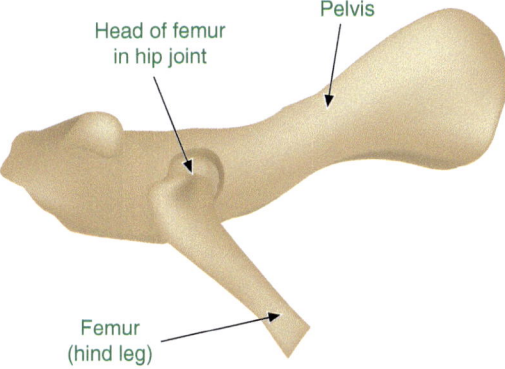

Figure 3.47 Ball and socket joint.

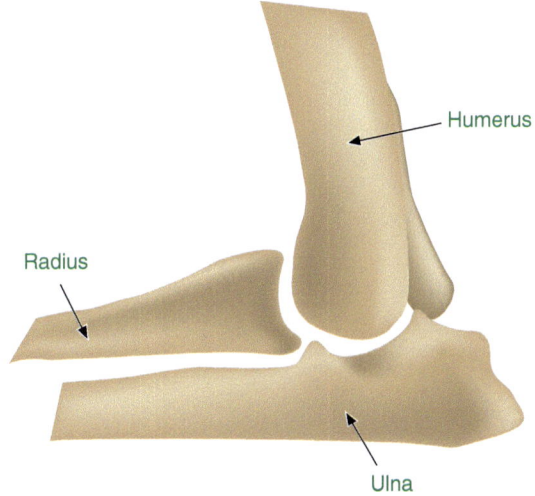

Figure 3.48 Hinge joint.

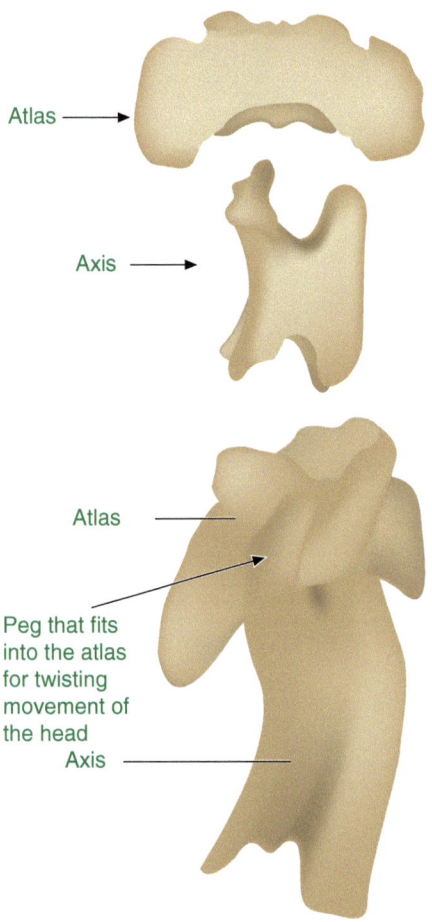

Figure 3.49 Pivot or rotatory joint showing the first two cervical vertebrae.

Atlas

Axis

Atlas

Peg that fits into the atlas for twisting movement of the head

Axis

The stability of all synovial joints is improved by:

i. Ligaments
ii. Surrounding muscles and tendons
iii. Well-shaped/fitting articular bone surfaces

Summary of the Skeleton

This essential system consists of:

- Bones and joints that are vital structures for physical integrity, mobility, and overall health.

The skeleton works to:

- Give support and structure to an animal.
- Protect the animal's vital organs.
- Enable movement through interaction with nervous and muscle tissue.
- Store minerals vital for health.
- Produce blood cells for defence, repair and supply of oxygen around the body.

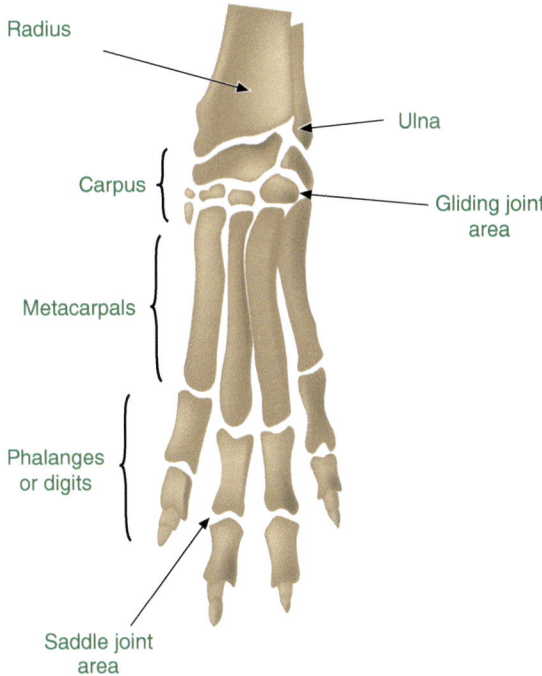

Radius

Ulna

Carpus

Gliding joint
area

Metacarpals

Phalanges
or digits

Saddle joint
area

Figure 3.50   Saddle and gliding joints – foot (foreleg).

The Reproductive System

Reproduction refers to the formation of more individuals, from one parent (*asexually*) or from two parents (*sexually*).

Different animal species have evolved different reproductive processes that ensure they can protect their offspring and ensure that their species can survive, even when the environment is challenging.

Mammalian reproduction is a sexual process, and the male and female reproductive anatomy is very similar (Figures 3.51 and 3.52).

The reproductive process

Every cell in every organism contains a set of instructions (genetic material) in chemical form for building the whole of the new organism. The set of instructions are called *chromosomes* and are situated in the nucleus of each cell. Reproduction is via special cells called *gametes*, produced only by the reproductive organs. Mammals have the most advanced reproductive systems in the animal kingdom. Not only do they have internal fertilisation, but they also have internal development as well. Birds lay eggs; therefore, the development of their offspring is external. Reptiles usually lay eggs but may also have live young.

Animals can be classified as:

- *Viviparous* – give birth to live young that have developed inside the parent
- *Oviparous* – lay eggs and young develop outside of the parent
- *Ovoviviparous* – produce eggs that hatch inside the body

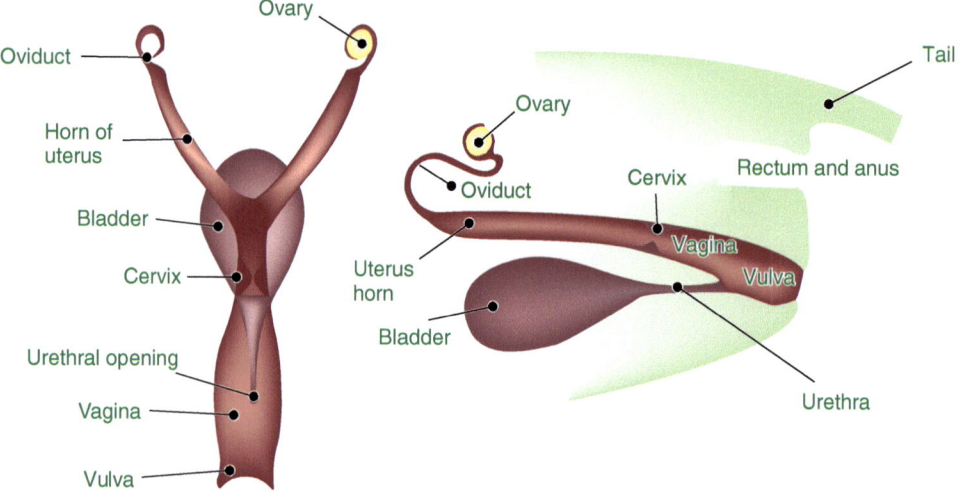

Figure 3.51 Female dog and cat reproductive anatomy.

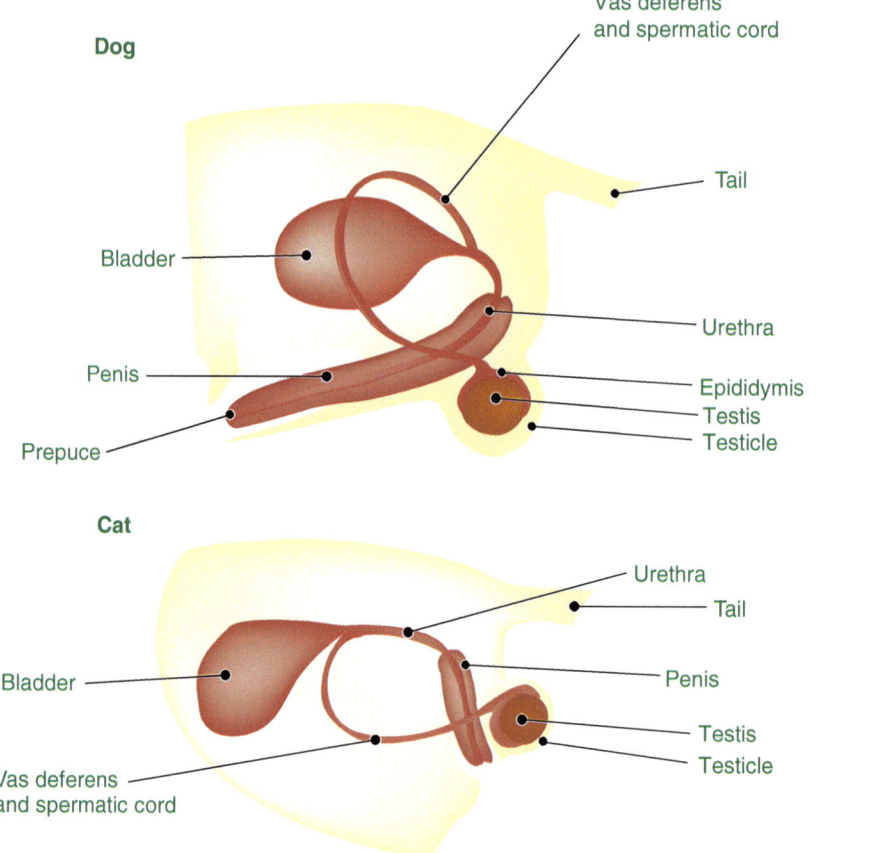

Figure 3.52 Male dog and cat reproductive anatomy.

Internal development has the advantage that the female mammal does not have to remain in one place, as birds do when they incubate their eggs, but can lead a reasonably normal life during the period of *gestation* (pregnancy). This also assists in the survival of a species.

The female reproductive system has the following functions:

- Produce the ova or egg.
- Receive the male gametes or sperm.
- Provide a suitable environment for the fertilisation of the egg by the sperm.
- Provide a safe place for the developing individuals/embryo.
- Provide food and nutrients to the developing individuals/embryo.

Production of ova (eggs)

The function of the ovary is to produce 'functional' eggs or *ova* and to act as an endocrine organ, producing the hormones *oestrogen* and *progesterone* to maintain reproductive functions in the female.

Cells in the ovary group together to form *follicles* and *follicular fluid* (Figure 3.53). Some of the follicles produce eggs. Their formation is like that of sperm in that *meiosis* occurs and each *ovum* will have only *half the required number of chromosomes*.

When the outer surface of the follicle ruptures, the follicular fluid and the mature ova are expelled. This is *ovulation*, and in some species, several ova are released at the same time. Eggs are passed into the *oviducts* or fallopian tubes which act as passageways to the *uterus* where, once fertilised by a sperm, the egg will implant and pregnancy (development of the embryo) takes place until the end of the *gestation* period and *parturition* (birth).

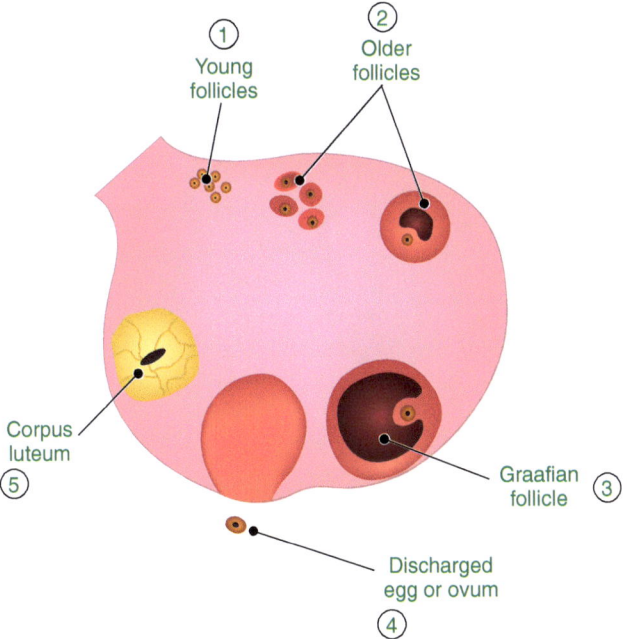

Figure 3.53 The stages of follicle development in an ovary.

Production of sperm

The anatomy of the testes is shown in Figure 3.54. In the testes, the walls of the *seminiferous tubules* consist of two types of cells:

i. Those which produce sperm (*spermatogenic cells*).

ii. Those which produce fluid in which sperm may be supported and supplied with nutrients (*Sertoli* cells).

The testicles also produce the hormone *testosterone*.

The spermatogenic cells divide and from these *spermatids* are formed. These in turn become sperm by undergoing a series of changes including the formation of a tail section for movement. At this stage, they detach from the sperm-producing wall in the tubule and move into the *epididymal duct* for storage and to allow the sperm to mature. This leads to a sperm duct or *vas deferens*, which directs the sperm into the *urethra*.

The urethra leads to the *penis*, which is made up of erectile tissue, supported and encased in a heavy fibrous capsule. The penis contains the end section of the urethra, which carries both urine and secretions containing sperm. It is the organ via which sperm is placed into the female reproductive tract.

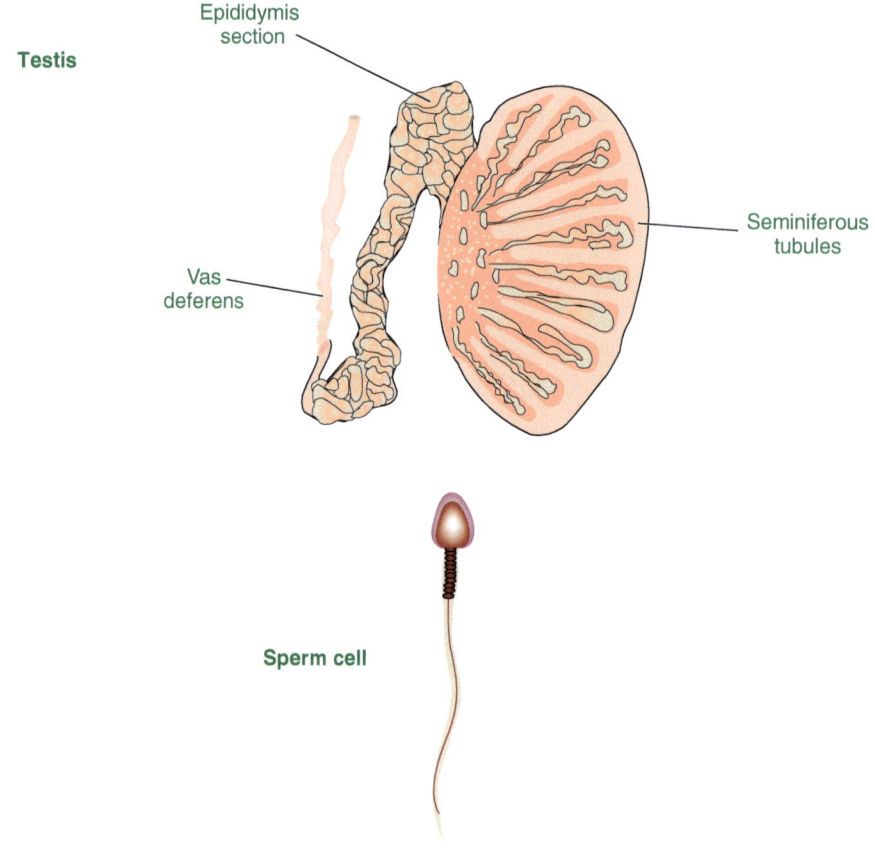

Figure 3.54   Testicle and sperm cell.

The breeding cycle

A female is said to be '*on heat*' or '*in season*', when she becomes attractive to the male, due to the secretion of pheromones (scent attractive to the male). Different species of animal will be in season at different times, so note must be taken of:

- The season – cats tend to have a breeding season from January to September; rabbits breed from January to November, ferrets breed from March to September
- Age
- Species variation

Table 3.5 provides breeding information for a range of species.

Oestrus

This is the *period of sexual receptivity* and, depending on species, may last from one to several days. During the rest of the *oestrous cycle*, the female does not accept the male's advances or allow mating. The cycle is made up of four or five stages, depending on the species and whether the animal is *polyoestrous* (cycles repeatedly like the cat, ferret, rat or hamster) or is *monoestrous* (cycles only once during the breeding season, like the dog).

The stages of oestrus

1. *Anoestrus* – the end of the breeding season, with no activity on the part of the reproductive organs.
2. *Pro-oestrus* – just before oestrus, *follicle stimulating hormone* (FSH) secretion causes the follicles to develop in the ovary. FSH stimulates the ovary to release increased amounts of *oestrogen*, causing changes to the reproductive tract and preparing for pregnancy.
3. *Oestrus* – will accept a male. The release of the ova (ovulation) occurs. FSH levels decrease and LH increases, causing the ripened Graafian follicles to rupture, releasing the ova.
4. *Metoestrus* – the period in which hormone activity fades and tissues are less active. If the ovum has been fertilised, the *corpus luteum* forms and produces *progesterone*, which is responsible for maintaining pregnancy. Oestrogen secretions decrease. If pregnancy does not occur, the corpus luteum decreases in size, reducing the production of progesterone. This is followed by anoestrus and the cycle starts once more.

Table 3.5 Species breeding data.

Species	Puberty	Oestrus	Gestation
Cat	6–10 months	Every 21 days	63–65 days
Dog	7–12 months	Twice yearly	63–67 days
Guinea pig	4–5 weeks	15–16-day cycle	60–72 days
Hamster	6–10 weeks	Every 4 days	15–22 days
Mouse	3–4 weeks	Every 4–5 days	19–21 days
Rabbit	3 months	Induced ovulation	30–33 days
Ferret	4–8 months	Seasonal until mated (March–September)	42–45 days
Rat	6 weeks	Every 4–5 days	20–22 days

Signs of heat/oestrus
- Increased vocalisation, especially in cats (known as calling)
- Behaviour changes, e.g. more affectionate or more aggressive
- Restless
- Seeking the male animal
- Rolling and appearing submissive
- Swelling of the vaginal area
- Discharge from the vaginal area

Summary of the reproductive system

This essential system consists of:

- The organs that are responsible for the creation and growth of offspring

The reproductive system works to:

- Ensure the survival of the species

Homeostasis

Homeostasis is the *state of equilibrium in the body* with respect to various functions and the chemical composition of fluids and tissues. The word 'homeostasis' means 'staying the same'. All body systems work together cooperatively to ensure homeostasis is achieved. Some of the factors that must be kept the same are:

- Chemical constituents like glucose and electrolytes (salts)
- Osmotic pressure and the movement of fluid (water) and substances carried by this water
- Levels of the waste gas carbon dioxide
- Body temperature

Other products must be eliminated from the body because of their harmful effect. The most important of these are the nitrogenous waste products arising from protein metabolism and toxic substances released by micro-organisms that live in the body.

Internal Environment

This refers to the immediate surroundings of the cells. The cells are surrounded by tiny channels and spaces filled with fluid, and the fluid can be identified by the following names:

- Intercellular (between)
- Extracellular interstitial
- Tissue fluid

The cells are provided with a medium in which they live, and this represents the organism's internal environment, which must be kept constant if the cells are to continue their vital functions. This fluid will return to the bloodstream eventually, either by osmotic pressure or via the lymph.

Other examples of homeostatic mechanisms in the body include the following:

- The regulation of sugar levels in the bloodstream. Sugar may be broken down and used as energy at the cellular level, stored in the liver as glycogen, converted to fat for storage, or released into the bloodstream to top up the circulating levels.
- Regulation cannot be achieved without the various hormone chemical messengers provided by the organs of the endocrine system.
- The nervous system receives information from the body about all products and whether they are at the correct levels. If not, it sends a message to the organs concerned to rectify the situation.
- To control homeostasis, the body has feedback mechanisms. The sense organs give back information to the brain, and from here, messages are sent to the relevant system or tissue for a response. The results of this response are then fed back to the brain, which decides on any subsequent action.

There is an important difference between homeostatic feedback and a voluntary or conscious control action by the body. In homeostasis, feedback is largely an unconscious activity – the animal is unaware that it is taking place as it usually needs the action to happen extremely quickly. Feedback mechanisms may be positive or negative. Examples of positive feedback mechanisms are childbirth, lactation, and blood clotting. Examples of negative feedback mechanisms include temperature regulation, blood sugar control, and thirst mechanisms.

Homeostasis is most highly developed in mammals and birds, probably because of their evolution. They can maintain a constant body temperature despite environmental temperature change. This is greatly assisted by feathers and fur for insulation.

Summary of homeostasis

Homeostasis is crucial for survival as organisms adapt to changes in both their internal and external environments to effect a change for maintaining optimal functioning.

All body systems are involved in homeostatic processes.

4

Basic Genetics

Learning goals

In this chapter, the learning goals are:

- To define the terms relating to basic genetics
- To identify the structure and function of chromosomes, genes, and DNA
- To identify and describe the stages of cell division – mitosis and meiosis

What Are Genetics?

Genetics is the study of heredity, i.e. how characteristics are passed from parent to offspring and subsequently down the generations.

Why Are Genetics Important?

Studying genetics allows us to identify dominant characteristics; it allows us to identify genes that cause specific diseases, and it allows us to map the genetic code (*genome*) for species. At this point in time, more than 51 species of animal have had their genome mapped, including dogs, chickens, chimpanzees, and turtles.

Important Events in the History of Genetics

Gregor Mendel (1822–1884) is said to be the father of modern genetics. A monk who lived in the nineteenth century, Mendel conducted many investigations on pea plants and made detailed notes about their inherited characteristics, which were published at the time through the Brünn Society for the Study of Natural History. At the time, his investigations were disregarded but became more important 40 years later after his death. Mendel's theories were brought forward by the Dutch scientist Hugo De Vries (1848–1935).

Mendel's investigations with pea plants culminated in him establishing two laws relating to inheritance and forming the basis of today's modern genetics. Mendelian genetics were the cornerstone to today's advances in genetics.

Animal Biology and Care, Fourth Edition. Emily Jewell.
© 2026 John Wiley & Sons Ltd. Published 2026 by John Wiley & Sons Ltd.
Companion Website: https://www.wiley.com/go/animal/biology4e/jewell

Mendel's first law

Mendel's first law is also referred to as the 'Law of Segregation'. This law states that every individual has a pair of *alleles* for any particular *trait* and that each parent passes a randomly selected copy of one allele to its offspring. The trait exhibited in the offspring will depend on which of the alleles received from the parents are dominant, e.g. colour of an animal's fur.

Mendel's second law

Mendel's second law is also called the 'Law of Inheritance'. It states that separate genes of separate traits are passed independently of each other from parent to offspring. Mendel stated that different traits shown in a species are inherited independently of each other. This is now known only to be true when genes are not linked to each other.

Chromosomes, Genes, and DNA

In Chapter 1, it was said that the nucleus of the cell contains chromosomes and that chromosomes are rod-shaped components containing DNA (*deoxyribonucleic acid*). DNA contains genetic code for the characteristics an animal possesses. It is due to this genetic code that DNA can produce exact copies of itself, and instructions can be passed on to new cells that form in the body. Chromosomes are always found in pairs in the nucleus.

The shape of the DNA molecule within the nucleus is one of its most significant features. It is known as the double helix and was discovered in 1953 by James Watson and Francis Crick and was one of the most notable discoveries of the twentieth century. The helix shape is brought about by two strands being linked across the middle to form 'stairs'. When stretched out, the DNA of a cell can stretch to 1.5 m in length (Figure 4.1).

Each linkage strand within the double helix structure is simply a long line of chemical units called *nucleotides*. A nucleotide consists of a sugar molecule and a phosphate molecule linked to a DNA base. There are four different types of DNA bases, which are represented by the letters A, G, C, and T. Each single strand of DNA can contain any sequence of these letters. On the opposite strand of DNA will be a similar sequence of the letters, and if one side of the strand is known, then the other side can be predicted as the *nucleotides always exist in set pairs*: A always pairs with T and C always pairs with G.

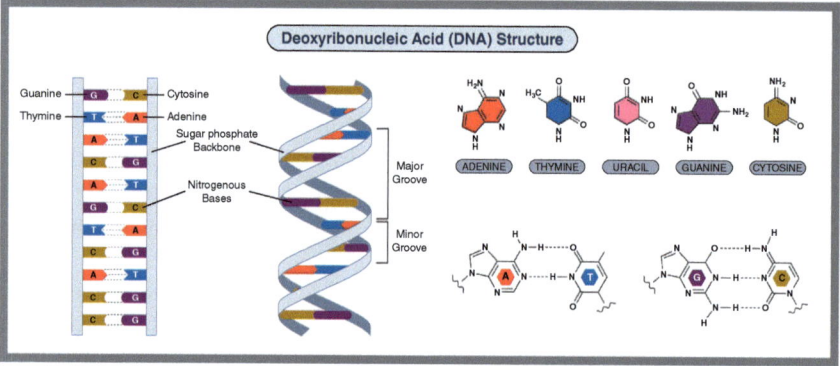

Figure 4.1 Structure of DNA.

Table 4.1 Number of chromosomes in different species.

Species	Number of chromosomes
Human	46
Chimpanzee	48
Horse	64
Dog	76
Cat	38

Therefore, if the code on one strand is:

AATCGCTAATGCCGGAT

then the code on the opposite strand is:

TTAGCGATTACGGCCTA

The base pairs are attached to a *sugar phosphate backbone*, which comprises the longitudinal strands on the helix. The base pairs are:

A = adenine   T = thymine
G = guanine   C = cytosine

As already mentioned, DNA is stored in the nucleus of a cell in structures called chromosomes. The number of chromosomes in each species of animal is different and specific to that species (Table 4.1).

The DNA on the chromosomes is split into specific segments called *genes*. Genes are the *single unit of heredity*. Many characteristics can be determined by a single gene. Genes control all aspects of the body, whether it is the coat, hair, or eye colour; rate of bone growth; or the ability of the blood to clot. Unfortunately, genes are responsible for many diseases and disorders as well, which are called inherited factors.

Each gene has its own allocated place on a particular chromosome called the *gene locus*. Genes exist in pairs, just like chromosomes. Therefore, each chromosome carries two copies of a gene. The copies may not be the same, and in this case, genes that occupy the same gene locus on a chromosome are called *alleles*.

Genetic Terms

Table 4.2 is a glossary of commonly used genetic terms.

Cell Division

There are two methods of cell division, depending on the cells involved.

Table 4.2 Genetics glossary of terms.

Term	Definition
Genetics	The science of heredity, i.e. how characteristics are passed on from parents to offspring.
Meiosis	Cell division process to form daughter cells containing half the original number of chromosomes – exclusive to sex cells.
Mitosis	Cell division process to form new cells containing the same number of chromosomes as the parent cell.
DNA	Deoxyribonucleic acid.
RNA	Ribonucleic acid.
Chromosomes	Structures within the nucleus of a cell that contain all the information for the characteristics of an individual.
Genes	The basic unit of inheritance for any characteristic – lengths of DNA that contain specific codes for particular proteins.
Locus	The specific location of a gene on a chromosome.
Allele	Different versions of the same gene occupying the same locus on the chromosome, e.g. coat colour.
Genotype	The genetic make-up of an animal.
Phenotype	The physical expression of genotype – i.e. the appearance of the animal, e.g. coat colour.
Dominant	Genes that are expressed in the phenotype even when only one allele is present. Dominant alleles suppress other alleles and are represented by capital letters, e.g. B in the genotypes BB and Bb.
Recessive	These alleles are only expressed in the phenotype when both alleles are present and are represented by lower-case letters, e.g. b in Bb and bb. The recessive characteristic will only be shown in the case of bb.
Co-dominant	Both alleles of a gene are expressed.
Homozygous	Both alleles of a particular gene are the same, e.g. BB or bb.
Heterozygous	Alleles of a particular gene are different, e.g. Bb.
Masked genes/ epistasis	Some genes have an overwhelming effect on other genes and can block the expression of alleles on a different locus, e.g. albino gene blocks the coat colour gene.
Mimic genes	This occurs when two or more distinctly different genes produce similar bodily effects. Mimic genes are often expressed in species that want to look like more toxic versions of themselves.
Rogue genes	Produce bad or life-threatening effects on the animal, e.g. extra toes, deafness in white gene animals, eyesight defects like the Siamese gene.
Lethal factors	Genes that are not compatible with life and so the animal dies if one of these genes is present.

Mitosis

Mitosis is the process of cell division that results in the production of two identical daughter cells, each containing an identical set of chromosomes compared to the parent cell. Mitosis occurs in all body cells (*somatic cells*) except the sex cells (*gametes*). The original number of chromosomes is known as the *diploid number*.

Figure 4.2 Mitosis. *Source*: Dorland's Medical Dictionary for Health Consumers (2007). Reproduced with permission of Elsevier.

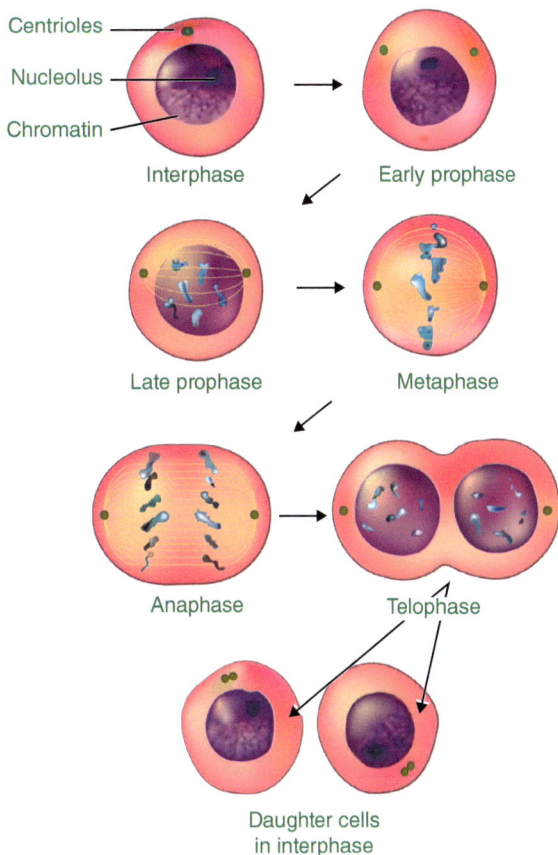

Centrioles

Nucleolus

Chromatin

Interphase

Early prophase

Late prophase

Metaphase

Anaphase

Telophase

Daughter cells in interphase

Before a cell divides, copies of each chromosome form alongside the originals and then separate from the originals. As a cell divides, a full set of chromosomes collects at each end to form part of the two new cell nuclei (Figure 4.2).

Meiosis

Meiosis is the type of cell division that results in the production of gamete cells. Meiosis only occurs in the ovaries or testes. Each daughter cell produced contains only *half the number of chromosomes* when compared to the parent cell. This half number of chromosomes is known as the *haploid number*. The result of meiosis is that each sperm and each egg contains one member of each pair of chromosomes. The union of a sperm with an egg at fertilisation produces a fertilised egg with the usual diploid number of chromosomes (Figure 4.3).

The phases of mitosis and meiosis can be remembered using the acronym IPMAT:

- I Interphase
- P Prophase
- M Metaphase
- A Anaphase
- T Telophase

The final division in both processes is known as *cytokinesis*.

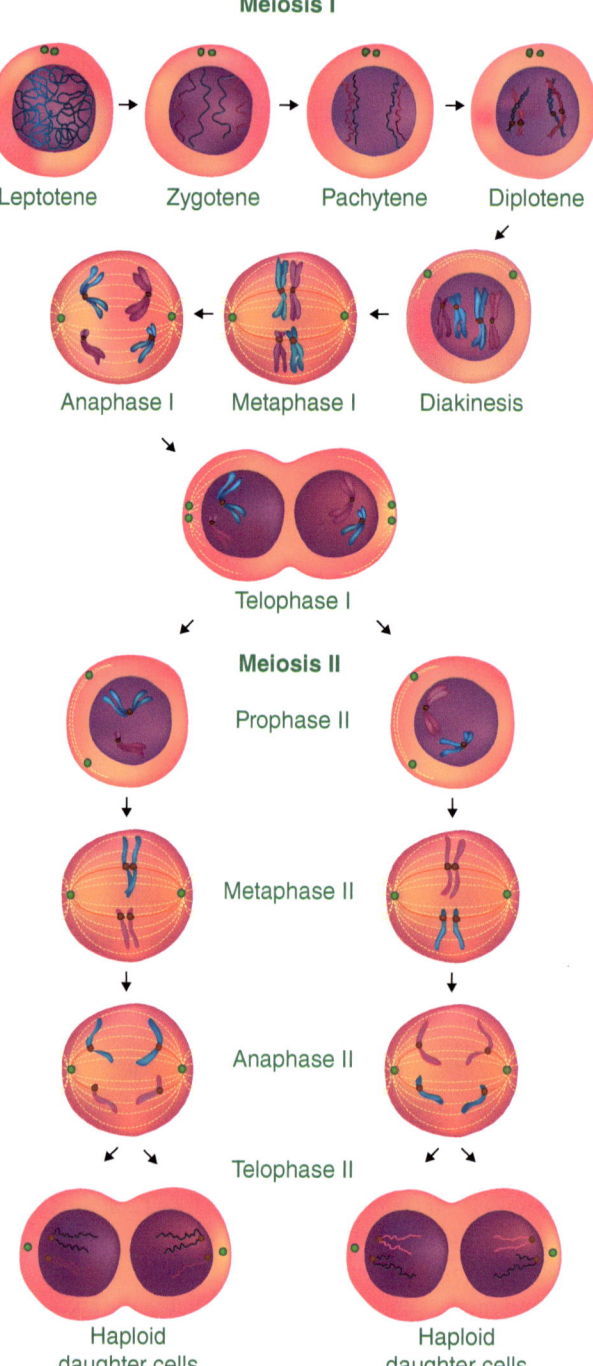

Figure 4.3 Meiosis. *Source*: Dorland's Medical Dictionary for Health Consumers (2007). Reproduced with permission of Elsevier.

Table 4.3 Comparison of mitosis and meiosis.

Mitosis	Meiosis
Division of a body cell to form new body cells.	Division of cells in the sex organs (testes or ovaries) to form sex cells (gametes).
The daughter cell carries identical gene information to the parent cell.	The daughter cells give each new cell half the number of genes present.
Both cells are referred to as diploid.	Both cells are referred to as haploid.
	Only occurs in the testes and ovaries.

Comparison of mitosis and meiosis

A comparison of mitosis and meiosis is presented in Table 4.3.

Breeding and Genetics

Genetic studies have become significantly important in relation to the breeding of pedigree animals. There is considerable focus in these times on inherited diseases that are completely avoidable if disease-free animals are bred from. Responsible breeders will test for these diseases and avoid breeding from affected stock. Examples of genetically linked diseases in dogs and cats include hip and elbow dysplasia, canine X-linked muscular dystrophy, progressive retinal atrophy (PRA), von Willebrand's disease, polycystic kidney disease (PKD), and hypertrophic cardiomyopathy.

Anyone considering breeding from an animal should research the animals and make careful choices in the selection of a mate to avoid producing offspring that are carrying inherited disease(s).

It is important to be aware of the following terms when discussing breeding:

- *Pedigree* – mother and father of the same breed with written pedigree from the owner tracing ancestors (pedigree chart).
- *Crossbred* – Mother and father are of different breeds. They may both be purebred, making the offspring a 'first cross' (*F1 generation*). This means the size and behaviour of the offspring are reasonably predictable; however, behavioural issues are being reported in some of these breeds. This type of breeding is becoming more popular to create fashionable/designer breeds, e.g. Labrador × Poodle – Labradoodle and Pug × Beagle – Puggle, Miniature Schnauzer × Poodle – Schnoodle. If two F1 generations are mated, then the resulting offspring are said to be *F2 generation*. F1 and F2 generations can be predicted using Punnett squares (Figure 4.4).
- *Mongrel* – If a female is mated with an already crossbred male, the offspring would be mongrels. The same applies if a male is mated with an already crossbred female. This means the size and behaviour of the offspring are unpredictable.
- *Inbreeding* – mating for specific characteristics. It involves mating individuals that are more closely related than animals chosen from other bloodlines, for example, father/daughter and brother/sister.
- *Line breeding* – It is a form of inbreeding, but animals are not so closely related. It is mating within certain family lines and maintains a relationship with a particular ancestor for specific characteristics.

Table 4.4 Glossary of breeding-related terms.

Term	Definition
Sire	The father.
Dam	The mother.
Seasonally monoestrous	An animal that has one reproductive cycle in a breeding season.
Seasonally polyoestrous	An animal that has more than one reproductive cycle within a breeding season.
Pro-oestrus	The first part of a reproductive cycle where a female starts to become attractive to males but does not mate.
Oestrus	The second part of the reproductive cycle characterised by sexual activity in animals and ovulation.
Metoestrus	Period after ovulation where corpora lutea are formed and produce progesterone for maintaining pregnancy.
Interoestrus	The short period of time between each reproductive cycle in one breeding season.
Anoestrus	A long period of reproductive inactivity between reproductive cycles in between breeding seasons.
Season	The time at which an animal is ready to mate, i.e. oestrus.
Puberty	The time at which an animal is sexually mature and able to breed.
Adolescence	The growth phase prior to puberty usually equating to teenage years.
Misalliance	A mating that has occurred that is unplanned/unwanted.
Gestation	Pregnancy.
Pseudopregnancy	False pregnancy.
Parturition	Labour and birth.
Dystocia	Difficulty/problems giving birth.
Lactation	The period of milk production in mammals.
Neonate	Newborn animal.
Colostrum	The first milk produced by the mother that contains antibodies.
Weaning	The process of transferring young onto solid foods from milk.

- *Outbreeding* – breeding individuals that are less closely related, typically chosen at random from available animals.

Table 4.4 identifies a glossary of terms relating to breeding.

Punnett Squares

Punnett squares are a tool used in genetics to determine the possible offspring of two parents. They are commonly used in breeding experiments to predict traits of the offspring, such as coat colour. They are easy to use for simple traits but can become complex as the genetics becomes more complex.

Trait:

- White head (H) is dominant.
- Non-white head (h) is recessive.

Punnett square for F1 generation:

	H	H
h	Hh	Hh
H	Hh	Hh

F1 generation results:

- Of the offspring, 100% will be Hh (white head) as H is dominant over h.
- No ratios apply.

Punnett square for F2 generation:

	H	h
H	HH	Hh
h	Hh	hh

F2 generation results:

- Of the offspring, 75% will have white heads as H is dominant over h – this includes HH (homozygous dominant) and Hh (heterozygous) genotypes.
- Of the offspring, 25% will not have white heads as h is recessive – this includes the hh (homozygous recessive) genotype.
- Genotypic ratio is 1:2:1   (HH:Hh:hh)
- Phenotypic ratio is 3:1   (White head:Not white head)

Figure 4.4 Worked example of a basic Punnett square for F1 and F2 generations.

Here is an example of a Punnet square (Figure 4.4), using the characteristic of head colour in Hereford cattle for F1 and F2 generations. The white head of Hereford cattle is a dominant trait (H).

For a simple monohybrid cross (one trait), one parent has the genotype HH (homozygous dominant) and the other has hh (homozygous recessive), the Punnett square would show that all offspring will be Aa (heterozygous), expressing the dominant trait.

Ratios can be used to express the results.

Genotypic ratios refer to the gene expression.

Phenotypic ratios refer to what is seen.

Genetic mutations

Sometimes changes occur to the DNA code and a genetic mutation can occur. These are entirely natural events. Mutations may have positive or negative effects, and in most cases, they are hardly noticeable as they do not affect the phenotype.

Mutations may be caused by:

- Errors when replicating (copying) the genetic code.
- Environmental factors such as chemicals or radiation.
- Inherited mutations from parents.

Types of mutation include the following:

- *Point mutations* – a base pair has a simple change, which can lead to a different protein being synthesised.
- *Insertion* – an additional base pair can be added to the DNA sequence, thereby altering the protein synthesised.
- *Deletion* – one or more base pairs can be missing from the DNA sequence, and therefore, the protein synthesised is altered.
- *Chromosomal mutation* – These are larger changes that can affect entire chromosomes.

Gene interactions

Gene interactions shape the characteristics of an animal. Genes can work together in several different ways:

- *Co-dominance* – Both alleles in a heterozygous individual are fully expressed, e.g. A black cow (BB) is crossed with a white cow (WW) and their offspring (BW) are a pattern of black and white rather than grey.
- *Incomplete dominance* – The traits blend together in the offspring – this is evident in Royal Pythons and their different colour morphs.
- *Multiple alleles* – Some traits are controlled by more than two alleles and an example of this is blood types in humans and coat colour in rabbits.
- *Lethal genes* – Unfortunately, some combinations of genes can lead to death either before birth or shortly after. In Manx cats and Mexican hairless dogs, this is an important consideration when breeding as the homozygous dominant genotype is lethal in both cases. The heterozygous and homozygous recessive genotypes are not lethal for these examples.
- *Sex-linked traits* – These are linked to genes located on the X or Y chromosome. XX is female and XY is male. An example in cats is where the orange coat colour gene is carried on the X chromosome as is the black coat colour gene. Male cats can be black or orange as they are XY, but females can be black, orange, or tortoiseshell as they are XX. The majority of tortoiseshell cats are female. Male tortoiseshell cats are rare, but they can exist.
- *Epistasis* – One gene can mask the expression of another gene, or two genes can control the same phenotype. For example, in Labrador Retriever dogs, two genes control coat colour. The B gene (black or brown in colour) and the E gene (allows colours to show). If a dog has two recessive ee genes, then the dog will have a yellow coat, even if it carries B or b alleles, because the E gene masks the B gene.

Summary of Genetics

Genetics is a complex topic, and this chapter is a basic introduction to the concept.

- Be aware of the technical terms associated with genetics and how to use a Punnett square to predict F1 and F2 generations.

- The structure and function of chromosomes, genes, and DNA is critical to the continued breeding success of any species.
- Meiosis is the process that occurs in gametes and produces daughter cells with a haploid number of chromosomes.
- Mitosis is the process that occurs in all cells for growth and repair and produces cells with a diploid number of chromosomes.

5

Veterinary Terminology

Learning goals

In this chapter, the learning goals are:

- To identify parts of the body using veterinary terminology
- To be able to define commonly used prefixes and suffixes used in veterinary terminology
- To identify the different body cavities and their boundaries
- To identify the main organs of the different body cavities

When describing the location of a part of the body, it is helpful to be able to identify more accurately the part of the body using veterinary terminology.

Veterinary Terminology

Most terms referring to the body systems and medical conditions are developed from Greek or Latin. Most of these terms are a combination of two or more word parts. When they combine to become a word, they usually indicate some or all of the following:

- Body tissues involved
- What has gone wrong
- Quantity (a lot or very little)
- Levels of infection or inflammation
- Colour or substance
- Fluid involved

It may be helpful to practise defining the components of the words separately and then combining them to find out the meaning of the complete word.

Certain syllables are commonly used as the beginning or ending of medical terms, in many cases being added to a word stem that refers to a particular organ or part of the body:

- *Prefix* – beginning of a word stem
- *Suffix* – ending of a word stem

Learning veterinary terminology is, in many ways, no different from learning a new language, and by memorising the common beginnings (prefixes) and endings (suffixes), the rest can be worked out. It is always helpful, however, to have a veterinary dictionary for the less frequently used terms and words.

Common prefixes

- **A** - or **An** – lack of, e.g. anaemia (lack of blood cells)
- **Dys** – difficult or defective, e.g. dysphagia (difficulty swallowing)
- **Endo** – within, e.g. endoscope (equipment used to look at working organs)
- **Ex** – out, e.g. excision (to remove)
- **Haema** or **Haemo** – refers to blood, e.g. haemorrhage (loss of blood)
- **Hyper** – excess of, e.g. hyperthermia (high body temperature)
- **Hypo** – lack of, e.g. hypothermia (low body temperature)
- **Poly** – many or much, e.g. polydipsia (drinking a lot)
- **Pyo** – pus, e.g. pyometra (pus-filled uterus)
- **Sub** – beneath or under, e.g. sublingual (under the tongue)

Common suffixes

- **ectomy** – surgical removal or excision of a body part e.g. splenectomy is removal of the spleen
- **itis** – inflammation, e.g. arthritis (inflammation of a joint)
- **logy** – science or study of, e.g. dermatology (study of the skin)
- **osis** – pathological condition or process e.g. haematosis means disease of the blood
- **otomy** – surgical incision – e.g. craniotomy – incision into the skull, osteotomy – incision into a bone
- **pathy** – affected by disease e.g. cardiomyopathy – heart disease
- **penia** – deficiency, e.g. leucopenia (deficiency of white blood cells)
- **phagia** – eating, e.g. coprophagia (eating faeces)
- **rrhoea** – increased discharge, e.g. diarrhoea (increased discharge of faeces)

Examples of prefix and suffix use

The following common words may help to illustrate the prefix/suffix idea:

- *Nephritis* – **neph** refers to the specialised cell of the kidney, known as the nephron; – **itis** refers to the inflammation of a tissue. The meaning of this word is kidney cell inflammation.
- *Arthritis* – **arth** refers to a joint; – **itis** means inflammation. The meaning of this word is joint inflammation.
- *Hepatitis* – **hepat** refers to the specialised cell of the liver known as the hepatocyte; – **itis** means inflammation. This word means inflammation of the liver cells.
- *Haematoma* – **haem** refers to blood; – **toma** refers to a lump or swelling. The meaning of this word is blood-filled lump or swelling.

These words are descriptions, not diagnoses, and simply refer to a tissue type or organ and what is happening to it.

Terms linked to body organs and systems

- *Cardio or cardiac* – relating to the heart
- *Cranial* – relating to the brain

- *Cutaneous* – relating to the skin
- *Cys* – relating to the bladder
- *Digit* – relating to the phalanges
- *Entero* – relating to the intestines
- *Gastric* – relating to the stomach
- *Hepatic* – relating to the liver
- *Nasal* – relating to the nose
- *Neph* – relating to the kidneys
- *Ocular* – relating to eyes
- *Oral* – relating to the mouth
- *Osteo* – relating to bones
- *Ot/Oto* – relating to ears
- *Pulmonary* – relating to the lungs

These terms are all examples of terminology linking to body systems.

Anatomical Directions

Anatomical directions are used to describe areas of the animal body (Figure 5.1).

The first four words are another way of saying above, below, front, and back and are in common use when recording information about patients in the veterinary world:

- *Dorsal* – towards the top or back surface of the body
- *Ventral* – towards the underside, lower surface, or facing the ground
- *Cranial or anterior* – situated at the front of the body or towards of within the head
- *Caudal or posterior* – situated towards the back end of the body or towards or within the tail

Words to indicate side, middle, or near the nose are as follows:

- *Lateral* – to the side (left or right) or away from the middle of the body
- *Medial* – a term describing something that lies nearest to the midline of the body
- *Rostral* – on the head but towards the nose

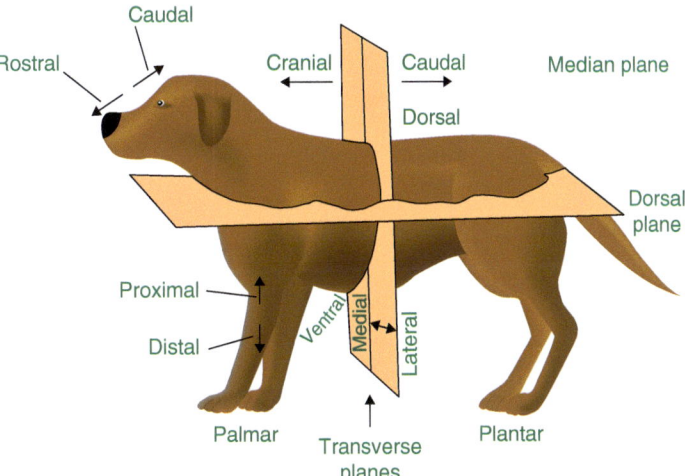

Figure 5.1 Anatomical directions. *Source*: Adapted from McBride, D.F. (1996) Learning Veterinary Terminology. Reproduced with permission of Elsevier.

Words indicating near or far from a named body structure (especially limbs) are:

- *Proximal* – near to the body trunk/centre of the body or closer to a named structure, e.g. the part of the femur bone closest to the hip joint would be called the proximal end of femur.
- *Distal* – away from the body trunk or further from the centre of the body, e.g. the part of the femur bone nearest to the knee or stifle would be called the distal end of femur.

Words that describe where on a limb, surface, especially lower limb, surfaces are:

- *Palmar or volar* – indicating the caudal or back surface of the forelimb, below the carpus or wrist area
- *Plantar* – indicating the caudal or back surface of the hindlimb, below the tarsus or hock area

Words indicating inside or outside are:

- *Internal* – inside the body
- *External* – outside or on the surface

Limb movements

These terms relate to the movement of a whole limb in relation to the rest of the body:

- *Protraction* – movement of a limb towards the head (cranially).
- *Retraction* – movement of a limb towards the tail (caudally).
- *Elevation* – movement of a limb up and nearer the body (proximal to body).
- *Adduction* – movement of a limb towards the middle of the body (midline).
- *Abduction* – movement of a limb away from the middle of the body (away from the midline).

Body Cavities

There are three main sections to the body known as cavities (Figure 5.2):

- *Thoracic*
- *Abdominal*
- *Pelvic*

When describing physical locations within the body, it is useful to know which body cavity the organs are located in. Each cavity has boundaries that separate it from the next cavity.

Thoracic cavity

The thoracic cavity is found within the chest. Its boundaries are as follows:

- *Cranial or anterior* – the thoracic inlet through which the trachea and oesophagus pass
- *Dorsal* – the thoracic vertebrae and joining muscles
- *Ventral* – the sternum
- *Lateral* – the ribs and intercostal muscles
- *Caudal or posterior* – the diaphragm

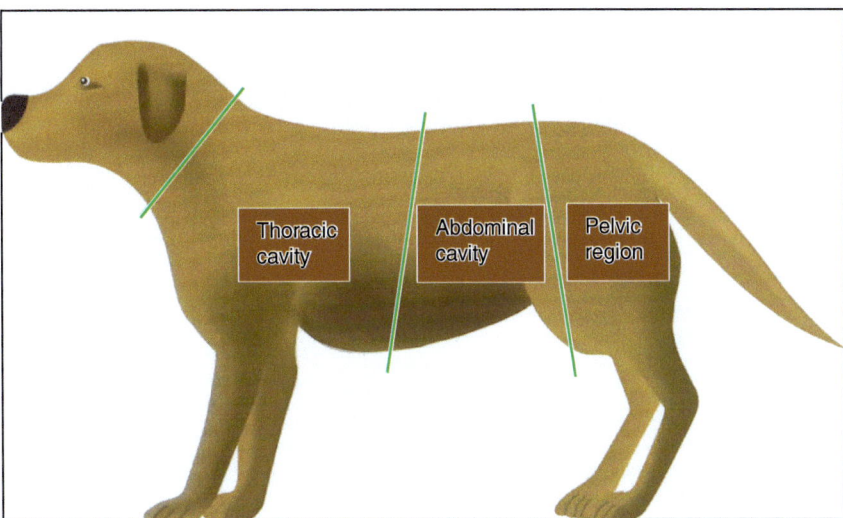

Figure 5.2 Body cavities.

The heart and lungs are located within the thoracic cavity. The heart is surrounded by the *pericardium*, which is a double-membrane layer designed to protect the heart.

Abdominal cavity

The abdominal cavity is found between the thoracic cavity and pelvic region of the animal. Its cranial boundary is the diaphragm, and its caudal limit is the pelvic opening. Dorsally are the lumbar vertebrae and the diaphragm. Lateral and ventral boundaries are the abdominal muscles. The abdominal cavity contains the stomach, liver, gall bladder, intestines, pancreas, and kidneys.

Pelvic region

There is no physical barrier that splits the abdominal cavity and the pelvis; hence, this area is often referred to as the pelvic region. Its cranial opening is the pelvic inlet, and the caudal opening is the pelvic outlet. Dorsally are the bones of the pelvis (pubis and ischium), and the lateral boundaries are muscles or ligaments. The pelvic region protects the bladder, the sex organs, and the rectum.

Cavity linings

Body cavities are lined with a *serous* membrane. This is a smooth, shiny membrane that produces a watery fluid to lubricate between two tissue surfaces and prevent friction:

- In the thoracic cavity, the lining is the *pleura*. If the pleura becomes inflamed, then the animal is suffering from *pleurisy*.
- In the abdominal and pelvic cavities, the lining is the *peritoneum*. If the peritoneum becomes inflamed, then the animal is suffering from *peritonitis*, which can be extremely serious.

Summary of Veterinary Terminology

Knowing the body cavities and the commonly used prefixes and suffixes is essential when working with animals as it helps to understand the veterinary notes and discussions.

- Practice defining the commonly used prefixes and suffixes to strengthen your knowledge.
- Incorporate veterinary terminology in daily discussions and notes to feel more confident with its use.

Section 2

Animal Health

6

Animal Welfare and Legislation

Learning goals

In this chapter, the learning goals are:

- To be able to define the term animal welfare
- To describe how to assess animal welfare through identification of the good and poor indicators of animal welfare
- To identify key pieces of animal welfare legislation
- To describe the main rules of the Pet Travel Scheme
- To identify types of animal welfare organisation
- To briefly examine the concept of animal rights

Animal welfare is a term that is frequently used within the animal industry and regard for an animal's welfare must be paramount for anyone caring for or working with animals. There are many important strands to animal welfare, and it is important to know what the term means and how the welfare of an animal can be promoted and enhanced.

Definition of Animal Welfare

> Animal welfare is the physical and psychological state of an animal as regards its attempt to cope with its environment.
>
> Professor Donald M Broom (1991), Colleen Macleod
> Professor of Animal Welfare, University of Cambridge, UK

It logically follows that the factors that affect an animal's welfare are not only the environment in which it lives but also the treatment it receives from its owners/carers/keepers and the ultimate quality of the animal's life.

Consider the following cases which could occur.

Case 1

A 6-year-old brood bitch is kept in the house of her owner, is provided with a nice warm bed, is given the best diet for her breed, always has access to fresh water, is sufficiently exercised every

Animal Biology and Care, Fourth Edition. Emily Jewell.
© 2026 John Wiley & Sons Ltd. Published 2026 by John Wiley & Sons Ltd.
Companion Website: https://www.wiley.com/go/animal/biology4e/jewell

day, and is played with to stimulate her mind. The owner has bred from her every year for the past 4 years and plans to continue to do so. Consider whether the bitch's welfare needs are being met in terms of quality of life.

Case 2

A small rescue centre has been given a pair of female ferrets at a weekend when there is minimal staffing and several volunteers. One of the volunteers has been told to find some housing until the manager is in work on Monday. The volunteer places the ferrets in an empty hutch and run that is large enough for the ferrets. The hutch that the ferrets are in is opposite a bank of hutches that currently houses rabbits. Consider how the welfare of (a) the rabbits and (b) the ferrets is affected by the actions of the volunteer.

Case 3

A young couple own a Bengal cat. The cat was the centre of their world until recently a baby was born. The cat is fed each day and has access to water, but the food bowl is often overflowing, and the water is not always replaced each day. The cat has access to a litter tray and to outside if necessary, but the litter tray is not always cleaned on a daily basis. The cat used to sleep on the owner's bed prior to the arrival of the baby and is now only allowed in a certain area of the house. Consider how the cat's welfare has been affected by the arrival of the baby.

Case 4

An elderly man owns two Shih Tzu dogs. His wife passed away 1 year ago. The dogs are middle-aged and have daily walks for approximately 30 minutes. The dogs are fed wet food each day and have access to water. The owner takes the dogs for grooming at a salon every 3 months. On the last couple of occasions, the salon owner has noticed that the dogs are coming in knottier and more matted than usual and has found signs of fleas on them. Consider how the dogs' welfare has been affected by the loss of the man's wife.

How Is Animal Welfare Assessed?

To assess the welfare of an animal, it is important to consider the whole animal and consider the good and bad aspects of welfare.

Indicators of good welfare

- A variety of normal behaviours shown
- Physiological indicators of pleasure
- Behavioural indicators of pleasure

Good welfare can be difficult to assess as an animal's behaviour can sometimes mask how it is really feeling. Most assessments of animal welfare tend to focus on the poor indicators of animal welfare.

Indicators of poor welfare

There are two types of indicators related to poor welfare:

1. Indicators relating to a failure to cope:
   i. Reduced life expectancy
   ii. Reduced ability to grow or breed
   iii. Increased disease
   iv. Reduced survival of offspring
   v. Reduction in production output (e.g. milk, eggs)
2. Extreme efforts involved in coping or attempting to cope:
   i. Extreme changes in physiology – the stress response is put into action.
   ii. Changes in behaviour – abnormal behaviours displayed and reluctance to perform normal behaviours.

It is important to remember that animal welfare affects both the physical and psychological status of the animal.

Animal Welfare Legislation

The law acts as a framework of guidelines for people to work within to uphold professional standards in relation to society. It is the responsibility of all people who work with animals to maintain a practical and working knowledge of the law relating to the animals and the industry in which they are working and always working within that law. The legislation in the United Kingdom refers to both Acts of Parliament and Regulations.

Laws (also known as *statutes*) – are created by the UK Parliament. They are first presented before Parliament as draft legislation in the form of a bill, after which they are debated initially in the House of Commons and the House of Lords. They are then considered by a specifically formed parliamentary committee, before finally receiving the Monarch's signature to become law and being placed on the Statute Book as an Act of Parliament.

Regulations (orders) – These detail the technical implications of laws. The relevant government minister adds regulations to the legislation. This information is a supplement to the existing law and must have approval of Parliament.

Welfare codes – must also have parliamentary approval. Failure to comply with the provisions of a code is not in itself an offence but could be used in evidence if prosecuted. Codes of practice are issued by Department for the Environment, Food & Rural Affairs (DEFRA) and, at the time of writing (2024), exist for farmed species of animals (cattle, sheep, goats, deer, pigs, rabbits, goats, and gamebirds reared for sport) as well as dogs, cats, and equines.

The purpose of any animal-related legislation is to:

- Ensure the health, welfare, and protection of the animals through setting minimum husbandry requirements.
- Protect the public.
- Set standards and provide a framework of guidelines for the control of licensing in certain areas of the animal industry.

It is important to note that some pieces of legislation do not apply to the whole of the United Kingdom. When this is the case, the name of the country that the piece of legislation applies to will be included in the title of the legislation, e.g. Welfare of Animals Act (Northern Ireland) 2011.

In 2020, the United Kingdom left the European Union (EU), which is an international organisation aimed at uniting the economies and political powers of the member states that have signed up to it. The United Kingdom had been a member since 1973 and during that time, much EU legislation was linked to UK legislation. Any EU legislation that applied to the United Kingdom (directly or indirectly) prior to 11 p.m. on 31 December 2020 has been retained in UK law under the European Union (Withdrawal) Act 2018. Since 2023, any retained EU law is now known as assimilated law under the Retained EU Law (Revocation and Reform) Act 2023. Details of all legislation applying to the United Kingdom can be found on the Government's website www.legislation.gov.uk (at the current time – December 2024).

Several pieces of legislation relating to animal welfare have been identified in this chapter, but it is not an exhaustive list as there are more in existence.

Animal Welfare Act 2006

The Animal Welfare Act (AWA) 2006 was without doubt the most significant piece of legislation concerning animal welfare to be published this century. It took several outdated pieces of legislation such as the Protection of Animals Act 1911 and the Abandonment of Animals Act 1960 and brought them together with additional information to produce a piece of legislation more relevant to today's society.

The AWA applies to all vertebrate animals with the exclusion of humans. One of the most important aims of the act is that it relates specifically to pet owners to ensure that they have a legal duty of care to meet the five animal welfare needs of their pet(s). The AWA is also applicable to all people who work with animals and keep animals for breeding or working purposes whether in a zoo, aquarium, circus, farm park, rescue centre, kennels, or veterinary practice.

The Five Animal Needs were previously known as the Five Freedoms of Animal Welfare. The Five Freedoms were created in 1963 in relation to farm livestock, and over the years, they have been applied to all animals kept in captivity. In 2006, they were amended to be known as the Five Animal Needs to be incorporated into the new AWA 2006. By meeting the five welfare needs, it is ensured that people are caring for those animals properly and are promoting responsible pet ownership.

The Five Animal Needs

1. An animal should have a suitable environment in which to live.
2. An animal should have a proper diet, including fresh water.
3. An animal should have the ability to express normal behaviour.
4. An animal should have its needs to be housed with, or apart from, other animals met.
5. An animal should have protection from, and treatment of, illness and injury.

When establishing how the needs for an animal can be met, an owner should think about what the animal would have in its natural environment in terms of housing, feeding, and how it relates to other animals (*see* Table 6.1). By meeting these basic needs, the animal should be able to display the normal behavioural repertoire for that species. Since animals are kept in captivity, whether as pets, working animals, production animals, or visitor attractions, owners/carers/keepers of those animals have a responsibility to ensure that the animal(s) remain healthy and protected against illness and disease, and this includes preventative treatments as well as reactive treatments.

The five welfare needs are important to animal welfare as they provide a framework on which to provide advice and guidance to owners/carers/keepers.

The five welfare needs provide a framework for organisations, such as the Royal Society for the Prevention of Cruelty to Animals (RSPCA), to step in prior to animal suffering occurring, which was not possible under any previous legislation. Environmental Health Officers also now have

Table 6.1 Factors to consider for each animal welfare need.

Animal welfare need	Factors to consider

Need for a suitable environment	Aquatic or terrestrial
	Climber or burrower
	Endotherm or ectotherm
	  • Temperature
	  • Lighting
	  • Humidity
	  • Ventilation
	Housing
	  • Size
	  • Materials
	  • Substrate provision
	  • Bedding provision
	Location of environment
	Security
	Numbers in accommodation (i.e. stocking density)
	Animals nearby
	Life stage
	Illness

Need for a proper diet, including fresh water	Food:
	  • Type
	  • Quality
	  • Quantity
	  • Presentation
	Supplements
	Treats
	Feeding plans
	Life stage
	Adaptation for chronic disease

Need to express normal behaviour	Exercise requirements
	  • frequency
	  • type
	  • duration
	Food presentation
	Housing needs
	Social needs
	Stereotypical behaviours and their prevention

Need to be housed with, or apart from, other animals	Solitary or social animals Other animals in the location Interactions with other animal species

(Continued)

Table 6.1 (Continued)

Animal welfare need	Factors to consider
Need to be protected from pain, injury, suffering, and disease	Grooming requirements
	Environment safety
	Health checking
	Weight monitoring/condition scoring
	Routine veterinary care
	Preventative treatments
	Prevention of stress
	Biosecurity
	Quarantine procedures
	Isolation procedures

powers to issue improvement notices and prosecute if an animal is being mistreated. The AWA allows improvement notices to be issued prior to seizure of any animals, and therefore, owners/carers/keepers have a chance to resolve any situation in the first instance.

The key areas addressed by the AWA are that animals may not be sold or given as prizes to children aged under 16 years and that separate sections have been incorporated to address the contentious and emotive issues of tail docking, animal fighting, mutilation, and animal poisoning.

A person or persons who are successfully prosecuted under the AWA may be disqualified from owning/keeping/dealing in/transporting a specific type of animal (e.g. dogs) or be disqualified from owning/keeping/dealing in/transporting all animals, depending upon the nature of the offence. They can also face up to 5 years in prison and/or an unlimited fine. These penalties were increased in 2021 by the Government of the time following a survey of the general public who voted to make sentences tougher in the case of animal cruelty.

The AWA was amended in 2019 with the addition of the Animal Welfare (Service Animals) Act 2019. This Act was introduced to ensure service animals, such as police dogs, have protection in law if deliberately injured while undertaking their working duties. The legislation is also known as "Finn's Law as it was brought in following the serious injuring of an on duty police dog named Finn."

Animal Welfare (Licensing of Activities Involving Animals) (England) Regulations 2018

The Animal Welfare (Licensing of Activities Involving Animals) (England) Regulations 2018 set out the requirements for licensing various activities involving animals to ensure their welfare.

The key points are:

1. Licensable activities:
   - Selling animals as pets (Schedule 3)
   - Providing boarding for cats and dogs (Schedule 4)
   - Hiring out horses (Schedule 5)
   - Dog breeding (Schedule 6)
   - Keeping or training animals for exhibition (Schedule 7)

2. General conditions:
   - Suitable environment and diet
   - Ability to exhibit normal behaviour
   - Handling and interactions
   - Housing needs
   - Protection from pain, suffering, injury, and disease
3. Licensing process:
   - Local authorities are responsible for granting licenses.
   - Inspections are conducted to ensure compliance with welfare standards.
   - Licenses can be granted for up to 3 years, with risk-based inspections determining the frequency with which inspection take place.
4. Specific conditions:
   - Each activity has specific conditions outlined in the regulations to ensure higher welfare standards.
   - These regulations aim to promote and protect the welfare of animals involved in the named activities by setting clear standards and ensuring regular oversight.
   - The Animal Welfare (Licensing of Activities involving Animals) (England) Regulations 2018 replaces the following previous pieces of legislation:
     - Breeding of Dogs Acts 1973 and 1991 as amended by the Breeding and Sale of Dogs (Welfare) Act 1999
     - Riding Establishments Acts 1964 and 1970
     - Animal Boarding Establishments Act 1963
     - The Performing Animals (Regulation) Act 1925
     - The Pet Animals Act 1951 amended 1983

Microchipping of Cats and Dogs (England) Regulations 2023

The *Microchipping of Cats and Dogs (England) Regulations 2023* makes the microchipping of cats and dogs compulsory to improve their welfare and assist with their return if lost.
   The key points are:

1. Mandatory microchipping:
   - All cats must be microchipped by the age of 20 weeks.
   - All dogs must be microchipped by the age of 8 weeks, except for certified working dogs.
2. Database registration:
   - The microchip must be registered with the keeper's contact details on an approved database.
3. Import requirements:
   - Imported cats and dogs must be microchipped within 30 days of entry into England.
4. Exemptions:
   - Animals can be exempted from microchipping if a veterinary surgeon certifies that it would harm their health.

Penalties for non compliance:

   - Owners who fail to microchip their pets may face fines of up to £500.

These regulations aim to ensure that lost or stray pets can be quickly reunited with their owners, thereby enhancing animal welfare across England.

Pet Abduction Act 2024

The Pet Abduction Act 2024 is a new piece of legislation introduced in recognition of the emotional bond between owners and their pets. It is now a criminal offence to abduct dogs and cats. This is one of the few pieces of legislation that specifically recognises cats in law.

The key points are:

- It is a criminal offence to take or detain a dog or cat from its lawful owner.
- Acknowledgement of the emotional trauma caused to both the pet and the owner during abductions/thefts.
- Recognition that cats and dogs have an emotional value and are no longer just viewed as property.
- There is potential to extend the legislation to cover other pets in the future.
- Pet owners must ensure their pets are microchipped and that the details are kept up to date.

Penalties for offences:

- Offenders can face up to 5 years in prison for pet abduction.

Control of Dogs Order 1992

The *Control of Dogs Order 1992* in the United Kingdom was established to help with the easy identification of dogs if they are lost so that they may be more easily returned to their owners. The Microchipping of Cats and Dogs (England) Regulations 2023 augment this order.

Key points are as follows:

- All dogs in public places must wear an identification collar/tag with the owner's name and address inscribed on it.
- Working dogs, such as guide dogs and those used for sporting purposes, are exempt from this requirement.

Penalties for non-compliance include:

- Fine of up to £2000
- Imprisonment for up to 6 months (or longer if a severe incident)

This act has not been significantly updated since 1992 but the following pieces of legislation are linked to it:

- These orders replace the Dog (Fouling of Land) Act 1996 and can be put in place on an area of land to control:
  - Dog fouling
  - Restricting access of dogs to certain areas of land (e.g. beaches)
  - Stating specific areas where dogs must be kept on a lead
  - Stating specific areas where dogs must be put on a lead if asked to do so
  - Walking multiple dogs in specific areas
  - Dog Control Orders can be put in place by local authorities or parish councils. If an order is broken, then a fine of up to £1000 can be issued
- The Dog Control Orders (Prescribed Offences and Penalties, etc.) Regulations 2006
- Microchipping of Cats and Dogs (England) Regulations 2023

Note: The Dog (Fouling of Land) Act 1996 was incorporated into the *Clean Neighbourhoods and Environment Act 2005, Part 6.*

Dangerous Dogs Act 1991

The UK Government introduced the Dangerous Dogs Act 1991 (DDA) after an increase in the number of dog attacks on people in the 1980s. The DDA legislation was intended to make it more difficult to own and import specific breeds of dogs into the UK; however, a review in 2012 found this not to be the case and recommended a greater focus on all breeds of dogs. The Act was amended in 2023 with the introduction of the Dangerous Dogs (Designated Types) (England and Wales) Order 2023, which added the XL bully to the list of prohibited breeds.

Key points include:

1. It is against the law to own, breed, sell, or exchange specific breeds listed under the act
   - American Pit Bull Terrier
   - Japanese Tosa
   - Dogo Argentino
   - Fila Brasileiro
   - XL Bully (added in 2023)

If any of these specific breeds are owned, then there are specific rules that owners must follow:

- Notify the police of ownership
- Obtain a certificate of exemption from the police, which is only issued once the dog has been neutered and permanently identified with a microchip and tattoo.
- The dog must be covered by third-party liability insurance
- In public places, the dog must always be on a lead and muzzled
- The dog must not be solely taken out by anyone under 16 years of age
- The dog should not be sold, exchanged, or abandoned; otherwise, prosecution can occur
- It is an offence to breed from these dogs

Penalties for non-compliance:

- Fines of up to £5000
- Prison sentence of up to 14 years depending on the severity of the attack
- Seizure and destruction of the offending dog
- Banned from owning dogs in the future

Since the 2012 review of the DDA, it is now important to note that any dog dangerously out of control and a risk to the public comes under the remit of this act. There is now greater focus on education, responsible pet ownership, and the behaviour of individual dogs rather than specific breeds (although the rules around the listed prohibited breeds still apply).

Guard Dogs Act 1975

The Guard Dogs Act 1975 exists to ensure that dogs used to protect property are used safely and are under control so as not to put the public at risk.

Key points are:

- Notices must be displayed advising that guard dogs are on the premises, especially at the entrance to the premises.
- Guard dogs should only be off the lead if a person capable of controlling the dog is present.
- Guard dogs should not be left to roam freely on the premises without supervision being present.
- The person who is responsible for the dog must hold the relevant Guard Dogs Kennels Licence.
- The act does not cover dogs kept to protect agricultural land.

- Owners of guard dogs can be liable for any injuries to people under the Animals Act 1971 unless they are covered by an exemption under this act.
- This act was last reviewed and amended in 2015.

Dangerous Wild Animals Act 1976, Amended 2010

The Dangerous Wild Animals Act (DWA) 1976 aims to ensure that private individuals who keep dangerous wild animals do so safely in a way that creates no risk to the public. The act was introduced due to the desire of the public to begin keeping more exotic animals, and there was a concern for the welfare of the animals and the safety of the public. Animals kept under the DWA are also subject to protection under the AWA 2006.

The key points are:

1. Licensing
   - Individuals must obtain a licence from their local authority to keep any animal listed in the Act's schedule, which is available on the Department for Environment, Food & Rural Affairs (DEFRA) website. The government may amend the list at any time, and it is the responsibility of animal owners/carers/keepers to keep themselves familiarised with the Schedule.
   - Inspections are carried out by authorised veterinary surgeons who then report to the local authority as to whether a licence should or should not be issued.
   - Any person that holds a licence must:
     ○ Be 18+ years of age
     ○ Hold sufficient liability insurance
     ○ Meet the welfare needs of the animal
   - In March 2010, the DWA was amended under the Legislative Reform (Dangerous Wild Animals) (Licensing) Order 2010 with the main changes being:
     ○ A licence will be valid for a maximum of 2 years instead of 1 year.
     ○ New licences will come into force as soon as they are granted.
2. Husbandry conditions
   - The license inspection assesses how well the establishment applies the five animal needs for the animals being kept as well as inspecting security in place, emergency procedures, and biosecurity arrangements.
3. Exemptions
   - Zoos, circuses, and pet shops are exempt from this Act as they are covered under The Animal Welfare (Licensing of Activities Involving Animals) (England) Regulations 2018.
   - Premises covered under Animal (Scientific Procedures) Act 1986 (ASPA) are exempt.

Penalties for non-compliance:

- Keeping a dangerous wild animal without a licence can result in fines or imprisonment.
- Authorities can seize and dispose of animals kept without a licence without having to provide any form of compensation.

Convention on International Trade in Endangered Species of Wild Fauna and Flora (CITES) 1973

The Convention on International Trade in Endangered Species of Wild Fauna and Flora (CITES) is also known as the Washington Convention.

The treaty is an international agreement that aims to protect the world's endangered species of animals and plants by controlling their export and import on a worldwide scale.

Animal and plant species are listed on appendices based on a risk of extinction level and the protection that they need:

- Appendix 1 – Those species threatened with extinction. Trade is only allowed in exceptional circumstances.
- Appendix 2 – Those species likely to become threatened unless trade is closely controlled.
- Appendix 3 – Species may be protected in at least one of the member countries and they ask other member countries for help in controlling trade.

The treaty is voluntarily signed by countries who then agree to follow a framework to ensure that the CITES guidelines operate at a domestic level within that country. At the current time (2024), there are 184 countries that are signed up to CITES.

CITES regulations are reviewed and amended at the annual Conference of the Parties (CoP) summits.

Penalties for non-compliance may include:

- Fines (amount depends on severity of offence)
- Imprisonment (length depends on severity of offence)
- Seizure of illegally traded species
- Bans on future trade

Zoo Licensing Act 1981

The Zoo Licensing Act 1981 (ZLA) sets out how zoos in Great Britain are inspected and licensed to ensure that zoos are safe for the public to visit, that high standards of animal welfare are implemented, that zoos contribute to the conservation of wildlife, and that zoos play a role in the education of the public. Zoos are required to follow the Standards of Modern Zoo Practice for Great Britain as published by the Secretary of State for the Department of Environment, Food and Rural Affairs (DEFRA) in the United Kingdom. These were updated in May 2025. European Council Directive 1999/22/EC is also implemented in the United Kingdom through this piece of legislation and it has been upheld in law since the United Kingdom left the European Union in January 2020.

The key points are:

- The term 'zoo' refers to a collection of wild animals that are on display to the public for educational purposes.
- If such a collection opens to the public for seven or more days in any 1 year, then they must apply for a zoo licence.
- Local authorities are responsible for issuing licences to zoological collections, following an inspection of the premises with an authorised Secretary of State Zoo Inspector.
- Licences are renewed on a six yearly basis with interim checks during the period that the licence is held (Note, the first licence is only valid for 4 years).
- Any vertebrate animals kept in zoos are also subject to protection under the AWA 2006.

Penalties for non-compliance:

- Improvement notices issued
- Fines
- Imprisonment
- Zoo closure

Veterinary Surgeons Act 1966

The Veterinary Surgeons Act 1966 is the key piece of legislation in the United Kingdom that regulates the practice of veterinary surgery.

The key points are:

- The Act defines veterinary surgery as the diagnosis, treatment, and surgery of animals.
- Only individuals registered with the Royal College of Veterinary Surgeons (RCVS) are permitted to practice veterinary surgery.
- Schedule 3 of the act enables registered veterinary nurses (RVN), veterinary students, and animal owners to perform specific procedures under certain conditions. For example, RVNs can carry out minor surgery providing that it does not require entry into the body cavity of the animal. RVNs can also treat an animal medically providing they are under the direction of the registered veterinary surgeon.
- Schedule 3 also allows animal owners, keepers, or employees of the owner to administer certain medications to their animals.
- Anyone under 17 years undergoing instruction in animal husbandry procedures either directly supervised by a veterinary surgeon or at a recognised institute of education under direct supervision may carry out specific husbandry procedures.
- Other procedures that can be carried out include:
  - Emergency first aid to maintain life and prevent suffering
  - Castration or tail docking of lambs
  - Removal of dewclaws in a dog before its eyes are open
- Schedule 3 was reviewed in 2015 to include the work of animal physiotherapists.

Penalties for non-compliance include:

- Fines can be issued for practising veterinary surgery without being registered with the RCVS.
- Individuals may be removed from the RCVS register for either a specific time or permanently.
- Imprisonment is an option depending on the severity of the non-compliance.
- A person calling themselves a veterinary surgeon but not being registered is being non-compliant and penalties can be applied.

Protection of Animals (Anaesthetics) Act 1954, amended 1982

This act decrees that any animal undergoing any procedure/operation that involves sensitive tissues or bone must be provided with anaesthetic to prevent pain.

There are several exemptions to the act:

- Emergency first aid situations
- Docking of the tail of a dog before its eyes are open
- Removal of dewclaws in a dog before its eyes are open
- Castration of a male animal before a specified age (further details on the DEFRA website)
- Minor procedures that are usually carried out by a veterinary surgeon or veterinary nurse. They are usually performed without anaesthetic as they are deemed to be painless, e.g. injections involving hollow needles
- Home Office–licensed procedures under ASPA 1986
- The act does not apply to birds, fish, or reptiles

This act has been amended by the Welfare of Farmed Animals (England) Regulations 2007 (or other specified country, e.g. Scotland).

The Animal (Scientific Procedures) Act 1986

The *Animal (Scientific Procedures) Act 1986* (ASPA) regulates the use of animals in scientific research in the United Kingdom. ASPA covers all living vertebrates (except humans) and cephalopods. Embryonic forms are covered once they enter their last third of the gestational period.

Regulated procedures covered by the act include those for scientific or educational purposes that cause an animal 'a level of pain, suffering, distress or lasting harm equivalent to, or higher than, that caused by inserting a hypodermic needle according to good veterinary practice'.

Guidance on the operation of the ASPA is available on the UK Government's website.

There are three types of licences as part of the act:

- Personal Licences – Required for individuals conducting procedures.
- Project Licences – Required for specific research projects, detailing the scope and purpose.
- Establishment Licences – Required for institutions where research is conducted.

Licences are issued by the Home Office in England, Scotland, and Wales.

Any research undertaken must have passed an *ethical review process* that assesses the potential benefits against the harm to animals.

The act emphasises *the principles of replacement, reduction, and refinement* (the 3Rs) to minimise animal use and suffering during procedures – i.e. can something be achieved without the use of the animal.

There are further protections for primates, cats, dogs, and horses and specific requirements for the housing, care, and humane killing of animals.

Annual inspections occur and strict compliance requirements are in place. Penalties for non-compliance include fines and revocation of licences.

The ASPA aims to ensure that animal research is conducted responsibly and ethically, with a strong and vital emphasis on animal welfare.

Penalties for non-compliance:

If the ASPA is not followed, then non-compliance is reported to the Home Office and an investigation will occur to determine the severity of non-compliance. Potential consequences can include:

- Issuing of compliance notices
- Adding conditions to the licence
- Revoking of the licence
- Criminal prosecution

Wildlife & Countryside Act 1981

The Wildlife & Countryside Act 1981 (WCA) is designed to protect and conserve wild animals and their habitats.

Key points are:

- All wild birds, their nests, and eggs are protected from being taken, damaged, or destroyed, especially during breeding seasons.
- Specific wild animals (e.g. all bat species, otters, red squirrels, great crested newts) are protected from being killed, injured, or taken.

- Certain wild plants (e.g. Bluebells and certain orchid species) are protected from being uprooted or destroyed.
- Restrictions on the release of non-native species into the wild, which may compromise populations of native species in wild habitats.
- Enhanced protection of Sites of Special Scientific Interest (SSSIs), which are crucial for conservation.

Amendments are in operation relating to specific parts of the United Kingdom (e.g. Scotland, Northern Ireland).

Penalties for non-compliance can include:

- Fines of up to £5000 and/or 6 months in prison for killing or taking protected species
- Fines and restoration orders for damage to SSSI areas.

Animal Health Act 1981

- Includes the Rabies (Importation of Dogs, Cats and Other Mammals) Order 1974 and subsequent amendments.
- Includes the (Zoonoses) (England) Order 2021, which lists two new organisms – *Coxiella burnetti* and Severe acute respiratory coronavirus syndrome 2 (SARS-CoV-2).

The Animal Health Act 1981 covers a range of situations relating to animal health including biosecurity, cleaning and disinfection, identification of animals, movement of animal carcasses, animals entering the food chain, transport of live animals, identification of dogs in public places (must wear a collar with an identity tag stating name and address of owner), and a National Contingency Plan relating to specific diseases and import and export of animals.

The Animal Health Act 1981 makes provision for dealing with notifiable diseases named in Section 88 of the act. Any person that is in possession of an animal that is suspected or confirmed as having a notifiable disease must report to the police.

The Animal Health Act also allows the appropriate authorities to deal with suspect or confirmed rabies cases, under the Rabies (Control) Order 1974. It allows government officers to remove affected or suspected animals and those that have been exposed to the infection. The orders and regulations covered by the Rabies (Control) Order 1974 include:

- Reporting of suspected or actual cases of rabies to the DEFRA, the local authority, and the police.
- Declaring the place where the suspected animal is identified as an infected area. This can also result in control of movement on and off the premises and prevent any gathering of animals in the local area.
- Destruction of an infected animal by authorised veterinary personnel.

The Rabies (Importation of Dogs, Cats and Other Mammals) Order 1974 also provides the Secretary of State with the power to extend the quarantine period of any animal detained at quarantine premises if:

- An outbreak of rabies occurs at quarantine premises.
- An animal in quarantine is suspected of being infected by rabies.
- The Rabies (Control) Order 1974 also applies to suspected cases in quarantine premises. Movement of animals into and out of the premises would stop, including those animals covered by the requirements of the Pet Travel Scheme (PETS).

The Animal Health Act 2002 amendment provided additional guidance on foot-and-mouth disease and other diseases as required and provided additional powers for dealing with transmissible spongiform encephalopathies such as bovine spongiform encephalopathy (BSE) and scrapie. Amendments were made to powers of enforcement and further guidance on biosecurity was issued following the Foot & Mouth outbreak of 2001.

The Act was last reviewed and updated in 2021.

Animals Act 1971

This act covers civil liability for damage that has been caused by animals, including damage, death, and injury caused to people, property, and livestock.

Key points include:

- Owners of a dangerous animal must take precautions to ensure that there is no opportunity for the animal to inflict damage as stated by this law.
- If a dog kills or harms farm animals, farmers are entitled to protect the stock in their care. For example, if a dog is found harming sheep, the farmer may kill the dog but must report the incident to the police.
- If the owner of the animal is under 16 years, then the parent of the owner becomes liable. The owner is classed as the person in possession of the animal at the time of the incident that caused injury to livestock.
- There are exemptions from this act in certain circumstances such as if the person suffering the injury was proven to be at fault, or if the livestock harmed had strayed on to land where the dog was authorised to be present by the owner of the land.
- The term livestock under this act also includes captive game birds as well as farm livestock. Horses were included in the act under the Control of Horses Act 2015.

The Pet Travel Scheme

The PETS is the system that allows pet animals (dogs, cats, and ferrets) to travel from and to Great Britain without going into quarantine, providing that they comply with the rules of the scheme.

- The animal must be fitted with a microchip.
- The animal must be vaccinated against rabies (providing they have met the minimum age for vaccination). Subsequent rabies boosters must be kept up to date. The final vaccination must have been administered at least 21 days before the date of re-entry to the United Kingdom. The day of vaccination is counted as day 0. The 21-day wait for re-entry was introduced in January 2012.

The country that the animal is travelling to may have its own requirements.

Travelling to an EU country from Great Britain

- Tapeworm, flea, and tick treatment between 24 and 120 hours before leaving the outgoing country.
- Tapeworm treatment 1–5 days after entering the ingoing country.
- Additional vaccinations may be required, e.g. Kennel Cough against *Bordetella* species.
- Rabies Titre test – a blood test that indicates the level of rabies antibody in the circulating bloodstream of the animal.

- Animal Health Certificate issued by a veterinary surgeon. The certificate is valid for 10 days for entry into an EU country or Northern Ireland and for 4 months for onwards travel in the European Union or re-entering the United Kingdom. Travel to the Isle of Man and the Channel Islands does not require an animal health certificate pet passport.

Travelling to a non-EU country from Great Britain
- An export health certificate is required.
- An export application form needs to be completed.
- An official vet must be nominated who will complete the export health certificate.
- Check the specific rules for the country you are travelling to for all their requirements.

When bringing a pet into the Great Britain, a carrier and route must be used that is approved by the Animal Health and Plant Agency (AHPA).

Penalties for non-compliance:
Up to 4 months in quarantine if the rules are not followed.

The pet travel rules exist to keep the United Kingdom free from rabies and certain other exotic diseases. Although the United Kingdom has been free of rabies for many years, certain parasitic diseases are on the increase, and it is vital that there is an effective system in place to monitor animals entering the United Kingdom.

Up-to-date information relating to pet travel can be found on the UK Government DEFRA website, and this should always be checked thoroughly prior to travel as rules vary according to the intended country of travel or re-entry. The scheme also applies to assistance dogs, such as guide dogs and hearing dogs, although exemptions can be made.

If animals are permanently moving for sale, rehoming, or transfer of ownership, including rescue animals, then the Balai Rules apply as the animals are treated as commercial imports.

The Balai rules also apply if:

- you are bringing in more than five pets (and not attending a competition, show, or sporting event).
- you cannot accompany your pets 5 days before or after they arrive in Great Britain.

Details of the Balai rules and the animals that are covered can be found on the UK Government DEFRA website.

The Windsor Framework (Non-Commercial Movement of Pet Animals) Regulations 2024 comes into existence in 2025 and covers the non-commercial movement of pet animals from Great Britain to Northern Ireland.

Animal Welfare (Import of Dogs, Cats and Ferrets) Bill
This bill is currently progressing through Parliament. It aims to restrict the importation and non-commercial movement of dogs, cats, and ferrets to prevent illegal puppy farming and improve animal welfare.

Animal Welfare Organisations

There are a large number and wide variety of animal welfare organisations in existence, both in the United Kingdom and internationally, that represent the interests of animals. These organisations may be specifically interested in the welfare of all animals or specific animals only.

Table 6.2 Animal welfare organisations.

Health and welfare	Conservation	Sport	Registration bodies
RSPCA	RSPB	British Field Sports Society	The Kennel Club
Blue Cross	National Trust	The League Against Cruel Sports	Governing Council for the Cat Fancy
Dogs Trust	RBST	British Horse Society	British Rabbit Council
PDSA	County Wildlife Trusts	The Kennel Club	Weatherbys
The Donkey Sanctuary	WWF	Countryside Alliance	RBST
Animal Health Trust	IUCN		RCVS
British Veterinary Association	British & Irish Association of Zoos and Aquaria		
International Fund for Animal Welfare	National Parks		
International League for the Protection of Horses	Flora and Fauna International		

The interests can be widely grouped under the following headings:

- Health and welfare (including rescue and rehoming)
- Conservation
- Sport
- Registration bodies

Due to the sheer volume of animal welfare organisations in existence, examples can be provided, but there are too many to describe their work and do sufficient justice to them. Examples of national/international organisations relating to each area can be found in Table 6.2.

Information about varying organisations can usually be acquired by either contacting the organisation directly or by looking at their website.

Animal Rights

This term relates to the belief that animals should be entitled to the same considerations as human beings, and it is wrong to use them otherwise, for example, in recreational practices, such as racing sports, in fishing, in hunting, in product testing and as part of production processes.

Many people support animal rights and choose not to buy certain products, eat certain foods or attend certain sporting events. Some parts of society will actively demonstrate against such activities involving animals as they believe them to be cruel and unethical. These people are known as activists, and they will freely call for the abolition of such animal activities.

Key beliefs include:

- Animals should have the ability to live as they wish.

- Animals are sentient beings, capable of experiencing emotions and pain and as such should be treated with respect.
- Opposition of animal exploitation.

The issue of animal rights will always be an emotive one, but it is generally agreed that animals do have rights; it is simply a question of what rights they have and to what extent these rights are invoked.

In 2022, the *Animal Welfare (Sentience) Act 2022* was brought into law, and this recognises animals as sentient beings. The Act required the formation of an Animal Sentience Committee whose responsibility is to review and report on the work that the UK Government with regard to animal welfare.

Summary of Animal Welfare and Legislation

Providing for the needs of captive animals (farmed species, animals in a collection, or as domestic pets) is an essential part of upholding its animal welfare.

Using the Five Needs is a framework to help assess an animal's welfare status.

There is a vast array of legislation in existence that applies to animals.

It is the responsibility of keepers, carers and owners to keep up to date with relevant legislation and seek out advice from professionals with regard to its implementation.

If working in one of the countries of the United Kingdom that is not England, there may be specific legislation that applies, e.g. Scotland, Wales, or Northern Ireland.

There is a wide range of animal welfare organisations each with their stated purpose. Some focus on one species, others focus on a range of species.

Animal rights focus on the concept that animals should have their own individual rights.

7

Basic Animal Nutrition

Learning goals

In this chapter, the learning goals are:

- To identify the basic components of animal nutrition:
  - Proteins
  - Carbohydrates
  - Fats
  - Vitamins
  - Minerals
  - Water
- To identify how nutritional needs vary with life stages in animals

Food or nutrients are required by the body to produce energy. Energy is necessary to drive the essential processes and systems in the body:

- Breathing
- Circulating the blood to tissues and cells
- Maintaining body temperature
- Muscle movement throughout the body
- The materials for repair, growth, and reproduction
- General health

Nutrients are food substances that provide nourishment that support life. There are six major nutrient groups:

- Those that can supply energy:
  - Protein
  - Carbohydrates
  - Fats/lipids
- Those needed for health and growth:
  - Vitamins
  - Minerals
  - Water

Animals eat to satisfy their energy needs. In the wild, when animals have eaten enough food to meet the body's energy demands, they will stop. However, in captive environments, due to the

Animal Biology and Care, Fourth Edition. Emily Jewell.
© 2026 John Wiley & Sons Ltd. Published 2026 by John Wiley & Sons Ltd.
Companion Website: https://www.wiley.com/go/animal/biology4e/jewell

improved taste of foods, scraps from the human table, and 'treats', some companion animals will eat more than their body's needs, resulting in obesity and other linked diseases. Many animals have a sedentary lifestyle with owners unable to provide sufficient exercise, which means that the excess nutrients consumed will be converted to storage as body fat (*adipose tissue*).

Proteins

What are proteins?

Proteins are large molecules, consisting of hundreds of single units called *amino acids*, which join to form chains. Protein in the animal diet is broken down during the digestive process into its formative amino acids. There are a total of 20 amino acids (Table 7.1) that combine to form specific proteins with *peptide bonds*. Animals need all 20 amino acids to maintain their own body protein. Some of these amino acids are obtained from the food they eat and are described as being *essential*, and some are made within the body from the dietary protein. For example, dogs require 10 amino acids to be supplied by their diet but can create or synthesise the remainder. Cats require 11 amino acids to be supplied via the diet. The extra one needed in cats can only be obtained from animal protein.

Where does dietary protein originate from?

Protein in an animal's diet can originate from either animal or vegetable sources:

- Animal origin
  - Meat
  - Fish
  - Eggs
  - Milk
- Vegetable origin
  - Soya and other pulses/beans
  - Cereals

Table 7.1 Essential and non-essential amino acids.

Essential amino acids • Must be supplied in the diet	Non-essential amino acids • Can be manufactured in the body from the essential amino acids
Arginine	Alanine
Histidine	Asparagine
Isoleucine	Aspartic acid
Leucine	Cysteine
Lysine	Glutamic acid
Methionine	Glutamine
Phenylalanine	Glycine
Taurine (cats cannot synthesise)	Proline
Threonine	Serine
Tryptophan	Tyrosine
Valine	

What is the function of protein?

- Energy (only used as an energy source if in excess or other energy sources are not available)
- Growth
- Body proteins, e.g. muscle, fur, claws, hooves
- Repair of tissues
- Immune system antibodies to protect from disease
- Assisting metabolic reactions (enzymes and hormones)

What are the signs of protein deficiency in the diet?

- Poor growth
- Weight loss
- Disease
- Dull appearance

Many tissues in the body rely on protein as a major component, e.g. hormones, enzymes, plasma proteins, and antibodies. The quantities of protein required in the diet by an animal will vary according to:

- Species
- Age
- Sex
- Quality of the protein

The higher the biological value of a protein (in other words, the easier it is for the body to use), the smaller the quantity required. High-value protein includes:

- Egg
- White meat (chicken)
- Fish

After digestive disturbance or operations, it is usually recommended that high-value proteins are fed for a few days as they are easier to digest for the animal. Low-value protein includes:

- Soya bean and other pulses
- Cereals

Excess protein in the diet is converted by the liver to energy and nitrogenous waste (urea), which is removed from the body by the kidneys. Excess protein cannot be stored in the body.

Carbohydrates

What are carbohydrates?

Carbohydrates are needed to provide most of the energy required by the body. They are broken down in the digestive tract into *simple sugars* and *starches*. If simple sugars are unavailable as a nutrient, the body can divert some amino acids to become an energy source. Simple sugars can be converted into a temporary stored form called *glycogen*. This is stored in the liver and muscles and converted back to simple sugar whenever its energy is needed by the body. Starches provide a long-term energy supply over time.

One simple sugar molecule is called a *monosaccharide*, e.g. *glucose* and *fructose*.

Two monosaccharide molecules joined together are known as *disaccharides, e.g. sucrose* and *lactose*.

A chain of monosaccharides is called a *polysaccharide*, e.g. starch.

Where does dietary carbohydrate originate from?

Carbohydrate in an animal's diet can be from animal or vegetable sources:

- Animal origin
  - Mammalian milk
- Vegetable origin
  - Cereal starches (e.g. oats, lentils, rice)
  - Root vegetables (e.g. potatoes)

Carbohydrate can be divided into *digestible* (starches) and *indigestible* (dietary fibre or *cellulose*). *Dietary fibre* is found in plants and cereals and provides bulk to faecal materials. Fibre assists in regulating bowel function and the movement of undigested nutrients through the digestive tract. Starch is the main source of carbohydrate in the *monogastric* animal diet.

What is the function of carbohydrates?

- Energy – short term and long term
- Provision of dietary fibre to maintain function of the large intestine

What are the signs of carbohydrate deficiency in the diet?

There are no related problems provided that other energy providing nutrients are available in the diet (i.e. fats or proteins).

If the diet contains more carbohydrate than required for its energy needs, the surplus carbohydrate is converted into body fat and stored as *adipose tissue*. This can lead to *obesity* in pets and captive animals if they are overfed.

Fats/Lipids

What are fats?

Fat is also called *lipid*. It is made up of *glycerol*, with attached *fatty acid* molecules. Fatty acids are a very concentrated form of energy compared to protein or carbohydrates and are essential to good health in animals.

Including a good level of fat in the diet helps to:

- Improve energy density
- Improve feed quality
- Reduce dust in feed
- Increase palatability of the food
- Improve the passage of food through the digestive tract

Fats are classified as *saturated* or *unsaturated* and this is down to their chemical structure. Saturated fats are more solid in nature than unsaturated fats that are more liquid, e.g. oils.

Where does dietary fat/lipid originate from?

The sources of fat/lipid in an animal's diet can be of either animal or vegetable origin:

- Animal origin
  - Milk and other dairy produce
  - Fish oil
  - Fat of body origin (attached to meat)

- Vegetable origin
  - Nuts
  - Seed oils, i.e. sunflower, oil-seed rape and linseed
  - Margarine

What is the function of fats/lipids?
- Energy (a very concentrated form)
- Improved taste to the diet
- For the absorption, transport, and storage of the fat-soluble vitamins – A, D, E, and K
- Provide essential fatty acids (EFA) for body use – termed essential as they must be provided in the diet as they cannot be made in the body from other dietary fats.

In the dog and cat, there are three EFA:

- Linoleic
- Arachidonic
- Linolenic

Dogs and cats require linoleic and linolenic acids in their diet.
Cats require arachidonic acid in their diet.
Cats are *obligate* carnivores. They cannot maintain full health without sources of animal tissue in their diet as a source of ready-made essential fatty or amino acids.

What are the signs of fat/lipid deficiency in the diet?
- Reproduction problems
- Impaired wound healing
- Poor coat condition
- Dry skin

Body fat (adipose tissue) is created from a combination of fatty acids and simple sugars. If either is in excess in the diet, this can cause obesity in the animal, which in turn can cause further health problems in the animal.

Vitamins

What are vitamins?
Vitamins are chemical compounds needed in very small amounts in the body. They are essential to metabolic processes in the body.
There are two classification groups for vitamins:

- *Fat-soluble vitamins* – A, D, E, and K (Table 7.2).
  - Fat-soluble vitamins are stored in adipose tissue and in the liver.
  - Excess storage of some of these vitamins can be toxic, e.g. A and D.
  - These vitamins are involved in the digestion and absorption of dietary fat/lipids.
- *Water-soluble vitamins* – *B complex group and vitamin C* (Table 7.3)
  - Water-soluble vitamins are not stored in the body.
  - They must be supplied daily in the diet.
  - They must be supplemented where there is considerable fluid loss from the body, e.g. in cases of vomiting and diarrhoea.

Table 7.2 Fat-soluble vitamins.

Vitamin	Source	Function
A (retinol)	Fish oils, liver, egg, and cereals	Night vision, body cell division, reproduction, bone and tooth development, and enhancement of plumage colour in birds
D (cholecalciferol)	Liver, fish oils, egg, and cereals can be synthesised from cholesterol	Regulates calcium and phosphorus levels and bone growth and repair
E (tocopherol)	Vegetable oils, egg, and cereals	Supports tissues and cells around the body as an antioxidant and aids immune function
K	Green vegetables and synthesised in the intestines (no need for dietary source)	Assists in blood clotting

Table 7.3 Water-soluble vitamins.

Vitamin	Source	Function
B1 (*thiamine*)	Cereals, organ meat, green vegetables, and dairy products	Assists metabolic reactions, i.e. converts sugars to fatty tissues
B2 (*riboflavin*)	Organ meats and milk	Use and release of energy by cells
B3 (*niacin*)	Synthesised in the body from tryptophan, except in cats when must be provided in the diet	Metabolism of carbohydrates
B5 (*pantothenic acid*)	Green vegetables, cereal grains, meat, eggs, and dairy products	Metabolic processes
B6 (*pyridoxine*)	Cereals, meat, and yeast	Metabolism of amino acids
B7 (*biotin*)	Produced by gut bacteria and found in egg yolk	Assists metabolism of lipids and carbohydrates
B9 (*folic acid*)	Organ meats, fish; synthesised by gut microbes	Blood cell production in bone marrow and cell replication
B12 (*cyanocobalamin*)	Synthesised by gut microbes	Supports the function of folic acid and nucleic acid synthesis
C (*ascorbic acid*)	Green vegetables; created in the body	Creates collagen for tissues and supports bone cells

- Excess water-soluble vitamins are excreted via the kidneys in urine.
- An animal can become quickly deficient in water soluble vitamins.
- These vitamins aid metabolic processes in the body.

Most species can synthesise vitamin C in the liver, but primates, fish, and guinea pigs cannot and must receive a dietary source of vitamin C either as fresh fruit and vegetables or as supplements.

In ruminants and other hind-gut fermenters, the microbes of the rumen and caecum can synthesise the B vitamins required by the animal. Monogastric animals must have daily provision in the diet.

Table 7.4 Signs of vitamin deficiency.

Vitamin	Signs of deficiency
Vitamin A	Poor growth, poor repair and growth of skin and mucosal linings, night blindness, dryness of eyes, diarrhoea, kidney stones, and reproductive failure
Vitamin D	Rickets, poor bone growth (*osteomalacia*), and milk fever
Vitamin E	Deterioration of skeletal and cardiac muscle fibres and reduced immunity
Vitamin K	Poor wound healing/clotting, bruising, and increased bleeding time. Deficiency is rare in ruminants and hind-gut fermenters
Vitamin B complex	
B1 – Thiamine	Nervous system irregularities
B2 – Riboflavin	Poor growth, anorexia, lesions in the mouth, and hair loss
B3 – Niacin	Black tongue disease (dogs) and poor feather growth (birds)
B5 – Pantothenic acid	Reduced growth and nerve degeneration
B6 – Pyridoxine	Reduced immunity
B7 – Biotin	Reduced growth, skin lesions, and skeletal problems
B9 – Folic acid	Reduced growth, reduced immunity, and reproductive problems
B12 – Cyanocobalamin	Digestive issues, anorexia, and reduced immunity
Vitamin C	Scurvy, poor wound healing, leaky capillaries, poor bone growth, and anaemia

What are the signs of dietary vitamin deficiency?

Signs of vitamin deficiency depends on the vitamin.

- Reduced productivity.
- Reduced immunity.
- Diseases associated with deficiency of a specific vitamin (Table 7.4).

Minerals

What are minerals?

Minerals are inorganic chemical elements that are essential for an animal's physiological functions and metabolic processes.

Minerals are often referred to as ash on containers of animal food.

Provided the animal is fed a balanced dietary product, minerals do not normally need to be supplemented (Table 7.5).

Minerals are divided into two groups:

- *Macro-minerals* (needed in large or regular amounts):
  - Calcium (Ca)
  - Chloride (Cl)
  - Magnesium (Mg)
  - Phosphorus (P)
  - Potassium (K)
  - Sodium (Na)

Table 7.5 Minerals.

Mineral	Food source	Function
Calcium	Milk, cheese, meat, and bone	Nerve cell repair, muscle, and bone formation
Sodium	Salt and cereals	Nerve and muscle activity and fluid balance in the body
Magnesium	Bone, cereals, and greens	Bone formation and synthesis of protein
Phosphorus	Milk, meat, and bones	Bone and teeth formation
Copper	Bones and meat	Red blood cell formation – haemoglobin
Iodine	Milk and fish	Formation of hormones from thyroid gland
Iron	Meat, eggs, and greens	Red blood cell formation – haemoglobin
Selenium	Fishmeal, meat, and cereals	Synthesis of vitamin E
Zinc	Meat and cereals	Tissue maintenance and aids digestion of food

- *Trace element* minerals (needed in only small amounts):
  - Cobalt (Co)
  - Copper (Cu)
  - Iodine (I)
  - Iron (Fe)
  - Manganese (Mn)
  - Molybdenum (Mo)
  - Selenium (Se)
  - Zinc (Zn)

Where do dietary minerals originate from?

The sources of mineral salts in an animal's diet can be of either animal or vegetable origin:

- Animal origin
  - Dairy products
  - Meat
  - Egg
  - Bone meal
- Vegetable origin
  - Cereals
  - Green vegetables
  - Salt

What is the function of minerals?

Minerals are important for a variety of functions in the body:

- Assist in the maintenance of pH balance in the body.
- Maintain the body's fluid balance.
- Essential for the function of muscle tissues and conducting nerve impulses.
- Help regulate the body's metabolism (via enzymes and hormones).

Table 7.6 Signs of mineral deficiency.

Mineral	Signs of deficiency
Calcium deficiency or calcium–phosphorus imbalance	Rickets, poor bone growth (*osteomalacia*), lameness, leg weakness, abnormal gait, milk fever, and neurological signs
Magnesium	Neurological signs and muscular problems
Sulphur	Reduced feather growth, reduced wool growth, and weight gain
Sodium	Lethargy, reduced appetite, confusion
Potassium	Muscle weakness, lethargy and reduced appetite
Chlorine	Weight loss, reduced appetite, lethargy, mild polydipsia and mild polyuria
Trace elements	
Cobalt	Anaemia, reduced appetite, and reduced growth
Copper	Anaemia, changes in coat colour/pigmentation, skeletal abnormalities, neurological/muscular signs, and digestive issues
Iodine	Reduced growth rate, reproductive issues, hair loss, skin abnormalities, and swelling of thyroid gland (*goitre*)
Iron	Anaemia and fatigue
Manganese	Slow bone growth, skeletal abnormalities, joint swelling, reproductive issues, and beak issues in birds
Molybdenum	Deficiencies are rare
Selenium	Muscular dystrophy (linked closely to Vitamin E metabolism)
Zinc	Skin, feather, fur, wool problems, skin abnormalities, and impaired wound healing

What are the signs of mineral deficiency in the diet?

Some minerals have an extremely complex relationship in the body, and if one is out of balance, it can affect many metabolic processes (Table 7.6).

Mineral deficiencies are often associated with excess minerals being added to the diet, i.e. calcium deficiencies can be caused by phosphorus excess in the diet. This could happen in animals being fed an excess of dietary meat or organ tissues. If a good-quality diet (either commercial product or home recipe) is being fed, there should be no need to supplement vitamins and minerals to a normal healthy animal.

Water

Water is essential for all cells in the body and is found inside (*intracellular*) and outside all cells (*extracellular*); 60–70% of an animal's body weight is water. It is involved with most metabolic processes. As a result of the presence of water in the body, the following can take place:

- Transport of any material between tissues/cells
- Electrolyte balance
- pH balance
- Control of temperature

- Lubrication of all tissue cells
- A medium for blood and lymph

Water cannot be stored by the body and must be available all the time for all animals. Water input to the body is from:

- Food
- Drinking
- Chemical reactions (metabolism)

Water output from the body is via:

- The kidneys in urine
- The lungs in breathing
- The digestive system in faeces
- The skin via sweating

It is important to stress that fresh water must always be available for all animals. This must be emphasised to all animal owners/carers/keepers. Some water will be available from canned food, but if a dry diet is given, the animal should have access to fresh water to drink at all times.

Nutrition for Life Stages

As previously identified, the main dietary components are:

- Protein
- Carbohydrate
- Fats
- Vitamins and minerals
- Water

Protein, carbohydrates, and fats provide energy following their digestion and absorption. Fats provide twice as much energy as protein and carbohydrates. The quantities of these three main dietary components can be adjusted for any life stage so that the nutritional requirements of the animal are met (i.e. during growth phase, pregnancy, and lactation) provided that the basic rules are understood.

An animal's diet provides energy, but it is important that the nutrient content is balanced to the individual animal's requirements. The following stages need to be considered for animals:

- Young growing animals (from weaning to adult)
- Adult maintenance
- Working animals
- Senior/geriatric animals
- Pregnancy
- Lactation

Growing animals

Until they are weaned, young mammals are usually reliant on their mother for their nutritional needs to be met through her provision of milk. In some animals, however, this may fall to their owners/carers/keepers if they need to be hand-reared, and several formulated milk powders specific to species are available on the commercial market.

After weaning, young mammals need to be supplied daily with about 2–2½ times the nutrients required by an adult of the same breed/species. This is usually achieved through the provision of smaller, more frequent meals throughout the day. These increased requirements will gradually decrease as the animal becomes older and reaches adult weight.

Meals need to be frequent throughout the day (i.e. a 3-month-old puppy needs four to six meals), dividing the diet evenly between each one. The stomach size of young animals is too small to cope with only one or two meals a day. By 6 months of age, the frequency of meals is usually at two to three meals a day, down to one to two meals daily by 1 year of age for a dog. Cats tend to snack as adults and will often stay on two to three meals daily.

The time at which to reduce the frequency of meals is usually noticed by owners/carers/keepers when a young animal routinely does not eat a particular meal. The daily amount of feed should then be spread over one less meal until the adult routine is achieved.

When adult, a pet dog will be fed once or twice daily, and a cat will be fed two to three meals daily, as required. The type of food provided can affect the number of meals an animal required in a day. For example, animals fed on wet diets will usually have more meals during the day than animals that have regular access to dried food. An unlimited feeding method can be used in cats on dry diets, unless they are gaining too much weight.

Commercially formulated foods are available to meet the needs of growing animals. These diets are higher in protein and carbohydrate than an adult diet. Food size and texture is also important with young mammals as their deciduous teeth are not as strong as adult teeth.

Adult

Adult diets can be provided once an animal has reached maturity. Commercial diets give advice on feeding and quantities, but if part of the ration is always left uneaten, reduce the amount of food until everything is eaten at each meal. To maintain the animal's interest, many owners supplement the diet with meal scraps, gravy, etc. Cat foods are produced in many flavours, some owners using a different one for each day of the week.

The condition, energy levels, health status, and body weight of the animal need to be monitored to ensure that the diet suits the individual animal. If any change in the diet is considered, always introduce the new diet slowly over several days, overlapping it with the old diet to avoid any digestive upset.

Once established, feeding routines should not be altered in timing, place, or diet types where possible. Animals are creatures of habit, and any changes may be stressful to the animal. Feeding times should never be too late in the evening, because the animal may need to urinate or defaecate within 3–4 hours of eating, by which time it may be shut in and unable to access an outdoor toileting area.

Working animals

Depending on the training, working, resting times, and function, working animals may need different diets and feeding routines. For example, a working dog that runs long distances each day may need as much as two to three times the normal recommended adult ration of food, e.g. sheep dogs that may run more than 20 miles a day.

A dog that participates in agility competitions may need a diet with a higher carbohydrate level during training and competition season as they need increased energy for short durations.

Other working breeds that are active for long periods and in all weather conditions will need more energy for running and to hold the body temperature in extreme cold (sheep dogs and sledge dogs).

Increased fat in the diet is ideal for these animals. Protein in increased amounts may be useful for muscle development, but the energy requirements will come from carbohydrate and fat. Diets that have increased carbohydrate and fat levels are often referred to as 'active diets'.

Working dogs are normally fed only a small meal before work, leaving the main meal of two-thirds of the required daily intake to be fed after a rest period, allowing time for proper digestion.

Senior/geriatric animals

Older animals vary considerably in condition and health status. There are many commercial diets on the market to choose from. Depending on the health of the animal, some are for use with specific medical diseases; others are more generally restrictive of some nutrients for cases of obesity. Diets for obese animals are often referred to as light diets or reducing diets.

Older animals may have sight, taste, and smell losses, as well as poor appetite, poor teeth, and gum condition, all of which can make eating challenging. Many can have reduced gut passage time, leading to constipation problems.

To provide for the nutritional needs of these senior animals, consider:

- Improving the taste/smell of the food by warming it to body temperature
- Using a commercially available senior diet (seek veterinary advice first)
- Increasing fibre in the diet to prevent constipation, i.e. use of bran
  - Ensure fresh water is always available if fibre content is increased
- Using easily digested high-quality proteins, such as fish, poultry, and egg in the diet base
- Encouraging the animal to eat the daily ration by hand feeding initially if required
- Feeding small meals throughout the day (up to six), for the animal to eat the whole daily ration

For any animal, it is important to care for the teeth by preventing the build-up of tartar on the teeth. Also, check for loss of or loose teeth, gum disease, and inflammation. All these will affect the animal's ability to eat. Many dogs and cats will allow the owner to clean their teeth with a soft toothbrush or finger brush, but if this is not possible, a teeth de-scale and/or teeth removal by a veterinary surgeon may be required.

Mobility problems and joint disease in older animals may make bending to the food and water bowls difficult and so consider placing the food and water bowls on to a low box (Figure 7.1) with a ridge around the edge (to prevent the bowls falling off). These can be home-made or bought from most commercial outlets (Figure 7.2).

Pregnancy

For most of a mammalian pregnancy, it is not necessary to increase the quantity of food provided if a nutritionally balanced, good-quality foodstuff is being fed.

It is only during the final third of pregnancy that an increase in food intake is required as this is when most weight gain and growth in size occurs in the foetuses. Overfeeding before this stage of pregnancy may lead to fat deposits; weight gain as a result may lead to problems during *parturition* (birth process). A general strategy can be:

- Increasing the quantity of food by 10–15% per week during the last trimester of pregnancy (last third) until parturition. This increases total food intake to approximately 50% over maintenance levels of food being fed.

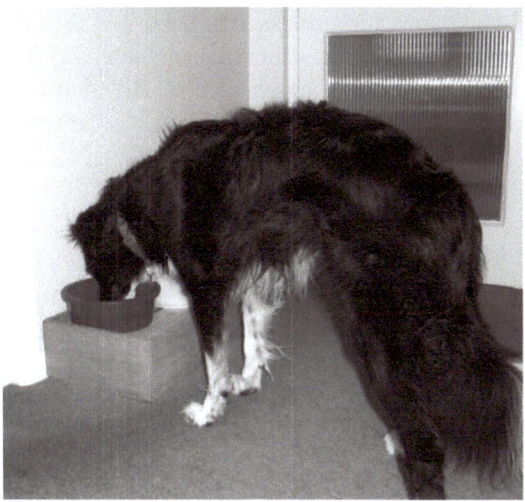

Figure 7.1 Food bowls on a low box.

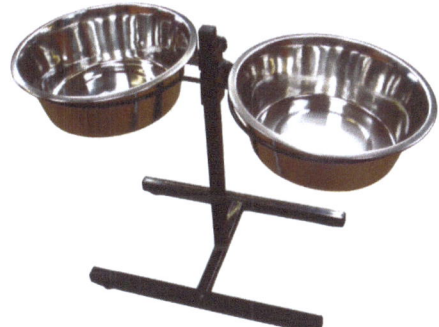

Figure 7.2 Raised bowl system.

- Using diets formulated for pregnancy and lactation needs – they are higher in fat and protein content.
- Feeding smaller meals more often in the final 2 weeks of pregnancy, to assist food intake.
- Always provide fresh drinking water.

Cats require an increase in food quantity once pregnancy has been confirmed. Diet quantities need to be increased for the pregnant cat to approximately 30% above maintenance amounts. Cats will rarely overeat; therefore, food can be constantly available as requirements increase (known as free choice feeding).

Lactation

Feeding young mammals is a very nutritionally demanding life stage and very energy consuming for the mother.

A high-quality diet should be provided that is easily digestible and both energy and nutrient dense to not only meet the demands of milk production but also maintain the mother's body condition.

Milk production is at its maximum a few weeks after birth, and therefore, the amount fed at this time should be approximately three times the usual adult diet quantity.

Once young animals have started the weaning process, the amount of milk provided can be reduced and the amount of solid food increased until they are eating solid food completely independently.

Summary of Basic Animal Nutrition

There are key animal nutrients that should be included in all animal diets:

- Proteins
- Carbohydrates
- Fats
- Vitamins
- Minerals
- Water

It is essential that owners/carers/keepers know the nutritional requirements for the species they care for as well as the amounts to feed, as both under- and overfeeding can lead to health problems for the animal.

The quantities of each nutrient required by an animal will depend on its life stage and this will change throughout its lifetime.

8

Basic Animal Health Care

Learning goals

In this chapter, the learning goals are:

- To identify how to assess an animal's health status using:
  - Behavioural indicators
  - Physical indicators including signs of pain
  - Physiological indicators
- To identify signs of health and suggest appropriate health routines
- To identify factors that affect the health status of an animal
- To identify prophylactic treatments for animals, including vaccinations, parasite treatments, and microchipping

An animal relies on its owners/carers/keepers to regularly check its health and provide any necessary treatments when needed. Only they will know what is normal for that animal. In order to ensure that three of the five animal needs (see Chapter 6) are being met, it is ideal to keep all animals in the best possible health. Early identification of potential health issues can prevent more serious problems from developing later in the animal's life.

Basic animal health care refers to the routine observations that are carried out by the owner/carer/keeper to assess the health status of the animal. Some assessments of the animal's health need to be carried out more frequently than others, and therefore, different routines can be put into operation according to the frequency of checks required.

When undertaking health checks, some animals cannot be directly handled, and as such, an adapted method will need to be used based more on observation at a distance. Restraint equipment may need to be utilised, and in extreme cases, sedation by a veterinary professional may be required to carry out a thorough examination.

Assessing the Health Status of an Animal

When assessing health status in animals, there are three types of indicators that can be used to get a complete picture of their health status:

- Behavioural indicators
- Physical indicators
- Physiological indicators

Animal Biology and Care, Fourth Edition. Emily Jewell.
© 2026 John Wiley & Sons Ltd. Published 2026 by John Wiley & Sons Ltd.
Companion Website: https://www.wiley.com/go/animal/biology4e/jewell

Behavioural indicators

Behavioural change in an animal is often the first sign that there is a problem. It is important to determine whether there are any changes to the animal's usual behaviour patterns.

Consider whether the animals:

- Are withdrawn
- Are non-communicative
- Appear fearful
- Appear to be in pain
- Are being actively aggressive
- Are not showing any change at all

Some animals (e.g. prey species) are very good at hiding when they are in pain, and so, behavioural indicators should not be the only type of indicator used to assess an animal's health status.

Physical indicators

Once the behaviour of the animal has been assessed, a full health check should be performed, as this will provide a clearer picture of the situation.

As well as performing a full health check (Figure 8.1), it is important to note if there are changes in the following:

Posture and locomotion	• Is the animal walking normally? • Is it weightbearing on all limbs equally? • Can it perform its usual range of movements, e.g. sitting to standing, standing to sitting?
Feeding habits	• Has appetite increased or decreased? • Is the animal vomiting?
Drinking habits	• Has water consumption increased or decreased? • Is the animal craving water?
Toileting habits	• Is the animal toileting more or less often? • What is the nature of the faeces produced? • What is the colour of the urine produced? • Is there a distinct odour to the urine produced?

Signs of pain

Signs of pain in an animal can include the following, but it will depend on the species of animal, and so, as an owner/carer/keeper, it is important to know the signs of pain for the species:

- Crying/whimpering
- Unusual body position, e.g. curled up
- The pupils of the eye are dilated
- Panting and heart rate are rapid
- Raised body temperature
- Not eating or drinking
- Unwilling to move or exercise

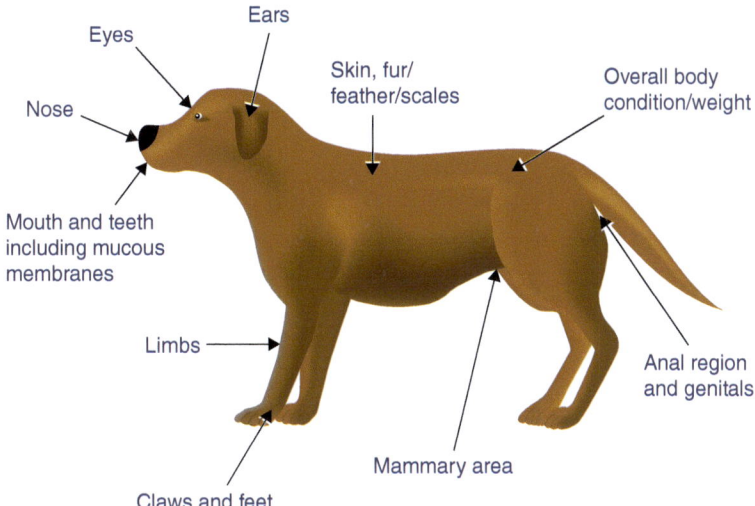

Figure 8.1   Areas to assess for a full health check.

Physiological indicators

Physiological indicators give a more representative picture of what is happening within the animal's body. Detailed physiological assessment can only be carried out by veterinary professionals (e.g. blood tests, urine analysis), but physiological indicators that can be checked by owners/carers/keepers are:

- *Temperature* – Is it raised or is it lower than normal?
- *Pulse rate* – Check pulse rate, regularity, and strength.
- *Respiration rate* – Check respiration rate, depth, and regularity. Note that one respiration is a single inspiration and expiration of air.

Combined together, this assessment is known as the *TPR assessment*. TPR assessments should only be done when the animal is resting but not sleeping and not straight after exercising, as both sleeping and resting can affect the individual parameters measured.

Signs of health in animals

For these purposes, a dog will be used, but the same health check process can be used in all species although some slight modification may be needed depending on species.

The health check should always be started at the head of the animal and finish at the rear end. An animal should be accustomed to this routine as early in life as possible as it means that examinations at a later age are easier because the animal is more tolerant, and therefore, the risk of any injury to the handler or animal is reduced.

Areas that should be checked on an animal when performing a full health check are shown in Figure 8.1. Signs of good and poor health are shown in Table 8.1.

It is also important to check:

- Posture, locomotion, and gait
- Temperature, pulse, and respiration rate
- Accommodation for signs of illness, e.g. blood, vomit, and diarrhoea

Table 8.1 Signs of good and poor health in animals.

Area of the body	Signs of good health	Signs of poor health
Eyes	Clear and bright	Dull, cloudy, discharge, redness, and swelling
Ears	Odourless and healthy colours	Excessive wax, discharge, redness, swelling, matted hair, cuts, and parasites
Nose	Normal for species	Swelling, soreness, nasal discharge, crusting, and abnormal for species
Mouth and teeth	Mouth, teeth and gums intact, healthy colour, and good capillary refill time for mucous membranes	Soreness of mouth, swelling, broken teeth, excessive tartar on teeth, blueness of mucous membranes, bleeding gums, signs of vomiting, and offensive odour
Skin, fur/feathers/scales	Shiny, glossy, good condition of coat/feathers/scales, and healthy colour to skin	Dull looking, matted coat, broken feathers, damaged scales, scratching, parasites present, soreness of skin, lumps, bumps, etc.
Overall body condition	Good body coverage, appropriate weight for the animal and its age	Excess or limited body coverage, obese, or anorexic for the animal and its age
Limbs	Ease of movement, no swelling, or obvious injury	Difficult or reluctance to move limbs, obvious injury, swelling, and hot to touch

What is being looked for in each area?

Suggested health routines

Having an identified health routine makes it easier for owners/carers/keepers of animals to notice more quickly if there is a problem. Suggested checks are listed in Table 8.2, but routines will differ according to the species, age, and existing health status of the animals.

It is worth noting that if an animal has an existing medical condition, is taking medication, is pregnant, or is elderly, then your veterinary practice can guide you on the frequency of veterinary checks required.

Working together with your veterinary practice promotes the best possible care for your animal(s). For animal collections, veterinary staff may assist in the creation of a health plan, which ensures that health can be tracked across the collection and routine treatments planned for the best time across the year. Any changes to the existing health of an animal should be recorded and monitored, with veterinary assistance sought if necessary.

Factors affecting health status

An animal's health status can be affected by many factors. Such factors may be animal related (Figure 8.3) or non-animal related (Figure 8.4). It is important to recognise that certain changes in an animal or its environment can affect the health status of the animal.

Hygiene

Good hygiene is essential when dealing with animals to remove a build-up of pathogens from the environment, which could otherwise cause illness in the animal. Again, splitting tasks into specific routines can help keep on top of things and minimise the risk of illness developing. The list in Table 8.3 is a suggested hygiene routine as routines will vary according to species and housing.

Table 8.2 Suggested health check routines.

Daily checks	Weekly checks	Monthly checks	Six monthly checks	Annual checks
Food and water consumption	Coat and skin condition	Check nail length	Seasonal requirements, e.g. changes to housing or moving location	Annual vaccinations as advised by official vaccination schedules
Urine output	Ears for odour, wounds, and wax	Check beak length in birds and chelonians	Parasite control – may be quarterly, depending on the product used	Veterinary health check – may or may not include blood samples May be 6 monthly in older animals or those with a chronic condition
Faecal output	Mouth, teeth, and gums (Figure 8.2)	Tooth length, e.g. rabbits, rodents, camelids, and equids		
Movement and exercise	Feel for lumps and bumps over the body	Overall weight and body condition		
General behaviour and temperament	Genital area for discharge, matts, and parasites			

Exercise provision

Exercise is essential to animal health. Each animal has its own specific exercise needs, and an owner/carer/keeper should endeavour to meet those needs to maintain good welfare in the animal. When choosing an animal, it is important to consider the exercise requirements for the animal and decide whether these can be accommodated into your lifestyle. Many pets, dogs specifically, are abandoned and/or rehomed because people cannot meet their exercise needs. The frustrations on behalf of the animal(s) then tend to manifest themselves as destructive or unwanted behaviours. For example, a breed such as the Border Collie has a high requirement for exercise, whereas a breed like the Pug has a much lower one. Breed-focused books clearly state requirements for exercise, temperament, and suitability for potential owners. Life stages and life span will also affect exercise needs, for example, older animals tend to need less exercise.

Plenty of exercise is necessary for animals used in the areas of:

- Working (including uniformed work and breeding animals)
- Racing
- Performance
- Agility
- Field trials

Less exercise is required for:

- Elderly animals
- Short-nosed breeds (brachycephalic)
- Some small breeds
- Animals with joint disease
- Animals with breathing and heart conditions

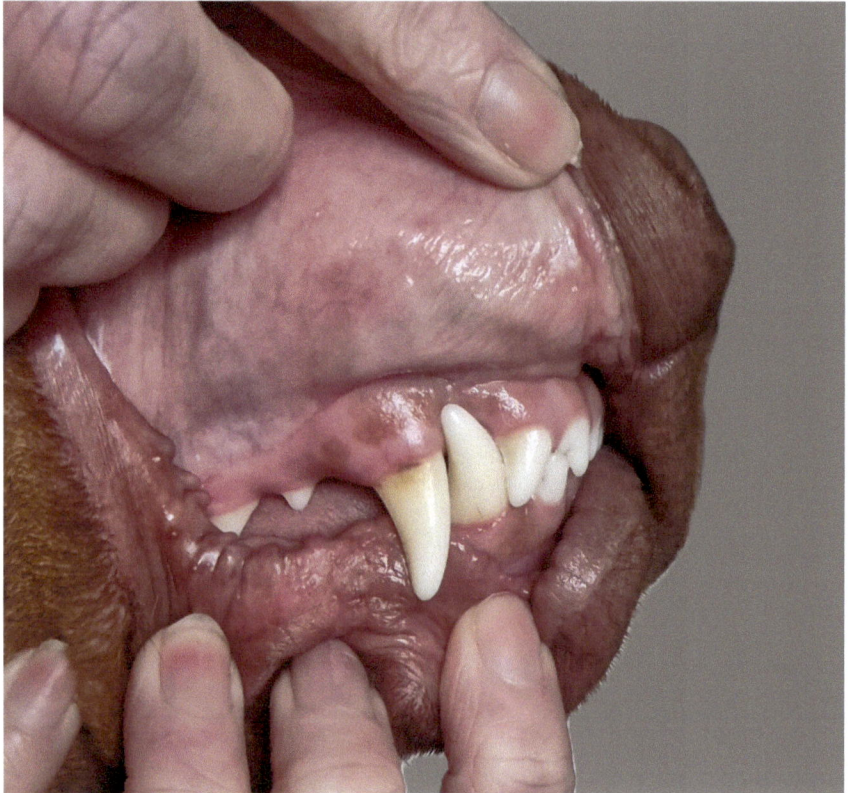

Figure 8.2 Checking the mouth, gums, and teeth.

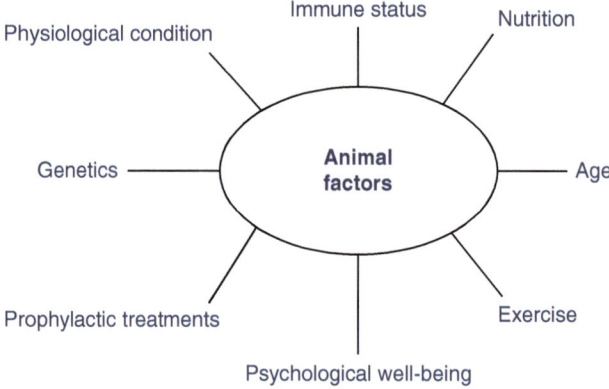

Figure 8.3 Animal factors affecting health status.

Some animals can 'self-exercise', but can be trained to walk on a lead, e.g. cats, ferrets, and rabbits. Small pets will exercise if they have enriched living areas with obstacles for climbing, toys and run areas, plus handling time, e.g. hamsters, guinea pigs, and rats. There are also exercise balls on the commercial market for small animals that can be used to increase the amount of daily exercise, but these are not suitable for all small animals.

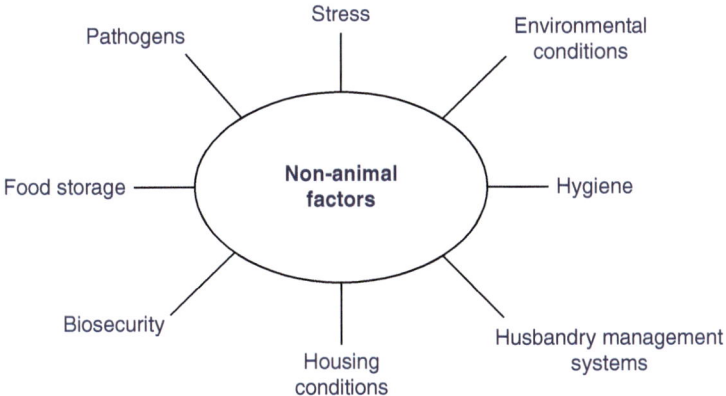

Figure 8.4 Non-animal factors affecting health status.

Table 8.3 Suggested hygiene routines.

Daily tasks	Weekly tasks
Wash food and water bowls/containers	Wash bedding
Remove 'normal' discharges from eyes, nose, and prepuce/vulva	Wash nylon harnesses or collars
Check coat/feather condition, groom as required (Figures 8.5 and 8.6)	Groom thoroughly
Check anus for faecal material on coat	Disinfect grooming equipment
Remove faeces from environment	Disinfect housing
Remove any urine-soaked bedding	
Spot clean where necessary	

Companionship

An important aspect of health care is time spent in the company of the animal. Owners, carers, and keepers can use this time to carry out health status checks. Dogs and cats are companion animals, and so, time must be spent with them to enhance their well-being – this also benefits human well-being. Some animals will respond badly to isolation, and this will usually be seen in their behaviour. Some breeds of cat and dog can suffer from separation anxiety, and all steps should be taken to reduce the amount of time that they are spent alone, where possible.

Signs of isolation response include:

- Temperament change
- Destruction of housing
- Being aggressive or withdrawn
- Fear

Of course, in some cases, this list could perfectly describe the normal behaviour of an individual. The only way to know if an animal is suffering from isolation response is to recognise what is normal for each animal, whatever the species.

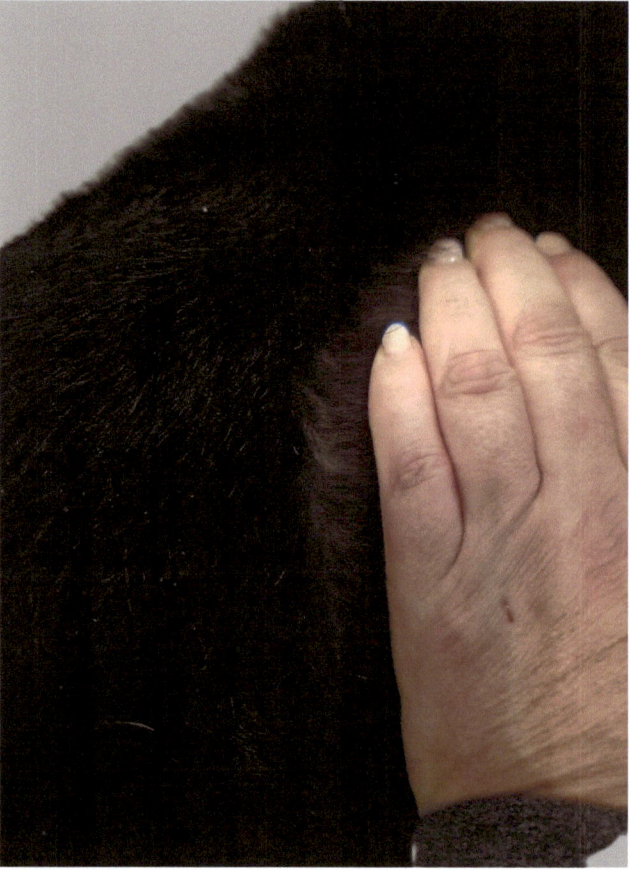

Figure 8.5 Checking coat condition.

Prophylactic treatments

Prophylaxis is the term given to a treatment designed to prevent the occurrence of a disease.

Vaccination

Vaccinations are treatments that are given to animals as a method of protecting them against potentially lethal disease(s).

A vaccine temporarily stimulates the immune system of the body and causes an immune response to the biological agent contained in the vaccine. The period of protection will vary depending on the species involved, the biological agent, the vaccine type, and the individual receiving the vaccine. It ranges in most cases from 6 months to 1 year, at which point the animal must receive a booster vaccination to protect it further. The owner/carer/keeper of the animal should know which vaccinations their animal(s) requires and how frequently they should receive them. If unsure, advice must be sought from veterinary professionals.

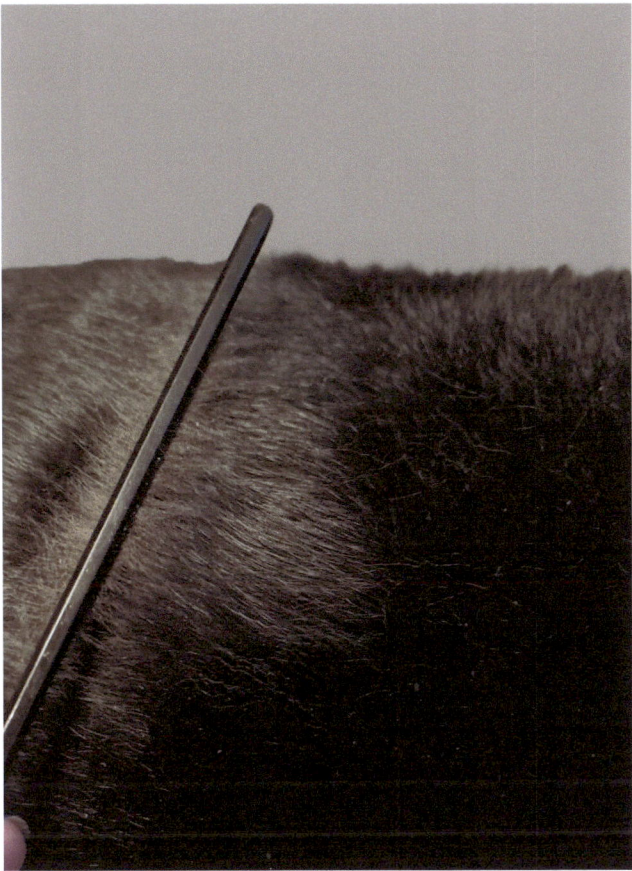

Figure 8.6   Groom out the dead hair.

Parasite treatments

Parasites may be internal or external and treatments vary according to that. Treatment of internal parasites is often referred to as 'worming' or 'drenching' and is in small animals, the most common internal parasites are roundworms and tapeworms.

The most common external parasites to be treated are fleas and ticks. The frequency of application depends on the species, the product being used, and the risk of reinfection.

As with vaccinations, an owner/carer/keeper should have knowledge of what anti-parasite treatments their animal(s) require and the frequency of application (Figure 8.7).

Microchipping

A microchip is a small electronic device, each containing a unique code. The chip is inserted through a needle into the most appropriate place on the animal for long-term existence and easy detection. In cats and dogs, this tends to be in the scruff. In bird species, it could be in the breast area, and in tortoises, for example, it may be implanted into the shell. The code is then logged with a registering database organisation.

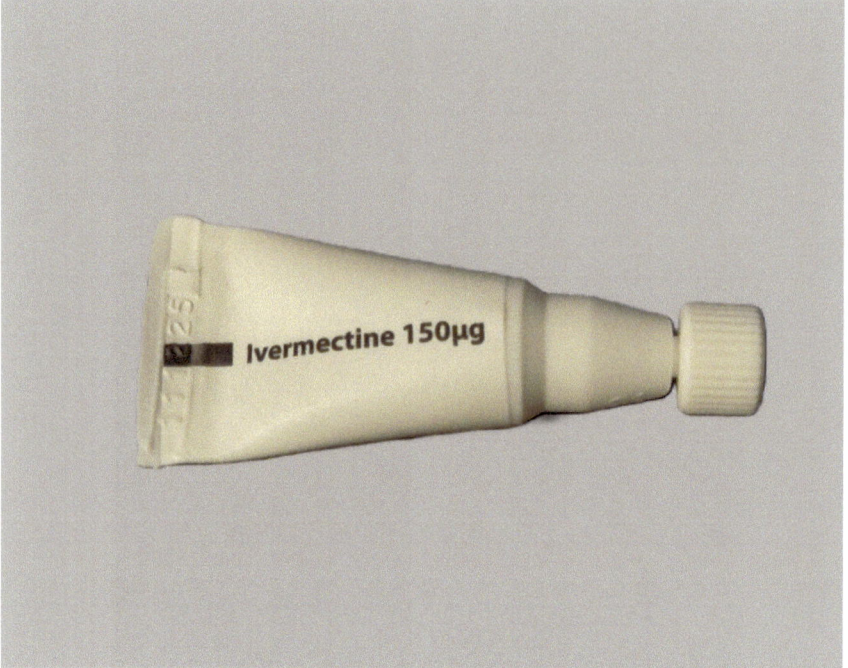

Figure 8.7   Ivermectin; frequently used for treating and preventing parasites.

Since 2016, it has been a legal requirement to ensure that all dogs are microchipped unless a veterinary surgeon identifies that the animal is exempt for health reasons. This requirement was updated in England in 2023 and extended to additionally cover cats under The Microchipping of Cats and Dogs (England) Regulations 2023. In Scotland and Wales, the current legislation is in place from 2016 (Scotland) and Wales (2015) and only applies to dogs at the current time.

The 2023 (England) regulations fall under the Animal Welfare Act 2006 and exist with the hope of reducing the number of strays and promoting the return of lost pets to their owners.

- The microchip must be inserted by a qualified professional, e.g. veterinary surgeon or trained implanter.
- Dogs must receive their microchip before they are 8 weeks of age.
- Cats must receive their microchip before they are 20 weeks of age.
- The microchip details, pet details, and keeper's details must be recorded with a microchipping database organisation, e.g. PetLog, Identibase, Animal Microchips, and Animal Tracker (company names as of January 2025).
- Owners are responsible for ensuring their details on the database are kept up to date, e.g. in the case of contact detail changes.
- Local council authorities are responsible for enforcement of the regulations.

If a missing/stray animal is found, then many organisations (e.g. Dogs Trust, Blue Cross, PDSA, RSPCA), veterinary practices, and dog wardens scan the animal to see if it has been microchipped. Sadly, it is often found that the details on the microchip database have not been kept up to date by the owner and it takes longer for the pet to be reunited with its family, if this happens at all.

Microchipping must be thought of as being an essential and routine part of responsible pet ownership in the same way that vaccination and parasite treatments are.

Summary of Basic Animal Health Care

Basic animal health care knowledge is vital in the responsible ownership of animals. Having a basic knowledge of behavioural, physical, and physiological indicators of health enables any concerns to be identified at the earliest opportunity. Having regular routines as part of animal health care plans is extremely useful when looking after several animals. Knowledge of prophylactic treatments available for a species is crucial in avoiding infection at a later stage.

9

Temperature, Pulse, and Respiration

Learning goals

In this chapter, the learning goals are:

- To identify methods for and describe the assessment of temperature, pulse, and respiration (TPR) in the animal
- To identify factors that can affect TPR assessments

Being able to monitor the temperature, pulse, and respiration (TPR) is a key skill to learn when caring for animals. Comparing normal behaviour against abnormal behaviour is involved in TPR monitoring as an animal may hold itself in a different position to relieve pain or it may behave in a slightly different way, which can affect TPR assessments. Knowledge of the animals in your care is vital and being able to recognise subtle changes in behaviour and temperament is crucial.

Many factors can cause changes in TPR measurements. External factors may, for example, include environmental changes, such as temperature, humidity, and noise levels. Internal factors can include exercise, stress, disease, and excitement. If an owner/carer/keeper is concerned about TPR measurements, then they should monitor the animal closely and consult their veterinary practice for advice.

Temperature

Mammalian species can regulate their body temperature to within a very narrow range, in response to internal and external environmental changes, due to the homeostatic process of thermoregulation. These processes may be disrupted when an animal is ill or injured, and this can affect their ability of warm-blooded animals to control their own body temperature. Normal body temperatures for a range of mammal species are shown in Table 9.1. Temperature assessments in cold-blooded species like reptiles is not useful due to their reliance on an external source of heat.

When an animal feels hot, they can adopt specific methods to lose heat from the body and these include:

- Sweating
- Panting
- Drinking water
- Position – spread out, seek a cold surface to lie on
- Vasodilation – surface blood vessels increase in size to lose body heat

Animal Biology and Care, Fourth Edition. Emily Jewell.
© 2026 John Wiley & Sons Ltd. Published 2026 by John Wiley & Sons Ltd.
Companion Website: https://www.wiley.com/go/animal/biology4e/jewell

Table 9.1 Normal temperatures of companion animal species.

Species	Celsius	Fahrenheit
Cat	36.7–39.2[a]	98.1–102.6
Dog	37.2–39.2[a]	98.9–102.6
Ferret	37.9–39.9[a]	100.2–103.8
Guinea pig	38.4–40.0	101.1–104
Hamster	36–38.0	96.8–100.4
Mouse	36.5–38.0	97.7–100.4
Rabbit	37.2–39.6[a]	99.0–103.3
Rat	37.5–37.8	99.5–100

[a]*Newly updated in recent literature (Hall, E. 2021).*

When an animal feels cold, they can adopt methods to preserve heat in the body that include:

- Shivering
- Position – curled up, tightly huddled in groups
- Vasoconstriction – surface blood vessels reduce in size to reduce heat loss through the skin

How Is Temperature Assessed?

The temperature of an animal is assessed by:

- Touching extremities
- Body position
- Taking a rectal reading with a thermometer
- Taking an ear reading with a digital thermometer
- Taking a non-contact reading with an infra-red thermometer

Thermometers

A thermometer is a device used for measuring temperature.
  Types of thermometers used to measure temperatures in animals include:

- Celsius or centigrade – with a scale reading of 35–43 °C (Figure 9.1)
- Digital
- Fahrenheit – with a scale reading of 94–108 °F (Figure 9.1)
- Infra-red thermometers
- Subclinical Celsius – with a scale reading of 25–40 °C

> The formula for converting Celsius to Fahrenheit is as follows:
>
> °F to °C – subtract 32, multiply by 5, and divide by 9.
> °C to °F – multiply by 9, divide by 5, and add 32.

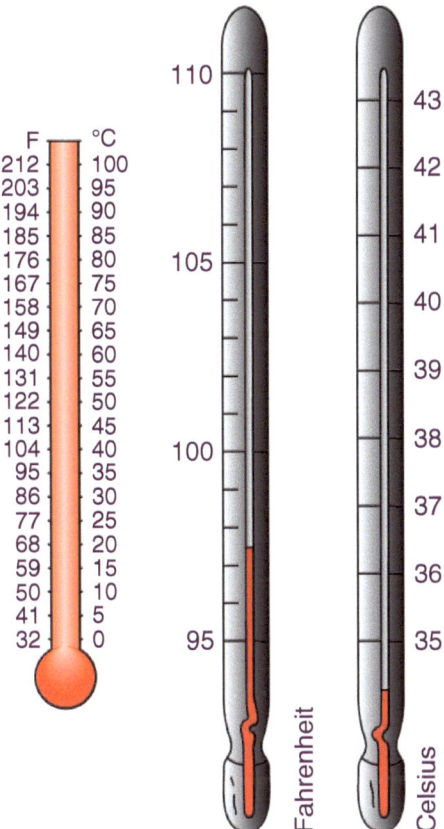

F	°C
212	100
203	95
194	90
185	85
176	80
167	75
158	70
149	65
140	60
131	55
122	50
113	45
104	40
95	35
86	30
77	25
68	20
59	15
50	10
41	5
32	0

Figure 9.1 Thermometer scales.

Thermometers containing mercury have been largely replaced by digital thermometers but may still be in use. It is vital that care is taken to avoid breaking the thermometer when shaking down the mercury in preparation for reading the temperature as mercury is toxic and broken glass is hazardous.

Differences between:

Clinical thermometer	Digital thermometer	Infra-red thermometer
Contains mercury	Digital readings of both scales	Digital readings of both scales
Triangular shape	Circular shape	Handheld
Scale difference	Fast, accurate readings using digital sensors	Fast, less accurate readings – more accurate readings from skin areas rather than fur covered areas
Constriction near bulb	Use disposable cover	
Needs to be shaken down before use	Check batteries charged	Check fully charged
Short shaft	Hygienic	Hygienic and safe as no contact with animal needed

Rules for assessing temperature are as follows:

- Take the temperature at least twice a day if you are monitoring an animal. The animal should be awake as body temperature is always lower after sleep.
  - Leave the thermometer in position for the correct amount of time advised on the instructions (usually 1–2 minutes).
- When taking a rectal temperature, tilt the thermometer to contact the epithelial wall lining the tract after insertion. This ensures that the thermometer is not placed into faeces in the rectum, which would give a false reading.
- When taking the temperature in the ear, do not poke the thermometer all the way down the ear canal, or the tympanic membrane may be damaged.

Equipment required for taking an animal's temperature with a clinical thermometer includes:

- Clinical thermometer
- Lubricant such as K-Y Jelly or medicinal liquid paraffin
- Small amount of cotton wool
- Antiseptic water-based solution
- Timing device

Procedure for taking an animal's rectal temperature with a clinical or digital thermometer:

1. Collect and prepare all required equipment.
2. Correctly restrain patient (second person restraining the head).
3. Prepare the thermometer to be ready to take the temperature.
4. Apply the lubricant to the thermometer.
5. Insert into the rectum for the correct length of time (do not reduce this time). A digital thermometer will usually beep once ready.
6. Remove, wipe with the cotton wool, and read.
7. Wipe clean using antiseptic solution.
8. Read and record the temperature, along with the time it was taken.
9. Ensure the animal is praised following the procedure.

After the temperature has been taken:

- Store the thermometer in a jar or container containing dilute water-based antiseptic solution.
- Always wipe clean of contaminating material before placing it in the jar or container.
- Protect the bulb of the thermometer by placing a layer of cotton wool at the bottom of the container.
- Never store or clean in a hot solution as this could damage the thermometer.
- Before using again, wipe clean of the antiseptic solution, which could irritate the rectal lining.

Procedure for taking an animal's ear temperature with digital thermometer:

1. Ensure the thermometer has been calibrated following the instructions provided.
2. Hold the dog's head still and if required, lift one of the ear flaps to expose the entrance to the ear canal.
3. Carefully insert the probe of the thermometer into the ear at a 90° angle to the dog's head.
4. Hold the probe in place for the correct length of time. The thermometer will usually beep once the recommended amount of time has passed.
5. Read and record the temperature displayed on the thermometer, along with the time of day.

6. Wipe the thermometer clean with antiseptic so that it is ready for using again.
7. Ensure the animal is praised following the procedure.

Increases in temperature may be seen at the following times:

- During infection or fever
- Following exercise
- If the animal is excited or afraid
- Heat stroke (*hyperthermia*)
- Hot weather

Decreases in temperature may be seen at the following times:

- In shock and severe bleeding
- In exposure cases (*hypothermia*)
- In hibernation
- During anaesthesia
- Before impending death (*moribund* animal)
- Immediately before *parturition* (giving birth)

Pulse

Measurement of the pulse is used as a means of checking the heart (*cardio*) and blood (*vascular*) function. With each heartbeat, artery walls expand and contract in size to allow the wave of blood created to pass and maintain its speed of flow. This is called the *pulse*. If there is a change in the heart function or the volume of blood, this will be reflected in the pulse rate (*speed or strength*). Normal pulse rates for a range of mammal species are shown in Table 9.2.

Words that can be used to describe the pulse include:

- Intermittent
- Thready – slow, soft pulse
- Irregular
- Strong
- Weak

Table 9.2 Normal pulse rates for companion animal species at rest.

Species	Pulse rate (beats per minute)
Cat	120–140
Dog	70–120[a]
Ferret	200–250
Guinea pig	230–320
Hamster	300–600
Mouse	450–750
Rabbit	180–350
Rat	250–400

[a] *The pulse range in dogs is due to the size variation from toy breeds (nearer the 180 end of the range) to giant breeds (nearer the 60 end of the range).*

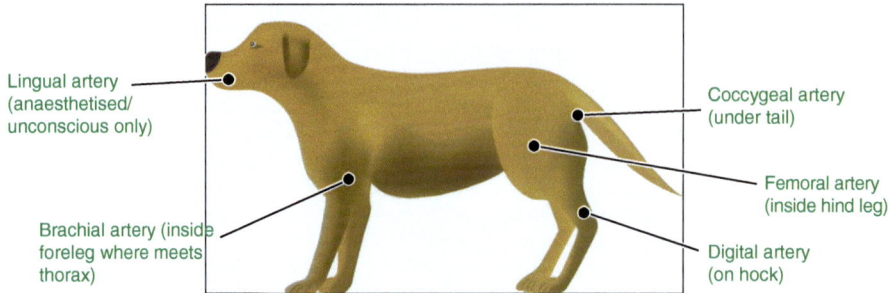

Figure 9.2 Sites for taking the pulse rate of an animal.

A normal pulse is described as being regular, strong, or firm. Regular practise in taking the pulse is essential for developing this skill and assessing the health status of an animal. It also dramatically decreases the time it takes to find the animal's pulse. The pulse can be taken where an artery runs close to the body surface. Each pulse detected corresponds with the contraction of the right and left ventricles of the heart.

Sites used for taking a pulse (Figure 9.2) include:

- *Femoral* artery located in the groin region on the medial aspect of the femur of the hind leg.
- *Digital* artery located on the cranial or anterior surface of the hock region of the hind leg.
- *Brachial* artery located under the forelegs.
- *Coccygeal* artery located on the ventral (underside) aspect of the base of the tail just above the rectum.
- *Lingual* artery located on the ventral (underside) aspect of the tongue. This site can only be used in unconscious or anaesthetised animals.

The most common site used to take the pulse is the *femoral* artery on the hind leg. Before taking the pulse, the animal must be suitably restrained, so two people make the task much easier.

Procedure for taking the pulse in an animal:

1. Ensure the animal is calmly but firmly restrained.
2. Once the animal is settled, take the pulse by placing the fingers over the chosen artery.
3. When properly located, using a watch with a second hand, count the pulse for 1 minute. Never shorten this period because the pulse can change quickly and a reading of less than 1 minute could be inaccurate and therefore useless.
4. Write down the pulse count at the end of the minute.
5. Relax the restraint and praise the animal.

Terms relating to pulse rate

- *Dysrhythmia* – indicates that the pulse and heart rate are not synchronised. The pulse is lower due to the heart pumping blood inefficiently.
- *Sinus arrhythmia* – the rhythm of the heart has been disrupted and is not regular, i.e. there is unequal amounts of time between beats. A fast heart rate is *tachycardic* and a slow heart rate is *bradycardic*.
- *Fast pulse* – occurs when the tissues are not getting enough oxygen, and the heart is compensating by speeding up to meet the body's needs. Fast pulse can be normal after exercise.

Factors that may cause a pulse increase include:

- Exercise
- Excitement or stress
- Heart/valve disease
- Shock or loss of blood
- Pain
- High temperature/fever

Factors that may cause a pulse decrease include:

- Sleep
- Unconsciousness
- Heart disease
- Other disease conditions

Respiration

Normal breathing is almost silent, although airflow may be heard in the airways. The breathing and cardiovascular systems are very closely linked, so a change in one is echoed in the other. If blood gas levels of oxygen or carbon dioxide become abnormal, this will be seen in the animal's colour, in its pulse rate and character, and in its breathing. There should be a regular rhythm to the breathing, i.e. the time between breathing in and out should be equal. The breathing can be varied using the skeletal muscles of the thorax.

Normal respiration (breathing) rates for a range of mammal species are shown in Table 9.3.

Certain breeds of dog and cat may, because of airway anatomy (short-nosed breeds), make considerable breathing sounds and this is normal. Geriatric animals can also make noisier breathing sounds due to loss of tone in the muscles of the airway.

The ability to voluntarily alter breathing means that the breathing rate can only be taken once the animal has settled. Any obvious restraint will cause the breathing rate to increase. The reading should be either taken on the breath in or the breath out (otherwise your reading is double what it should be!)

Table 9.3 Normal respiration (breathing) rates in companion animals.

Species	Rate (breaths per minute)
Cat	10–30
Dog	10–30
Ferret	30–40
Guinea pig	90–150
Hamster	35–127
Mouse	100–250
Rabbit	30–60
Rat	70–150

The respiratory rate should be taken when the animal is calm, awake, and settled comfortably. Do not take the respiratory rate when:

- The dog is panting
- The dog has been recently exercise
- The dog stressed by restraint procedures
- The dog is asleep

Procedure for taking the respiratory rate in an animal:

1. Decide whether counting the in-breaths or the out-breaths.
2. Comfortably restrain the animal and let it settle.
3. Count the breaths whilst timing for one minute, also taking notice of the depth of breaths being taken.
4. Record the respiratory rate.
5. Release and praise the animal.

Respiration rates can be increased by:

- Shock
- Bleeding excessively (*haemorrhage*)
- Recent exercise
- Pain
- Excitement or fear
- Heat stroke (*hyperthermia*)
- Infection/disease (especially of the respiratory system)

Respiration rates can be decreased by:

- Unconsciousness
- Sleep
- Poisons
- Low body temperature (*hypothermia*)

Terms relating to breathing:

- *Tachypnoea* – rapid, shallow breathing.
- *Hyperpnoea* – panting.
- *Apnoea* – no breathing taking place.
- *Laboured* breathing – irregular breathing accompanied by noises such as grunts or wheezes.
- *Agonal* breathing is a reflex breathing pattern (fast shallow breaths) that occurs when the brain is not getting enough oxygen and signals the impending death of the animal.
- *Dyspnoea* – difficulty breathing in or out and often painful.
- *Cheyne- Stokes* – abnormal breathing pattern (fast breathing followed by no breathing due to problems in the brain's feedback loop that regulates breathing) associated with heart failure and brain conditions.

Signs of breathing difficulties include:

- Forced breathing out
- Flaring of nostrils
- Extended head and neck

- Elbows rotated away from the chest
- Breathing through the mouth
- Exaggerated movements of the chest and abdomen
- Unusual sounds
- Unable to settle

Summary of TPR

Temperature, pulse, and respiration measurements give an assessment of what is happening in the animal's body. They should be carried out by experienced staff to get valid and accurate measurements.

All TPR measurements can be affected by extrinsic and intrinsic factors, and the animal must be as calm and settled as possible when taking measurements. If there are concerns about the measurements taken, then veterinary advice should be sought.

10

Disease Transmission and Control

Learning goals

In this chapter, the learning goals are:

- To identify the different methods of disease transmission including:
  - Vertical
  - Horizontal
  - Direct
  - Indirect – fomites and vectors (mechanical and biological)
- To identify disease transmission routes
- To identify methods of infection control
- To describe different methods of diagnosing disease
- To identify and describe types of basic animal treatments and their routes of administration

Disease in the animal body is caused by an infection. Infection is spread from one animal to another in different ways. Infections cause disease in the body through the effects that occur. The method and speed of infection transmission vary according to the type of microorganism that causes the disease. A disease-causing microorganism is known as a *pathogen*.

How Can Infection Be Transmitted?

When trying to identify how an infection is spread between animals, the following questions need to be asked:

- How does the infection leave the infected animal?
- How is the infection passed from one animal to another?
- How does the infection gain entry to a new host?

Infection transmission may be categorised as:

- Vertical
- Horizontal
- Direct
- Indirect

Vertical transmission

Vertical transmission occurs in pregnant animals when infection is passed from a mammalian mother (known as a dam) to her offspring while they are still *in utero*.

The effects on the offspring depend on the stage of pregnancy, e.g. if a pregnant queen (term for a female cat) becomes infected with 'feline parvovirus', then the effects can vary from abortion in early pregnancy to cerebellar hypoplasia later in pregnancy.

Horizontal transmission

Horizontal transmission may occur due to direct or indirect contact.

Transmission through direct contact

Transmission of infection by direct contact includes:

- Contact between one animal and another, e.g. through grooming, fighting, greeting, mating (*venereally*), biting, and being housed together
- Airborne over short distances, i.e. by aerosol infection also known as droplet infection, e.g. sneezing and coughing

The infectious agents (*pathogens*) that are spread by direct contact are often very fragile and cannot survive in the environment for long periods of time. Due to this characteristic, they are easily destroyed by light, heat, and disinfectants.

Indirect contact

Transmission of infection by indirect contact occurs when:

- Two or more animals are in contact with the same inanimate object – the time between periods of contact by the two animals may be long, e.g. ringworm – which can remain viable in the environment for long periods of time. Common contact points are food bowls and water bowls, bedding, and exercise areas.
- Two or more animals are in contact with the same animate object.

For indirect contact to occur, the pathogen must be able to survive away from the host for some time. Such pathogens tend to be hardy in their nature, and not easily destroyed, e.g. *anthrax*.

Transmission of infection by indirect contact is via:

- Inanimate objects – fomites
- Animate objects – vectors

Vectors may be mechanical or biological.

Mechanical vectors

A mechanical vector acts as a moving fomite as the infectious agent does not develop but is spread:

- e.g. insects carrying infectious agents on their mouthparts.
- e.g. *paratenic* hosts – a paratenic host is an intermediate host in a parasite lifecycle. The pathogen lives in the paratenic host without developing until it reaches its definitive host, e.g. *Toxoplasma gondii* larvae live in mice and only develop once a cat eats the mouse.

Biological vectors

A biological vector acts as an intermediate host for the infectious organism and some part of the organism's life cycle occurs in the biological vector; therefore, the vector is essential to complete the life cycle of the organism:

- e.g. Rabbits and sheep can act as intermediate hosts in the life cycle of various tapeworms.

How Does Infection Enter the Animal?

Routes by which disease-causing organisms may *enter* an animal are shown in Figure 10.1.

How Does Infection Leave the Animal?

Routes by which disease-causing organisms may *leave* an animal are shown in Figure 10.2.

It is important to realise that dead animals can also transmit infection, and therefore, there is strict legislation about the disposal of dead animals.

When disease-causing microorganisms are transmitted between animals, the infection can be transmitted by a *carrier animal* rather than an obviously infected animal. Carrier animals do not show clinical signs of disease but may be:

- Individuals that have had the disease and recovered, called *convalescent carriers*. These animals may not have fully excreted the microorganism and may remain infected for life.
- Individuals that never show clinical signs of the disease and are called *healthy carriers*.

Both types of carrier animal will excrete the disease-causing microorganism into the environment, putting other animals at risk.

Carrier animals can also be classified as *continuous excretors* or *intermittent excretors*.

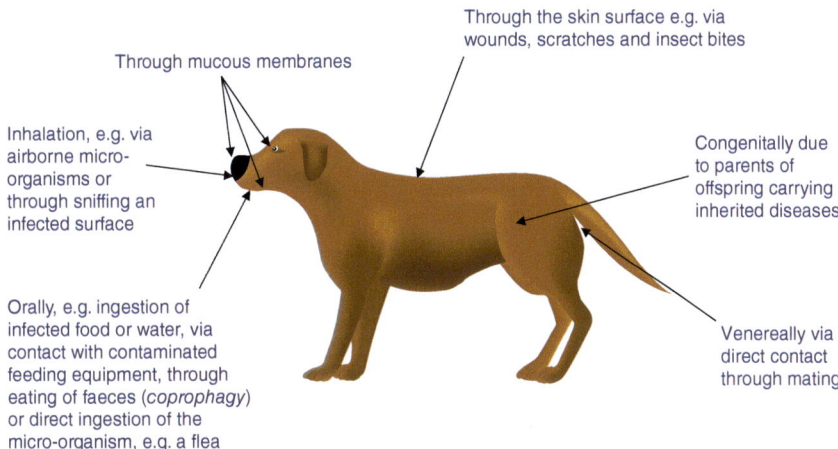

Figure 10.1 Routes by which disease-causing organisms may enter an animal.

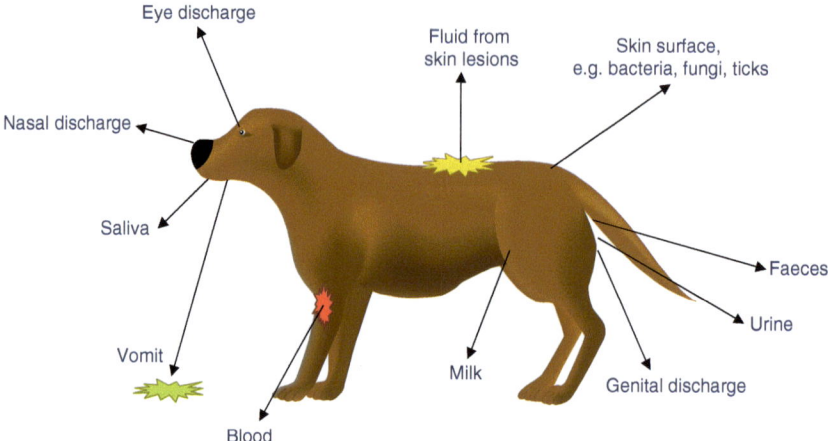

Figure 10.2   Routes by which disease-causing organisms may leave an animal.

Continuous excretors

- Animals continuously excrete the infectious organism.
- Can infect animals at any time.
- Easier to detect than intermittent excretors.

Intermittent excretors

- Animals that only shed the infectious organism at certain times, e.g. during stress.
- May be shed during parturition, lactation, rehoming, weaning, and when using steroid drugs.

Incubation of Disease

Incubation refers to the time between the host animal receiving the pathogen and showing clinical signs of disease. The incubation period will depend on:

- *Number of pathogens received* – If received via the respiratory and/or digestive tracts, secretions here and movement of particles will prevent microorganisms establishing, unless the animal is susceptible.
- *Immune status of the animal* – The animal may fail to mount an adequate immune response, allowing the microorganisms to move on to their target tissues and establish themselves.
- *General health* – If not good, then the animal is susceptible.
- *Age* – The immune response of the body is reduced with age.
- *Physiological state, e.*g. pregnancy can affect the immune system.

Infection

If the pathogen has entered the host animal and overcomes its resistance mechanisms, infection is more than likely to be established. Some infections are confined to a restricted area and are known as *local infections*, e.g. abscesses; other infections spread through the whole body via the bloodstream and are known as *systemic infections*.

Resistance to infection

Individual resistance of an animal to disease will depend on:

- Age
- Nutritional state (too thin or overweight)
- Health status, e.g. no wounds on the body
- Vaccination status
- Immune response and white cell activity

Methods of infection control

- Avoid direct contact with infected animals (use of isolation areas).
- High levels of hygiene/disinfection in the animal's environment.
- Reduce the number of animals kept within the same airspace or improve the efficiency of air movement to reduce aerosol transmission.
- Provide early and effective treatment of infected animals to prevent others being infected.
- Control parasites to prevent the passing of infection from one animal to another.
- Maintain vaccination status.

Infection terms

- *Subclinical infection* – has no clinical signs
- *Clinical* infection
- *Bacteraemia* – bacteria are present in the bloodstream
- *Viraemia* – viruses are present in the bloodstream
- *Pyaemia* – bacteria and white blood cells forming pus are in the blood
- *Septicaemia* – bacteria multiply in the bloodstream

Diagnosis of Disease

Once it has been identified that an animal has signs of ill health by performing a full health check using physical, behavioural, and physiological indicators, a veterinary surgeon will have arrived at a differential diagnosis. This is a list of possible diseases that the signs observed could indicate. To pinpoint the exact illness, there are a wide range of diagnostic tests that can be used to discover the underlying causes of disease and so begin an appropriate treatment. Diagnostic techniques may be *invasive* or *non-invasive*:

- An invasive technique retrieves samples from the body cavity, e.g. tissue biopsies and blood samples.
- Non-invasive techniques retrieve samples without invading the body cavity, e.g. urine samples and faecal samples.

There are five major categories of tests for diagnosing illness in an animal:

1. Biochemistry
2. Haematology
3. Bacteriology
4. Urine sampling
5. Faecal sampling

The test selected for use depends on the differential diagnosis reached by the veterinary surgeon and what is suspected as being the main underlying cause of the illness.

1. *Haematology* – involves taking blood samples from which a range of analysis tests can be conducted. The blood is usually collected into a tube that is treated with an anticoagulant to stop the sample from clotting.
2. *Bacteriology* – identifies the bacteria causing a particular illness. Samples are taken from blood, mucus, or skin scrapings, which are then used to create a smear slide. Common strains of bacteria identified are *Staphylococci* (Gram-positive bacteria associated with skin and urinary infections) and *Escherichia coli* (Gram-negative bacteria associated with digestive upsets).
3. *Biochemistry* – involves the analysis of body fluid – usually blood, for metabolite products, such as blood sugar, urea, and creatinine.
4. *Urine samples* – Urine can be collected from animals, and tests that can be performed on the urine include Clinistix tests, where a stick is dipped in urine and a colour change occurs according to the type of problem, e.g. diabetes. If a bacterial infection is suspected, then the sediment of the urine can be made into a slide and examined in the same way as for bacteriology.
5. *Faecal samples* – examining faecal samples is very useful if trying to detect the presence of endoparasites, such as roundworms and tapeworms, by undertaking an egg count. Worm eggs look like grains of rice in the faeces. Faecal sampling can also be undertaken to establish if the animal has an enzyme deficiency, bacterial infection, or digestive issues.

Once the results have been obtained from the diagnostic tests performed, then the veterinary surgeon can reach a final diagnosis and prescribe an appropriate course of treatment for the animal.

Basic Animal Treatments

Choice of medication

There are many different types of medication available to treat different problems in animals. The medicine chosen by the vet depends on:

- The part of the body the drug needs to target
- The speed at which the drug works
- The ability of the owner to give the drug

Types of medication

The sale and prescription of medications are strictly controlled to prevent misuse. The Medicines Act 1968 categorises medicines according to the level of control needed over the drugs. Each drug is labelled with its own category – see Chapter 20 for further information. Updates to the Act exist in the form of regulations and the most recent are:

- Veterinary Medicines (Amendment, etc.) Regulations 2024
- Veterinary Medicines Regulations 2013 (VMR)

Implementation and enforcement of the regulations is the responsibility of the *Veterinary Medicines Directorate (VMD)*.

Routes of drug administration

The methods by which medicines are given to animals are called routes. Routes of administration for animals include:

- By mouth – orally (Figure 10.3 and Table 10.1)
- On the body surface – topically (Figure 10.4)
- By injection – parenterally

Oral administration
Medicines to be administered orally are given to the animal via its mouth.

Topical administration
Topical medicines may be applied directly to the skin or to the eyes and ears. How the product is applied depends on its type. Some topical medications need to be rubbed directly into the skin, some need to be dabbed on gently, some need to be sprayed on, and some need to be applied in drop form.

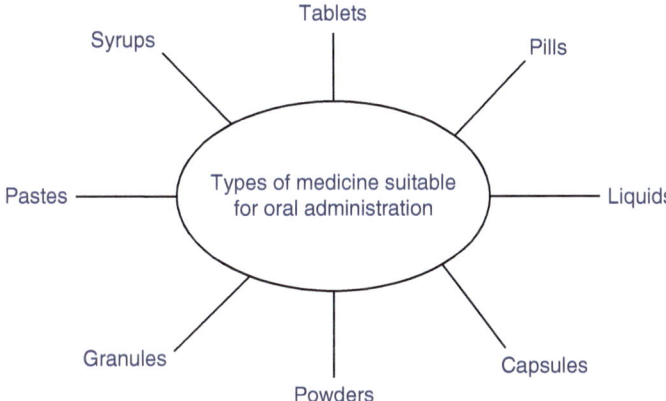

Figure 10.3 Types of medicines suitable for oral administration.

Table 10.1 Methods of administering oral medication.

Type of oral medication	How to give to animal
Tablets Pills Capsules	• Directly to back of mouth • Crushed or wrapped in food
Liquids Syrups	• By syringe into side of mouth • In drinking water
Powders Granules Pastes	• Mixed in food • Directly onto the animal's tongue

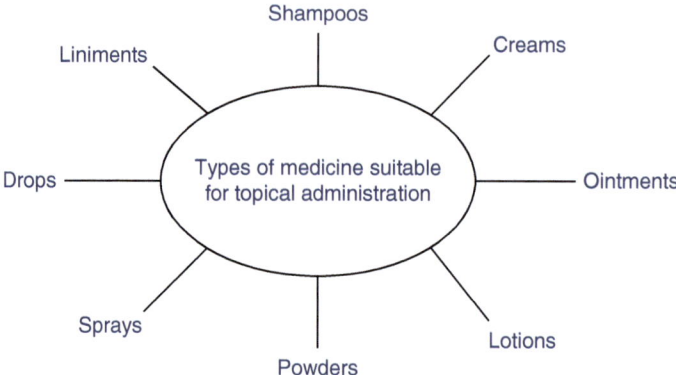

Figure 10.4 Types of medicines suitable for topical administration.

Parenteral administration

To administer an injection, you need a sterile syringe and a hypodermic needle of the correct size. The most common routes of injection are:

- *Subcutaneous* – under the skin – usually in the scruff or loose skin on the back.
- *Intramuscular* – into a muscle – the muscle in the front of the hind leg is the most common site.
- *Intravenous* – into a vein – veins usually used are in the neck, foreleg, and hind leg.

General Guidelines When Dealing with Medicines

You must take notice of the instructions that come with the medication in respect of:

- How the medicine is to be applied
- How often the medicine is to be given
- Any special instructions, e.g. wear gloves
- The dose rate
- The expiry date
- The batch number

Medicines should be stored in suitable labelled containers and put away in a lockable cupboard out of reach of children and animals.

Records must be kept regarding all medicines given to animals in terms of name of animal, date of treatment, product treated with, expiry date, batch number, withdrawal period, etc.

If medicines go past their expiry date, they should be returned to the veterinary surgery for disposal.

Summary of Disease Transmission and Control

This chapter is a basic introduction to disease transmission and control.

It is useful to know how an infection is transmitted so that control measures can be put in place to prevent further spread.

Once an animal is diagnosed with a disease, it is important to be able to administer the medications prescribed by the veterinary surgeon to counteract the infection.

When dealing with animal medicines, it is vital to use them only on the animal(s) they are prescribed for, to keep accurate records, and to store them safely in a locked cupboard.

11

Hygiene and Husbandry

Learning goals

In this chapter, the learning goals are:

- To define terms related to the term hygiene
- To explain the term hygiene
- To identify and describe the properties, effectiveness, and types of disinfectants and antiseptics available
- To explain relevant health and safety aspects related to the use of disinfectants and antiseptics
- To explain an ideal cleaning routine for animal housing
- To explain the use of alcohol gels in animal establishments

When working with animals, hygiene is of the utmost importance when aiming to prevent the build-up of pathogenic microorganisms and subsequent establishment of disease in the animal's environment. Keeping the environment that an animal comes into contact with clean and hygienic contributes to reducing the chances of disease. Using disinfectants and antiseptics helps towards this aim and contributes towards the *biosecurity* of an establishment.

What Are Disinfectants and Antiseptics?

Disinfectants and antiseptics are chemical compounds that play an essential role in maintaining the health, preventing infection, and promoting the recovery of an animal. Their use in basic hygiene for all small and domestic animal housing, veterinary practice, zoological collections, and on farms is important to the good hygiene of both the environment and living tissues.

Disinfectants are designed for use on the environment and non-living structures, including furnishings within an animal's housing, whereas *antiseptics are designed for use on living tissue*. As these products are both chemical compounds, if they are used incorrectly, such as at lower than advised concentration/dilution rate, then microorganisms may develop resistance, which reduces the value of the disinfectants and antiseptics to the upkeep of a hygienic environment. Advantages and disadvantages of disinfectants and antiseptics can be found in Table 11.1.

Animal Biology and Care, Fourth Edition. Emily Jewell.
© 2026 John Wiley & Sons Ltd. Published 2026 by John Wiley & Sons Ltd.
Companion Website: https://www.wiley.com/go/animal/biology4e/jewell

Table 11.1 Advantages and disadvantages of disinfectants and antiseptics.

Advantages	Disadvantages
Disinfectants	
More concentrated – increased efficacy	
Not so easily inactivated	Can be toxic, e.g. phenols
Broad spectrum of activity	Can damage surfaces
Added detergents to most	Expense versus economy
	May have long contact time
Antiseptics	
Rapid action	Inactivated by organic material
Tissue friendly	May irritate skin
Use on wounds and burns	Can be contaminated and so grow bacteria
Safe for operator	

Key Terms Relating to Hygiene

- *Antiseptics* – chemicals that kill or prevent infection without damaging living tissue. They will prevent organisms from multiplying, and therefore, infections cannot develop. Also called skin disinfectants as they are non-toxic and are applied to skin prior to operations or to damaged skin surfaces, i.e. to treat wounds, burns or surgical incisions.
- *Antisepsis* – preventing infection through use of antiseptics.
- *Asepsis* – is a state of being free from microorganisms.
- *Bactericidal* – kills bacteria.
- *Bacteriostatic* – inhibits growth of bacteria.
- *Biosecurity* – practice of reducing the impact of pathogenic microorganisms, thereby preventing spread of disease.
- *Cleaning* – the process of removing dirt (not necessarily microorganisms).
- *Detergent* – a water-soluble chemical substance that removes dirt and other impurities from environmental surfaces.
- *Disinfectants* – chemicals that kill microorganisms by killing or inhibiting growth. Usually too toxic to be applied to living tissues and so should only be used on hard surfaces, equipment, and instruments.
- *Disinfection* – the process of killing microorganisms.
- *Fungicidal* – kills fungi.
- *Fungistatic* – inhibits growth of fungi.
- *Hygiene* – conditions or processes that maintain health and prevent disease, through encouraging cleanliness.
- *Sterilisation* – the removal or destruction of all living microorganisms, including bacterial spores. Always used on surgical instruments.
- *Virucidal* – kills viruses.
- *Virustatic* – inhibits growth of viruses.

Disinfectants

Disinfectants should only be used in an animal's environment, on surfaces such as floors, walls, ceilings, exercise runs, and food bowls. Disinfectants are harmful to living tissues, and so, whenever disinfectants are being used, protective clothing should be worn – gloves, apron, and face mask if working in an enclosed area. Animals must always be removed from their enclosures when a disinfectant is being used.

What are the properties of an ideal disinfectant?

- Effective against a wide range of microorganisms.
- Non-toxic to humans or animals (through contact and aerosol transmission).
- Does not stain housing or clothing.
- Can wet the surface being disinfected easily.
- Penetrates through any organic matter on the surfaces being disinfected.
- Can be easily stored.
- Can be stored for a long time (long shelf life).
- Can be used in low concentrations for maximum effectiveness.
- Cheap to use.
- Readily available supplies.

Do disinfectants always work?

The operational activity of a disinfectant can be altered by:

- The presence of organic matter, e.g. faeces, blood, and pus.
- Other chemicals being used at the same time, e.g. detergents or antiseptics.
- Type of water – hard or soft.
- Temperature of water – hot or cold.
- Contact time, i.e. the time left on the surface.
- Material being disinfected, e.g. cork, rubber, plastic, and wood.
- Dilution rate of the disinfectant.
- The length of time the diluted product has been made up for.

Disinfectants are most effective when

- Used with hot/warm water rather than cold – check the instructions as if too hot, it may affect efficacy.
- Left in contact with surfaces for the correct amount of time (see instructions on label).
- Used at the correct strength.
- Freshly prepared (see instructions on label).
- Not mixed with other chemicals including soaps, detergents, and other cleaning agents.
- The amount needed is made up at any one time.

When choosing a disinfectant for environment cleaning, careful choice is needed. Some products are toxic to certain species of animals. The phenols or phenol-containing compounds are toxic to cats, rabbits, and rodents, so they tend to be used only in large animal and farming industry facilities. Products in this group are recognised as black, white, or clear. They normally have a strong and distinctive smell and will stain housing and bedding materials. Examples are Anigene, FAM 30, Jeyes Fluid, Virkon S, and Dettol.

When there is a notifiable disease outbreak, the disinfectant chosen must come from the Department for Environment, Food and Rural Affairs (DEFRA)-approved list under The Diseases of Animals (Approved Disinfectants) (England) Order 2007.

Which disinfectant to choose?

There is a wide range of disinfectants available for use. When choosing a disinfectant to use, you need to consider:

- Can it be used for the species you work with?
- Which microorganisms does it destroy?
- Is it low risk in terms of health and safety?
- How quickly does it work?
- What dilution is it used at?
- How should it be stored?
- Will it corrode the housing?
- How easy is it to dispose of?
- What effects does it have on the environment?
- What does it smell like?
- How much does it cost?

Depending on where you want to use the disinfectant, the manufacturer may provide different dilution rates. There are often different dilution rates for general use and specific use.

Disinfectants for general use often work against a wide range of microorganisms and so are called *broad-spectrum disinfectants*. Disinfectants that are used specifically against a particular type of microorganism are called *narrow-spectrum disinfectants*.

What types of disinfectant are there?

Disinfectants are split into different groups according to the active compound that they contain:

Phenols
- Phenols tend to be toxic to small animals and so are generally only used on farms and for large animal housing. Phenols may be black, white, or clear and have a strong, distinctive smell and a tendency to stain housing and beds. Phenols are effective against bacteria, fungi, and some viruses. Examples of phenols are Jeyes Fluid and Dettol. Phenol-based disinfectants should not be used for cats, rabbits, or rodents. They can also be irritating to skin and mucous membranes.

Aldehydes
- Aldehydes work against a wide range of microorganisms and are highly toxic to living tissue. When making or disposing of them, you must take strict safety precautions as they can give off fumes. They are usually used for sterilising surgical equipment. Examples include Formula H, Parvocide, and Vet-Cide.

Peroxides

- Peroxides are effective against a wide range of microorganisms. They are available as powders to be mixed with water for disinfecting housing and surfaces. Gloves and aprons should be worn when using this type of disinfectant as they can be irritating to eyes and skin. Once mixed, it is stable as a disinfectant for 5 days. Examples include Virkon S.

Halogens

- Halogens are only effective if the usage instructions are followed correctly as they can be inactivated by the presence of organic matter and incorrect dilution rates. They may irritate skin and so should be carefully prepared, used, and rinsed off surfaces thoroughly. Halogen disinfectants need to be made up frequently. Examples include bleach (sodium hypochlorite) and other chlorine-releasing products, e.g. Betadine. The product loses activity on exposure to air and light and so new dilutions should be made up frequently.

Quaternary ammonium compounds

Quaternary ammonium compounds (QACs) are highly effective against a broad spectrum of microorganisms, and they are relatively non-toxic and non-corrosive, but their effectiveness can be affected by the presence of organic matter and hard water. Examples include Kennel-Sol.

What precautions should be taken when using a disinfectant?

Precautions to be taken include:

- Wear protective clothing and avoid contact with skin – gloves, apron, and mask.
- Follow the safety instructions for using the disinfectant that can be found on the *COSHH* (Control of Substances Hazardous to Health) sheet produced by the manufacturer.
- Only use for the purpose recommended by the manufacturer.
- Use at the recommended concentration/dilution to achieve maximum effectiveness.
- Store the disinfectant in a secure location – preferably a lockable cupboard.
- Store the disinfectant in its original container with a tight-fitting lid to minimize the chance of leakage.
- Keep disinfectants away from children and animals.
- Wash hands thoroughly after use.

COSHH sheets

It is vitally important to follow the manufacturer's recommended instructions as much research will have been done on the chemicals before they are released onto the commercial market to determine the safest use of the disinfectant.

All disinfectants should have an associated COSHH sheet that should be read prior to use and stored in a safe place in case of emergency. All staff should be made aware of any potential hazards that may be caused when using the disinfectant.

Dilution rates

Manufacturers always recommend dilution rates for the disinfectant. There may be more than one rate, depending on the intended use and the pathogens that need to be destroyed. Often, a routine strength is recommended with stronger rates for specific disinfections. Too weak a solution will usually be ineffective and too strong a solution is wasteful, and it may also endanger the safety of the patients by causing irritation.

A dilution rate is usually:

- General cleaning strength=1:100 (10 ml disinfectant/litre of water)
- Broad-spectrum activity=1:50 (20 ml disinfectant/litre of water)
- Specific activity=1:25 (40 ml disinfectant/litre of water)

Communal areas such as offices, corridors, and reception areas should be cleaned using general strength dilution. Areas such as waiting rooms, consulting rooms, housing, and exercise runs should be cleaned using broad-spectrum strength. Where there has been exposure to specific pathogens, or an outbreak of disease, then a specific activity dilution rate should be used.

How do disinfectants work?

Disinfectants destroy the microorganism by disrupting its cell wall or contents in such a way that the microorganism will die (-*static*) or be killed by the chemical (-*cidal*).

The most resistant microorganisms to disinfectants are:

- Bacterial spores
- Unenveloped viruses
- Gram-negative bacteria
- Mycobacteria

The least resistant microorganisms to disinfectants are:

- Enveloped viruses
- Gram-positive bacteria
- Fungi, particularly yeasts

Disinfection and cleaning of the animal's environment

Animal housing and the surrounding environment can only be cleaned effectively if both *physical and chemical actions* are taken.

Physical action (scrubbing) is most important for several reasons:

- Removes foreign materials, such as blood, pus, and faeces, which are ideal breeding grounds for pathogens.
- Disinfectants must have direct contact with the pathogen to be destroyed to be effective.
- Disinfectants are effective only after all other debris has been removed.

What equipment is needed for cleaning animal housing?

- Dustpan and brushes
- Waste bags
- Scrubbing brushes
- Hot soapy water
- Buckets/hose pipe
- Clean water
- Disinfectant

To maximise the effect of the disinfectant being used and to prevent inactivation by organic materials, animals must be kept safe in alternative accommodation when disinfecting housing, surfaces, and furniture within enclosures.

What is the correct way to clean animal housing?

- Remove animal to a safe place or pen them into a safe area.
- Remove all food and water containers and enrichment/toys.
- Remove soiled bedding/waste substrate into waste container (bag, wheelbarrow or bin for example) and dispose of correctly.
- Soak all surfaces with hot soapy water.
- Scrub the soaked surfaces with scrubbing brush.
- Wash away all organic material and all soap with clean (preferably running) water.
- Apply disinfectant (made up at correct strength) and leave for the correct amount of time.
- Rinse off all disinfectant with lots of clean water if it needs to be.
- Leave to dry.
- Replace clean substrate/bedding.
- Replace all furniture for the enclosure after cleaning.
- Replace the animal safely into its usual accommodation, ensuring safety and security.
- Observe behaviour of the animal to ensure it is settled.
- Clean and disinfect the holding pen/cage and all equipment used to clean the accommodation, before storing away safely.

Antiseptics

Predominantly, antiseptics are used as cleansers for the skin and may be called skin disinfectants. When applied to skin or mucous membranes of living tissues, antiseptics stop or prevent the growth of microorganisms like bacteria and fungi but will not necessarily kill the microorganisms.

Antiseptics are non-toxic to living tissue and are used prior to operations, before handling animals to prevent transfer of microorganisms and after handling contaminated material. They are also used to disinfect the animal's skin pre- and post-surgery or after an injury where an open wound has resulted.

Antiseptics work very quickly, and although they are not generally toxic, some can irritate the skin, and so, it is important that they should only be used at their recommended dilution rate.

Which antiseptic to choose?

There are a range of antiseptics available, and choice will be affected by several factors in a similar way to disinfectants.

What types of antiseptics are there?

Quaternary ammonium compounds
There are two main types of QACs to choose from:

- Chlorhexidine plus a detergent property, e.g. Hibiscrub
- Cetrimide, e.g. Cetavlon, Savlon, or Vetasept

QACs are highly effective against microorganisms and have rapid action as an antiseptic. They are often used as a preoperative skin cleaner and as a surgeon's scrub. They have a low toxicity to tissues but cause irritation to some individuals. Recontamination by microorganisms is prevented for a time due to a residual effect. Use at recommended dilution and only on intact skin.

Iodophors – Iodine-based compounds (e.g. Povidine scrub, Betadine)

- Iodophors are effective against skin microorganisms, are non-irritant, and have low toxicity to tissues. Their action is slow, so the length of time that they are in contact with the skin surface is important. They can be inactivated by the presence of organic matter. These types of antiseptics usually stain the skin and any materials they are in contact with for a period of time following their use. Follow the manufacturer's safety instructions for use.

Alcohol Gel

Alcohol gels for hands are now routinely used in veterinary practices and other animal establishments as good practice in hand sterilisation prior to husbandry procedures occurring. Alcohol is a very effective agent against bacteria, viruses, and fungi, but has limited effects on the spores of these microorganisms. It is also effective against Methicillin-resistant *Staphylococcus aureus* (*MRSA*) (*see* Chapter 20).

Visitors to animal establishments, such as zoos and farm parks, are encouraged to use alcohol gels to sterilise their hands after handling animals or touching their enclosures, as a temporary measure until they can wash their hands thoroughly with soap and warm water.

Alcohol can also be used as a surface cleanser in surgical areas of the veterinary practice. Care must be taken when using alcohol as it is flammable and in excessive quantities can be an irritant. Repeated use can dry the skin, and so, those users who suffer from skin conditions, such as eczema, should take care in their use of alcohol gels and always use an effective moisturiser.

Summary of Hygiene and Husbandry

Any husbandry procedures carried out when working with animals should always be carried out with good hygiene in mind to prevent an increase in pathogens and potential disease outbreak.

There are several different types of disinfectants and antiseptics that may be chosen for use when working with animals to reduce/prevent pathogens and maintain good hygiene practices.

When working with disinfectants and antiseptics, it is vitally important to follow the instructions for use and the dilution rates recommended on the manufacturer's COSHH sheet, so that their use is most effective and does not cause other complications.

12

Basic Microbiology

Learning goals

In this chapter, the learning goals are:

- To identify the structure and function of:
  - Bacteria
  - Viruses
  - Fungi
  - Protozoa
- To identify and define basic terms relating to microbiology

What Is Microbiology?

Microbiology is the study and identification of microorganisms (also known as microbes). The main microorganisms to be considered are:

- Bacteria
- Viruses
- Fungi
- Protozoa

Microorganisms are measured in micrometres (µm): *1 µm = 1 thousandth of a millimetre (mm).* Microbes range from large protozoa to the smallest of viruses. Viruses can only be seen using an electron microscope and are measured in nanometres (nm): *1 nm = 1 millionth of a millimetre.*

Microorganisms live throughout all human and animal environments and are normally present on or within the body. Their presence on the body is usually balanced, but if the body's environment is out of balance, then some microbes may capitalise on this and overtake the body to cause infection.

Microbial Terms

- *Infection* – process by which microorganisms become established in the host.
- *Saprophytes* – live and feed on dead organic material.
- *Autotrophs* – synthesise (create) their own food.
- *Heterotrophs* – obtain nutrients from their environment.

Animal Biology and Care, Fourth Edition. Emily Jewell.
© 2026 John Wiley & Sons Ltd. Published 2026 by John Wiley & Sons Ltd.
Companion Website: https://www.wiley.com/go/animal/biology4e/jewell

- *Symbiosis* – the association between two different species living together.
- *Parasitic* – refers to the association between two different living organisms in which the parasite lives upon the host, taking food and shelter (host's own food or body fluids).
  Parasites fall into three groups:
  i. *Pathogens* – will harm the host animal, causing disease
  ii. *Commensals* – will not harm or benefit the host animal
  iii. *Mutualistics* – are of benefit to the host, e.g. help break down food in the intestine.

Bacteria

Bacteria range from 0.5 to 5 µm in length. They may be rod shaped (*bacillus*), round or spherical (*cocci*), or spiral shaped (*spirilla*), as shown in Figure 12.1.

Structure of bacteria

- *Cell wall* – for shape and protection (Figure 12.2).
- *Capsule or loose slime layer* – for sticking to surfaces, protection from its environment, and preventing destruction by phagocytic white blood cells.
- *Plasma membrane* – controls the passage of substances in and out of the cell.
- *Internal cell organelles* (cytoplasm, ribosomes, etc.) – to support the life of the cell.
- *Flagellum and pili* – hair-like structures for moving the cells along.

Bacterial reproduction

Bacterial reproduction takes place providing the following conditions are in place:

- Supply of *nutrients*
- Correct *temperature*
- Correct *pH* and *oxygen* levels, but it is important to note that not all bacteria require oxygen and are described as being *aerobic* or *anaerobic*:
  - *Aerobic bacteria* – only grow in the presence of free oxygen
  - *Anaerobic bacteria* – only grow in the absence of free oxygen

Bacteria reproduce first by growth and then by division of the cell. Most reproduce by an asexual method called *binary fission*. For many bacteria, this division takes 15–20 minutes.

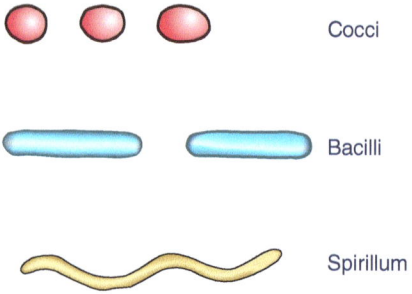

Figure 12.1 Shapes of bacteria.

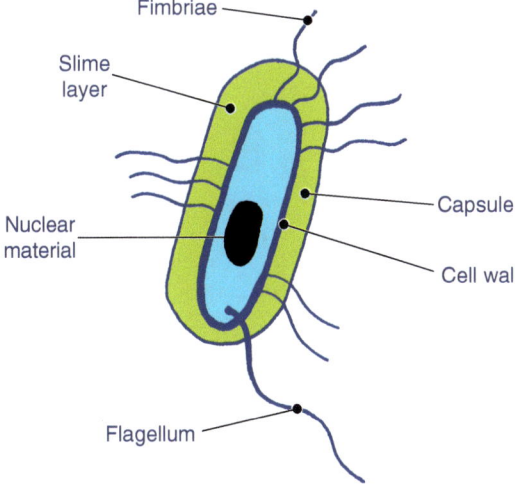

Figure 12.2   Bacterium in detail.

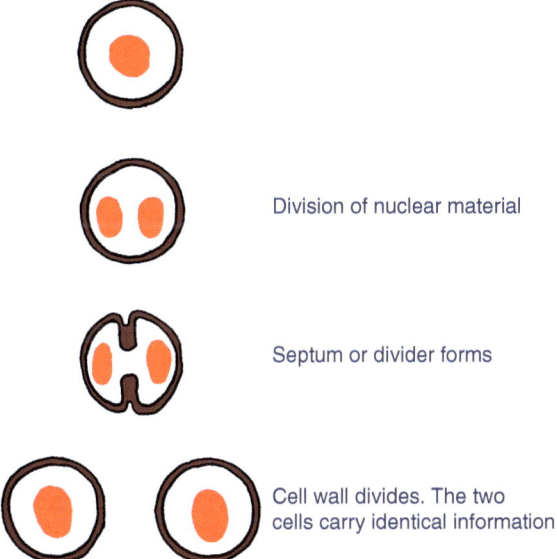

Figure 12.3   Binary fission.

Binary fission

One cell simply divides into two cells (Figure 12.3).

Conjugation or bacterial mating

Sexual reproduction refers to the passing of genetic material and information from a bacterial donor to a bacterial recipient. It is passed through a short tube called the *sex pilus* (Figure 12.4). This method passes part of the donor cell chromosome and extra genes, e.g. genes carrying an anti-biotic resistance factor, to another bacterium.

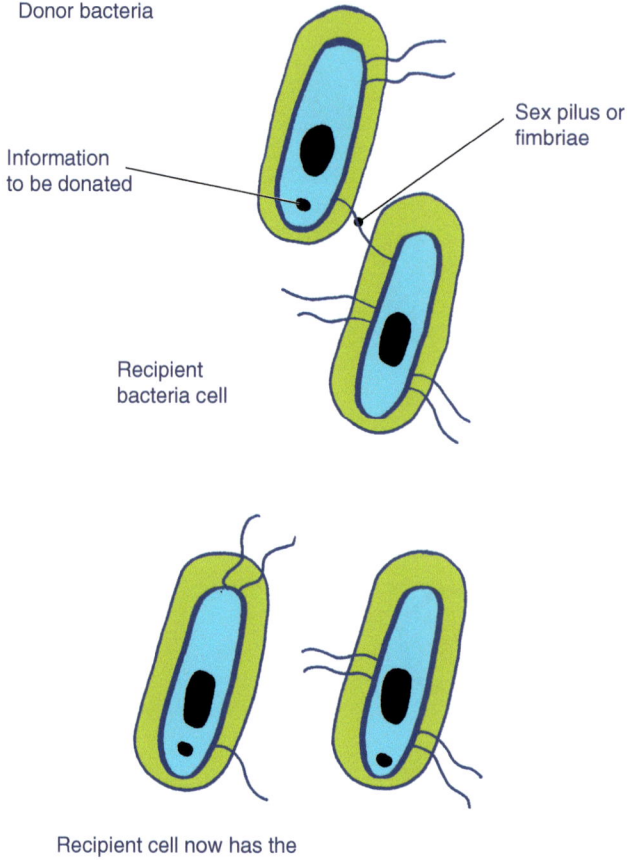

Donor bacteria

Information to be donated

Sex pilus or fimbriae

Recipient bacteria cell

Recipient cell now has the 'passed' information

Figure 12.4 Conjugation or bacterial mating.

Some bacteria produce a dormant spore (*endospore*). This process of spore production is like binary fission, but the septum or divider is nearer one end of the cell and grows to surround the genetic information. Spores tend to form when conditions for life are not favourable, e.g. the correct nutrients are not available. Once the spore forms, the original cell breaks down or *lyses*, releasing the spore into the environment to await improved conditions (Figure 12.5). This is not a form of reproduction but a means of survival.

Bacterial terms

- *Endotoxins – toxins produced within the bacteria and only released into the host animal when the* bacteria die. The toxins can cause signs of shock or fever and can be lethal.
- *Exotoxins – toxins secreted by the living bacteria which can also be harmful to the host animal's body.*

Examples of diseases caused by bacteria are *Salmonella infection* and *Kennel Cough*. See Table 12.1 for further information.

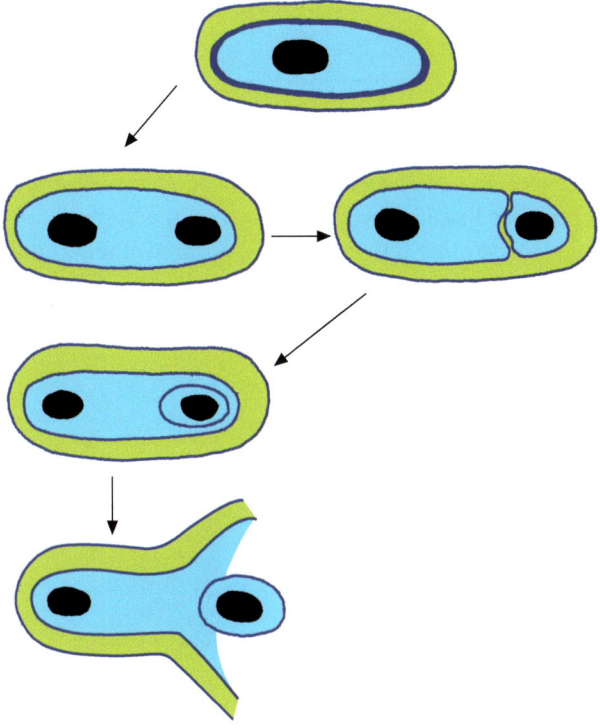

Cell finally ruptures to
release spore, which will remain
in this form, protected, until its
environment improves

Figure 12.5 Spore formation.

Table 12.1 Diseases produced by different microorganisms.

Micro-organism	Dog	Cat
Protozoa	Coccidiosis Toxoplasmosis	Coccidiosis Toxoplasmosis
Fungi	Ringworm	Ringworm
Bacteria	Kennel cough Leptospirosis	Salmonellosis
Virus	Distemper Infectious hepatitis Parvovirus Rabies	Panleukopenia Respiratory disease Infectious peritonitis Leukaemia Immunodeficiency Rabies

Viruses

Viruses are the smallest of the microorganisms (Figure 12.6). Viruses are always parasitic and reproduce by *replicating* (copying) themselves. This process happens after the viral DNA or RNA (genetic information) has entered a host animal's body cell. This strand of material takes over control of the host cell's metabolism and directs it to manufacture replicas of the viral material. When enough replicas have been produced, the virus will instruct the host cell to rupture, releasing the new viruses, which go on to use other host cells for the purpose of replicating (Figure 12.7).

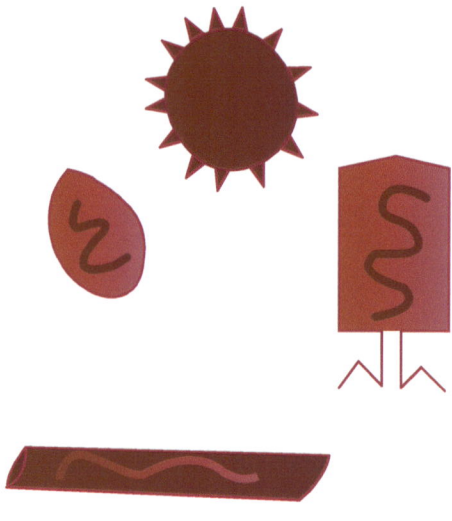

Shape variations with
DNA strand and protein coat
for protection

Figure 12.6 Examples of virus shapes.

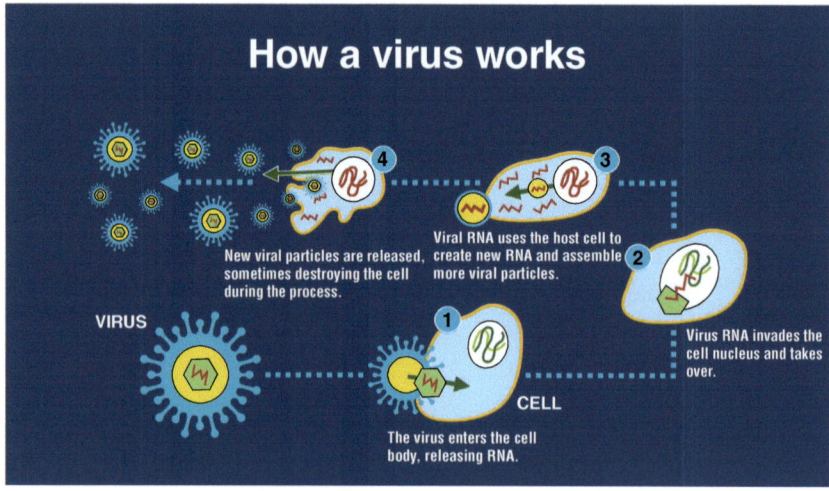

Figure 12.7 Virus replication. Dimitrios / Adobe Stock Photos.

The virus is not a cell. It is a protein coat around a DNA or RNA strand. Some viruses are also surrounded by a membrane known as an *envelope,* which may have structures like spikes on its surface for attaching to the host cell before entry.

In many cases, the cycle of viral infection causes no apparent harm to the host. Disease occurs when the host is harmed by the infection, which occurs when quantities of host cells have been destroyed.

Examples of diseases caused by viruses include *Parvovirus* and *Rabies*.

Fungi

Fungi are non-chlorophyll-bearing plants. They can be categorised as:

- *Moulds* – multicellular – often contain filament structures called *hyphae*
- *Yeasts* – unicellular

Fungi do not have the ability to create their own food and so must exist as parasites or saprophytes.

Distribution of fungal microorganisms is by spores (Figure 12.8).

Reproduction in fungi is sexual (hyphae from different strains unite into a survival spore form, awaiting favourable conditions), and there is also an asexual method (distribution of spores). Examples of diseases caused by fungi are *ringworm* and *dermatophytes*.

Protozoa

Protozoa are single-celled animals and range in size from microscopic to just visible to the naked eye. They have a cell membrane and have organelles for movement (flagella and cilia) (Figure 12.9).

Reproduction is asexual by binary fission.

Nutrition is *holozoic* (capture and assimilation of organic material in their environment). Protozoa are capable of pursuing prey by following a chemical trail, or they can be stimulated by movement, particularly in water.

Protozoa will form a *cyst* at some point in their life cycle. This is the form which passes from host to host and allows temporary survival outside the host. Diseases caused by protozoa include *Toxoplasmosis* and *Coccidiosis*.

Diseases are covered in more detail in Chapter 13.

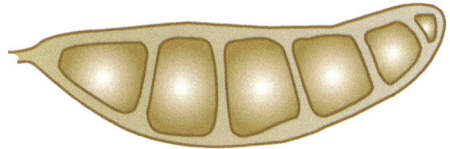

Spindle-shaped cells make up the spore, as seen in *Microsporum canis* (ringworm)

Figure 12.8 Fungal spore.

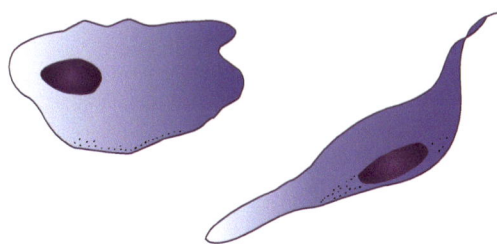

Figure 12.9 Protozoa forms.

Summary of Basic Microbiology

There are many microorganisms in existence that have the potential to cause infection and subsequently disease in an animal. These microorganisms are called pathogens.

Microorganisms are categorised as:

- Bacteria
- Viruses
- Fungi
- Protozoa

Each microorganism has its own distinct features and characteristics.

Having a knowledge of the terms linked to microbiology aids understanding of veterinary diagnoses and discussions.

13

Diseases of Domestic Animals

Learning goals

In this chapter, the learning goals are:

- To identify types of immunity
- To identify and describe examples of diseases affecting animals routinely kept as pet species, covering cause, signs, treatments, and prophylactic actions available

It is important that owners/carers/keepers of animals are aware of the diseases that may affect the animals that they are responsible for and ways that animals can be protected against them. Vaccination is an important disease control method that can help eradicate disease if most animals are vaccinated against that disease.

Immunity

Immunity refers to the body's natural protection against disease. It can be achieved by:

- Contracting the disease and recovering
- Vaccination

The immune system involves a complex network of cells, tissues, and organs that work together to defend the body against potentially harmful pathogens.

In immunological terms, any microorganism that the body recognises as being foreign is known as an *antigen*. A part of a virus or bacteria can be identified as an antigen and trigger an immune response, e.g. a surface protein.

In simple terms, a pathogen invades the body and causes disease, whereas an antigen triggers the immune response to fight the pathogen.

Cells of the immune system

There are many cells that can be involved in the immune system and the key ones are identified. More can be viewed in Figure 13.1.

Animal Biology and Care, Fourth Edition. Emily Jewell.
© 2026 John Wiley & Sons Ltd. Published 2026 by John Wiley & Sons Ltd.
Companion Website: https://www.wiley.com/go/animal/biology4e/jewell

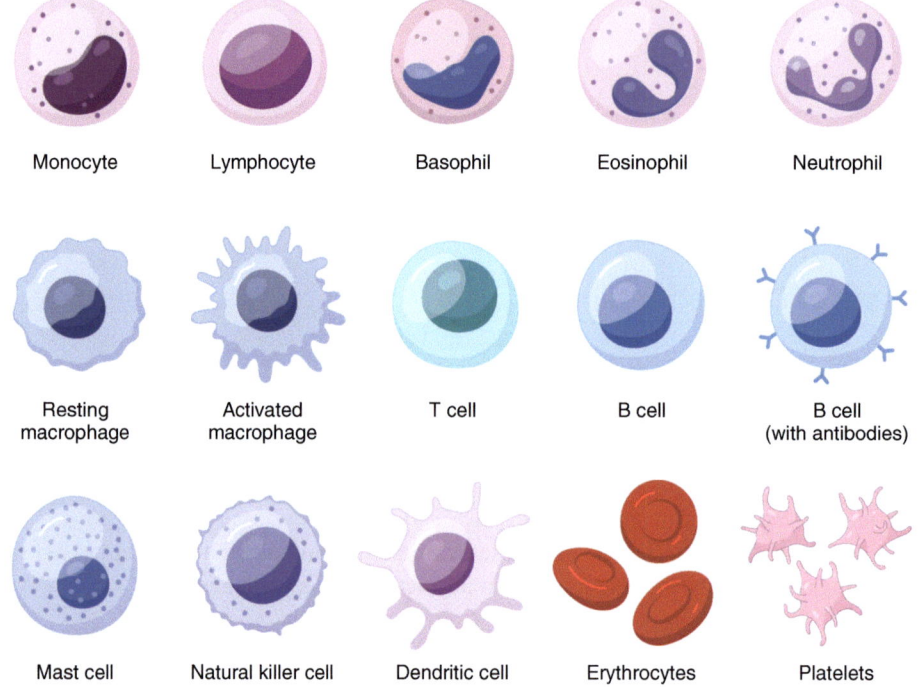

| Monocyte | Lymphocyte | Basophil | Eosinophil | Neutrophil |

| Resting macrophage | Activated macrophage | T cell | B cell | B cell (with antibodies) |

| Mast cell | Natural killer cell | Dendritic cell | Erythrocytes | Platelets |

Figure 13.1 Cells of the immune system. ONYXprj / Adobe Stock Photos.

- *T-Lymphocytes*
    T-cells originate from stem cells in the bone marrow and are matured in *thymus* tissue. The thymus is a small organ that is found behind the breastbone.
    T cells can be categorised into
    - helper cells (CD4$^+$) – release cytokines to stimulate other cells.
    - cytotoxic cells (CD8$^+$) – directly kill infected or cancerous cells.
    - regulatory cells – help regulate immune responses.
- *B-Lymphocytes*
    B-cells originate and mature in the bone marrow. They produce antibodies by binding to specific antigens and marking them for destruction by other cells of the immune system.
- *Natural Killer Cells (NK)*
    NK cells can destroy infected cells and tumour cells without having memory of them.
- *Phagocytes*
    A type of white blood cell that circulates in the bloodstream. Can be categorised as:
    - Monocytes – can differentiate into macrophages or dendritic cells in tissues.
        ○ Macrophages – engulf pathogens and cell debris. Present antigens to T-cells to stimulate an immune response.
        ○ Dendritic cells – Present antigens to T-cells to stimulate an immune response.

- Granulocytes
  - Neutrophils – most common white blood cell as they are first line responders to infection. Engulf and kill bacteria.
  - Eosinophils – combat parasites and control the allergic response.
  - Basophils – release histamine and other chemicals involved in allergic reactions.
- Mast cells – release histamine and other chemicals involved in allergic reactions.

Types of immunity

Immunity can be described as:

- Innate
- Adaptive
- Passive
- Active

Innate immunity

Innate immunity is the first line of defence in the body and is non-specific, i.e. it responds to all pathogens in the same way. The body's response is fast. Examples of innate responses are inflammation and fever.

Innate immunity (Figure 13.2) includes:

- Physical barriers – skin, mucous membranes
- Chemical barriers – stomach acid
- Immune cells – phagocytes and natural killer cells.

Innate immunity has no memory. It does not remember the pathogens that it is has previously encountered.

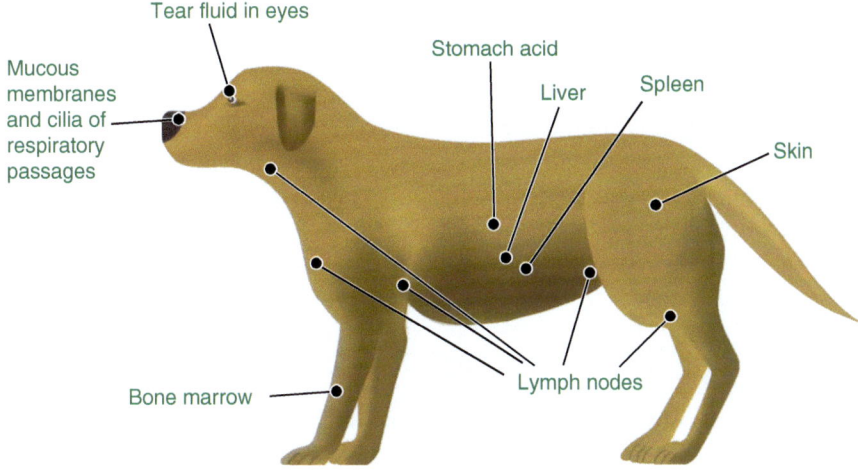

Figure 13.2 Physical and chemical barriers of the immune system.

Adaptive immunity

Adaptive immunity is the second line of defence. It is pathogen specific. Adaptive immunity has a slower response time.

Adaptive immunity involves:

- B-lymphocytes (B-cells)
- T-lymphocytes (T-cells)

Both B-cells and T-cells are antibodies that recognise specific pathogens and prevent or limit their ability to develop disease in the host animal.

Adaptive immunity has memory and can remember pathogens it has encountered before. If the same pathogen is subsequently encountered, an immune response is produced more quickly in the body.

How is immunity acquired?

Immunity may be acquired by passive or active means.

Passive immunity

Passive immunity results from the transfer of maternal antibodies to the newborn via the colostrum in the milk. The degree of immunity depends on the quantity of the first milk and the quality of the mother's own antibodies resulting from her own vaccinations. Passive immunity lasts between 3 and 12 weeks, depending on how long the antibodies remain active in the blood. After this time, the body will eliminate the antibodies. Passive immunity can also be acquired when blood products are given in transfusion processes.

Active immunity

Active immunity develops either because the animal is infected with a microorganism, develops the disease and recovers, or from a vaccination. Both cause the body to react in a similar way by stimulating the production of antibodies that are specific to pathogens. Active immunity is long lasting.

Vaccination

The purpose of vaccination is to prevent the disease by preventing or limiting the infection in a host animal. Vaccines cause stimulation of the immune system, which in turn produces antibodies.

The cells of the immune system responsible for producing this protection are the B-lymphocytes, and these in turn are assisted by the T-lymphocytes.

At the time of vaccination, the veterinary surgeon will fully examine the animal to ensure that any factors that may influence the body's response to the vaccine are not present, such as a high body temperature indicating infection.

There are many factors that influence an animal's ability to respond to vaccination. These include:

- The presence of colostrum antibodies from the mother's milk, which could interfere with the vaccine
- Vaccine type – live or inactive
- Route of administration – subcutaneous or intranasal
- Animal's age
- Medication that could interfere with the vaccine, i.e. anti-inflammatory drugs

- Diet
- Infection already present

Benefits of vaccination are:

- Prevent disease by previous preparation of the immune system.
- Reducing the spread of disease through the concept of herd immunity once a significant proportion of the population is vaccinated.
- Protection of vulnerable animals.
- Reduces the severity of disease encountered as symptoms tend to be milder.

Animal insurance companies require that routine vaccinations are kept up to date.

Summary of Immunity

There are many different cell types involved with providing immunity in the body.

There are different types of immunity that can exist.

Passive immunity is acquired, whereas active immunity is developed in response to pathogens.

Innate immunity provides a rapid, non-specific response to pathogens, while adaptive immunity provides a slower but more specific, long-lasting defence. The long-lasting defence is due to T-cells and B-cells developing memory cells allowing a faster, more effective response in case of future exposure to the same pathogen.

Terms Related to Disease

- *Infectious disease* – diseases caused by pathogens that enter the body from outside. They can be transmitted in various ways through direct and indirect contact.
- *Contagious disease* – a type of infectious disease that is easily spread from one animal to another via direct contact with infected individuals, their discharges or excretory products, and contaminated food and water bowls.
  Note: All contagious diseases are infectious but not all infectious disease are contagious.
- *Transmission route* – the way a pathogen is spread from one animal to another.
- *Incubation period* – the time between first exposure to a pathogen and signs of the disease appearing.
- *Zoonotic disease* – a disease that can be transmitted from animals to humans.
- *Anthropoonoses* – a disease that can be transmitted from humans to animals under natural conditions. Also called reverse zoonoses.
- *Notifiable disease* – a disease that must be reported by law to a UK Government agency, to closely monitor and control disease outbreaks.
- *Direct contact* – transfer of infectious microorganisms through direct physical contact.
- *Indirect contact* – transmission of infectious microorganisms through contaminated intermediate objects or surfaces.
- *Fomite* – any inanimate object that can carry and transmit infectious microorganisms. Examples include food and water bowls and accommodation surfaces.
- *Vector* – an organism that transmits a pathogen from one body to another – insects often have this role, e.g. mosquitoes are involved in the transmission of malaria.

- *Opportunistic pathogen* – a microorganism that is normally present in a species without any harm but can cause disease when the animal is under stress or is immune-compromised.
- *Carrier* – an animal that carries a pathogen without showing any signs of the disease. Despite having no signs of disease, the carrier animal can still transmit the pathogen to other individuals, therefore spreading the disease.

Bacterial Diseases

Canine leptospirosis

Canine leptospirosis is caused by a filament-like bacterium, *Leptospira icterohaemorrhagiae*, and is a zoonotic disease. A zoonotic disease is one that can be transmitted from animals to humans, and a number of precautions must be taken when dealing with animals that are infected with a zoonotic disease (see Chapter 14).

- The strains of the *Leptospira* bacteria that cause the disease in dogs are:
  - *Leptospira icterohaemorrhagiae* – (primary host is the rat) attacks mainly the liver.
  - *Leptospira canicola* – (primary host is the dog) attacks mainly the kidney.
- These bacteria are fragile and easily destroyed by sunlight, disinfectants, and temperature extremes.
- Transmission is by direct contact, bite wounds, or ingestion of contaminated food or water.
- Rodents such as rats are frequently carriers, shedding the bacteria in urine and thus contaminating water.
- The incubation period for leptospirosis is between 7 and 21 days.
- Clinical signs of leptospirosis may include:
  - High temperature
  - Shivering and muscle pain
  - Vomiting and diarrhoea
  - Dehydration
  - Shock
  - Jaundice (mucous membranes of mouth and eye appear yellow)
- Treatment may include
  - Antibiotics
  - Fluid therapy
  - Anti-emetics to control nausea and vomiting
  - Pain relief
  - Strict isolation
- Prevention can include:
  - Vaccination and annual boosters
  - High standards of hygiene in the environment
  - Avoiding stagnant water that may be contaminated
  - Reducing exposure to wild rodents
- Animals that recover from *Leptospira* infection shed the bacteria via the urine for some time after recovery. Both veterinary surgeons and doctors can provide advice and information to prevent a human owner/keeper becoming infected.
- Leptospirosis is known as Weil's disease in humans.
- An annual booster after initial vaccination is essential.

Salmonella infection

- Salmonellosis is caused by various strains of *Salmonella* bacteria.
- *Salmonella* infections are zoonotic diseases.
- *Salmonella* bacteria naturally exist in mammals, reptiles, and birds and are also shed in the faeces of these animals. When normal homeostatic balance in the animal is disrupted, then opportunistic bacterial strains can multiply and cause signs of disease.
- Salmonella is a hardy pathogen and can exist in the environment for long periods of time.
- Transmission is through ingestion of the *Salmonella* bacteria via contaminated food or water or transfer from fomites in the environment.
- Younger animals and pregnant animals tend to be more susceptible to the disease. Overcrowding and stress can also increase the risk of salmonellosis.
- Clinical signs of infection may include:
  - Diarrhoea
  - High temperature
  - Abdominal pain
  - Weight loss
  - Lethargy
- Treatment:
  - Antibiotics
  - Fluid therapy
  - Painkillers
  - When caring for animals with *Salmonella* infection, barrier-nursing techniques must be adopted – see Chapter 19 for further information on this technique.
- Prevention:
  - It is essential that good hygiene practices should be followed when working with all animals.
  - Thorough handwashing following any husbandry procedure with animals.

Campylobacter infection

- Campylobacter infection is caused by various strains of *Campylobacter* bacteria, e.g. *Campylobacter jejuni*.
- *Campylobacter* infection is zoonotic.
- Has been known to occur in dogs, cats, lambs, and ferrets amongst other animals. Birds are known to be carrier animals.
- Transmission from animal to animal or animal to human occurs when *Campylobacter* bacteria are ingested via contaminated food or water or fomites in the environment usually via contact with faeces.
- Clinical signs of infection include:
  - Vomiting
  - Haemorrhagic diarrhoea
  - Lethargy
  - Loss of appetite
- When caring for animals with *Campylobacter* infection, barrier-nursing techniques must be adopted – see Chapter 19 for further information on this technique.
- Treatment includes hydration to replace lost fluids and rest.
- It is essential that good hygiene practices should be followed when working with all animals with thorough handwashing occurring following any husbandry procedure.

Escherichia coli infection

- *Escherichia coli* infection is caused by various strains of *E. coli* bacteria, e.g. *E. coli 0157*, which can cause severe infection.
- *Escherichia coli* infection is zoonotic. In humans, *E. coli 0157* can cause major digestive disturbance, kidney failure, and death and so strict handwashing procedures must be followed.
- Has been known to occur in dogs, cats, and farm livestock amongst other animals. Birds and poultry are known to be carrier animals.
- Transmission from animal to animal or animal to human occurs through direct contact with faeces, which is why eating should never take place when undertaking routine animal husbandry procedures.
- Clinical signs of infection may include:
  - Haemorrhagic diarrhoea
  - Dehydration
  - Lethargy
  - Loss of appetite
- When caring for animals with *E.coli* infection, barrier nursing techniques must be adopted – see Chapter 19 for further information on this technique.
  - Treatment includes hydration to replace lost fluids and rest.
- It is essential that good hygiene practices should be followed when working with all animals with thorough handwashing occurring following any husbandry procedure.

Kennel cough

It is important to note that dogs do not just become infected from this disease in kennel environments. Any area where dogs frequently congregate or visit can be a potential source of infection. e.g. kennels, parks, doggy day care, etc.

- Caused primarily by the bacteria *Bordetella bronchiseptica* but can be impacted by the following viruses:
  - *Canine adenovirus type 2 (CAV2)*
  - *Canine distemper virus (CDV)*
  - *Canine parainfluenza virus (CPIV)*
- *Bordetella bronchiseptica*, CAV2, and CPIV are very contagious and commonly present when dogs are housed together, as dogs of any age can be infected. They cause nasal and tracheal inflammation lasting 5–14 days and then normally resolve, with the dog making a good recovery. During this time, the dog sheds the pathogens in its respiratory discharge.
- Clinical signs include:
  - Coughing with subsequent retching
  - Sneezing
  - Tracheitis
  - Rhinitis
  - Depressed but eating
  - Bronchitis
  - Pneumonia
- Risk of infection can be minimised by isolating affected animals and improving ventilation and good disinfection routines with a product that is effective against the relevant bacteria and viruses.

- Vaccination is recommended where dogs visit areas where a high number of other dogs visit, e.g. kennels, parks, doggy day care centres, and dog walkers where groups of dogs are walked together.
- Kennel cough vaccine boosters should be given annually to maintain protection against the disease.

Feline infectious anaemia

- Feline infectious anaemia (FIA) is caused by a group of organisms called *haemoplasmas*. Haemoplasmas live on the surface of the red blood cells and they cause direct loss of red blood cells, thereby causing anaemia to develop in the animal.
- There are three main haemoplasmas that can cause FIA:
  1. *Mycoplasma haemofelis* – causes severe anaemia.
  2. *Candidatus mycoplasma haemominutum* – causes mild infection often with no clinical signs observed.
  3. *Mycoplasma turicensis* – research is currently ongoing into the effect of this organism.
- Transmission can occur through fighting and from flea-infested cats.
- Cats of all ages can be affected. When the disease exists with Feline Leukaemia, white blood cell numbers are affected, and recovery of the animal is poor.
- The microorganisms responsible for FIA infection can be detected in a special blood smear examination in the laboratory or through a technique known as *polymerase chain reaction* (PCR), which serves to detect very small amounts of infection and allows differentiation of the haemoplasmas.
- The incubation period for FIA is up to 50 days, with recovered or carrier animals often shedding the organism for the remainder of their life.
- Antibiotics are currently used to treat FIA; products to safely remove fleas from affected households are required (e.g. Indorex), and other cats in the same household may need to be examined and treated. Further treatment may be required depending on the severity of infection. Your veterinary surgeon will advise on the most appropriate treatment plan.
- Clinical signs of FIA include:
  - Pale mucous membranes – mouth and gums
  - Breathing difficulty
  - Listless and loss of appetite
  - Third eyelid up as a sign of ill health
  - High temperature
  - Weight loss
- Currently, there are no preventative treatments for FIA.

Pasteurellosis

Pasteurellosis is a common disease found in rabbits.

- Pasteurellosis is commonly caused by the bacterium, *Pasteurella multocida*.
- It affects the respiratory tract of the rabbit and can be spread via direct contact and through airborne routes. Entry into the animal is via wounds or the nasal passages.
- Clinical signs include:

- Breathing difficulties
- Nasal discharge
- Inflamed, watery eyes
- Facial swelling/abscesses
- Occasionally, a rabbit may not show any clinical signs of infection but develop septicaemia and die.
- Treatment includes antibiotics over a 30-day period
- Preventative factors
  - Ensuring high levels of cleanliness in the enclosure
  - Good levels of ventilation in the enclosure (but not draughty)
  - Reducing stress for the rabbit
  - Ensuring enclosures aren't overcrowded

Wet tail in hamsters

Wet tail is the most common disease of hamsters, particularly young species and is often fatal. It is also known as *proliferative ileitis*.

- Caused primarily by the bacterium, *Lawsonia intracellularis*, but *Campylobacter* and *Clostridia* species may also be implicated.
- Clinical signs include:
  - Watery, sour-smelling diarrhoea
  - Wet fur around the anal area
  - Reduced appetite
  - Lethargy
  - Hunched posture
  - Sunken eyes due to dehydration from diarrhoea
- Treatment options:
  - Antibiotics may be prescribed
  - Fluids may be given
  - Euthanasia may be advised
- Prevention
  - Ensure the accommodation is regularly cleaned and fresh bedding is routinely provided to prevent buildup of bacteria in the environment.

Psittacosis

Psittacosis is a highly contagious bacterial infection of birds. It is also known as parrot fever or avian chlamydiosis. All birds can suffer from psittacosis.
Psittacosis is zoonotic and can be transmitted to humans.

- Caused by the bacterium *Chlamydia psittaci*.
- Transmission can be airborne or through direct contact.
- Incubation period is usually 1–2 weeks after exposure to the bacteria.
- Clinical signs include:
  - Nasal discharge
  - Sneezing
  - Breathing difficulties

- Eye discharge
- Lethargy
- Loss of appetite
- Weight loss
- Fluffed up feathers
- Diarrhoea that is lime green or yellow in colour
- Treatment includes:
  - Antibiotics for a minimum of 45 days
  - Hydration to replace fluids lost through diarrhoea
  - A warm, stress-free environment
- Prevention includes:
  - Regular cleaning and disinfection of cages and associated equipment such as food and water bowls.
  - New birds should be quarantined before being introduced or kept in the same environment as other birds in the collection.
  - Birds with signs of illness should be isolated to reduce transmission of the disease.
  - Avoid overcrowding of accommodation.

Mouth rot

- An infection commonly found in reptiles, which could be caused by any or all of the following bacteria species – *Pseudomonas, Aeromonas,* and *Klebsiella.*
- Also referred to as infectious stomatitis.
- Transmission can be through direct animal contact and fomites.
- Incubation period can be from 2 to 12 days following exposure to the causative pathogen.
- Clinical signs include:
  - Swelling of mouth and gums
  - Lesions in the mouth
  - Increased saliva production
  - Oral discharge which may include pus
  - Difficulty eating and reluctance to eat
- Treatment is via antibiotics. Oral swabs may need to be taken to identify the specific strain of causative bacteria so that the antibiotics can be more effective. Hydration and assisted feeding may be required. In severe cases, surgical intervention may be needed to remove dead tissue from the mouth.
- Prevention
  - Reduce stress in the environment
  - High standards of hygiene
  - High standards of husbandry ensuring the temperature

Viral Diseases

Canine distemper

Canine distemper is caused by a *paramyxovirus* that attacks several systems in the body, including the central nervous system, the respiratory system, the gastrointestinal system, and the integumentary system.

- The distemper virus is closely related to the measles virus of humans. The virus is inactivated by light, heat, and most disinfectants.
- Distemper is generally seen in puppies of 4–5 months as they are no longer covered by maternal antibodies. Distemper seasonally occurs in autumn and winter, as the virus is unable to survive in cold weather.
- An animal is infected with distemper via:
  - Respiratory tract due to aerosol (airborne) exposure
  - Mouth and eye mucous membranes
- The incubation period of the distemper virus is 3–10 days, during which time the virus replicates and travels via the lymphatic system to the lymph nodes, spleen, thymus, and bone marrow. Once in the lymph nodes, body temperature rises to between 39 °C and 40 °C for 2–4 days.
- About 50% of all puppies infected with distemper can mount an adequate immune response and produce antibodies that clear the infection. If this does not happen, then secondary infection can occur. If puppies survive, then the respiratory or gastrointestinal stage of the disease and the neurological signs develop up to 4 weeks later. Older dogs tend to present with just the neurological signs. Once neurological signs are displayed, the disease is usually fatal.
- Clinical signs of canine distemper may include:
  - Lack of appetite (anorexia)
  - Nasal and eye discharge
  - Coughing
  - Diarrhoea and vomiting
  - Hardening of the footpads
  - Incoordination
  - Paralysis
  - Epileptic-type fits
- Treatment may include:
  - Fluid therapy to replace lost fluids
  - Painkillers
  - Antiemetics
  - Anti-epilepsy drugs where seizures are observed
- After the initial vaccination course as a puppy, booster vaccinations are needed every 3 years.

Canine viral hepatitis

Canine viral hepatitis is caused by the *canine adenovirus type 1 (CAV1)*. It is a more serious disease in younger puppies than older dogs.

- Infection occurs through oral and nasal passages after exposure to infected materials.
- The hepatitis virus is highly resistant to destruction and survives outside the body for up to 11 days in bedding, feeding bowls, urine, and faeces. It can resist freezing, ultraviolet light, and most disinfectants but is destroyed by heat.
- The incubation period for canine hepatitis is 5–9 days. Following exposure, the virus replicates in the tonsils and lymph nodes of the animal. The virus then travels in the lymph and gains access to the bloodstream, where it replicates further in the liver and kidneys.
- The virus is shed from the body in urine and faeces, where it can be encountered by other dogs in the environment.
- Animals that recover from canine viral hepatitis can continue to shed the virus for several months afterwards, i.e. they are carriers of the disease.

- Clinical signs of canine hepatitis include the following signs:
  - In puppies:
    - High temperature
    - Death occurs within hours
  - In older dogs:
    - Survive the viraemic stage
    - Bloodstained vomit and diarrhoea
    - Acute abdominal pain
    - In some dogs, 'blue eye', a clouding of the cornea of the eye, occurs up to 3 weeks after acute infection.
- Initial vaccinations are required as puppies, followed by booster doses every 3 years to maintain immunity against canine viral hepatitis.

Canine parvovirus

Canine parvovirus is closely related to the *Feline panleukopenia* virus.

- The virus is very resistant to inactivation by most disinfectants except bleach and formalin-based chemicals and can survive for months in the environment.
- The route of infection is by faecal or oral contact. Damage to the bone marrow results in a lack of white cells, and the infection spreads from lymph cells of the intestinal tissues.
- Following an incubation period of 5–10 days, the virus replicates in lymphatic tissues and the intestinal epithelium lining. It is found in vast numbers in the faeces and vomit of infected animals and causes mild to severe *haemorrhagic enteritis* along with *myocarditis*.
- Clinical signs of canine parvovirus may include:
  - Being dull and depressed
  - Anorexia
  - High temperature (up to 41 °C)
  - Vomiting bloodstained gastric juice
  - Bloodstained diarrhoea 24 hours later
  - Becomes rapidly dehydrated
- Treatment may include:
  - Fluid therapy to replace lost fluids
  - Painkillers
  - Antiemetics
  - Anti-epilepsy drugs where seizures are observed
  - Antibiotics for any secondary bacterial infections
- Barrier nursing is essential.
- Initial vaccination as a puppy should be followed by boosters every 3 years for ensured protection, although this may be more often if there are high numbers of parvovirus cases in a particular geographical area.

Chlamydiosis (feline pneumonitis)

- Chlamydial infection in cats is caused by an organism that is similar to a virus but resembles a bacterium in its appearance.
- *Chlamydophila felis* affects the conjunctiva of the eye in cats, causing severe conjunctivitis, which may affect one or both eyes.

- *Chlamydophila* organisms are very fragile and cannot survive for any length of time in the environment.
- Transmission is via direct contact between animals.
- The incubation period is 3–10 days.
- Clinical signs of feline chlamydiosis infection include:
  - Initial watery discharge in one eye, spreading to both
  - Inflamed conjunctiva
  - Signs of eye discomfort
  - Sneezing
  - Nasal discharge
  - Fever
  - In kittens, diarrhoea can also occur
  - During pregnancy, chlamydia may cause abortion or stillbirth
- Chlamydiosis may last for 2–3 weeks or longer, especially as a part of the feline viral respiratory disease complex.
- Recovered animals may shed the responsible organism for several weeks, so any treatment usually continues for 3 weeks following recovery.
- The organism is killed by most disinfectants during routine cleaning.
- Antibiotics are usually the primary treatment along with topical eye drops.
- Vaccination is available against chlamydiosis with an annual booster required to maintain protection. It should be noted that this vaccine does not prevent infection but does reduce the severity of the disease.

Feline immunodeficiency virus

- Feline immunodeficiency virus (FIV) is a worldwide disease of cats with approximately 6% of healthy cats being infected.
- FIV is caused by a virus of the *lentivirus* group.
- There is often a long incubation period with anything from 4 weeks to several years following exposure to the virus; it is therefore unusual to detect infection in cats under 2 years of age. Once infected, the infection is life-long.
- FIV is carried in the saliva of the infected animal and is commonly transmitted by biting during fights. Therefore, cats that have access to outdoor life are more at risk than those housed completely indoors. Male cats are more commonly infected due to territorial fighting. The virus can also be passed on in cats that live in close social contact through grooming, sharing of food bowls, etc.
- Clinical signs of the disease are very similar to those of Feline leukaemia virus and include:
  - Conjunctivitis and nasal discharge
  - Enlarged superficial lymph nodes (lymphadenopathy)
  - Mouth and gum inflammation
  - Diarrhoea
  - Skin problems
  - High temperature
  - Neurological signs that include difficulty in walking and change in temperament
- FIV attacks the white blood cells, which in turn suppresses the immune system of the cat, leaving the cat more susceptible to other diseases.

- An animal may appear to recover from the disease as the clinical signs reduce, but due to gradual suppression of its immune responses, it will frequently suffer from recurring or ongoing infections of various kinds, often failing to respond to veterinary treatment. The cat will suffer weight loss, becoming inactive and listless.
- There is currently no treatment to eliminate an established FIV infection. Any treatment given is to reduce suffering and ease other signs displayed to promote a good quality of life.
- There is currently no vaccine available in the United Kingdom, so owners are advised to castrate male cats and limit exposure to other neighbourhood cats in order to avoid contact with an infected animal. Cats known to be infected with FIV should be kept indoors.

Feline infectious enteritis

- Feline infectious enteritis (FIE) is a highly infectious and contagious disease of cats, also called:
  - Feline parvovirus
  - Feline distemper
  - Feline panleukopenia
- The disease is caused by a parvovirus, similar to canine parvovirus. The disease can affect cats of any age but is mainly responsible for deaths in young kittens.
- The virus is hardy and can survive years in the environment and is resistant to most disinfectants.
- The incubation period is 5–9 days following direct contact with an infected animal, ingestion of the virus, or through contact with objects used by an infected animal (fomites).
- The virus targets rapidly dividing cells and tissues of the small intestines, lymph, and bone marrow. It is shed in saliva, vomit, faeces, and urine for up to 6 weeks following infection.
- Cats can also be infected by dogs that may be shedding parvovirus.
- Kittens can be infected across the placenta in pregnant queens during pregnancy. Kitten foetuses are affected by the virus targeting the brain tissue (cerebellum), causing death or abnormal nervous system development. Kittens show balance difficulties and incoordination at about 2–3 weeks of age if affected.
- Clinical signs of FIE include:
  - Diarrhoea, often bloodstained
  - Dull and listless behaviour
  - Abdominal pain
  - Fever and dehydration
  - Low neutrophil count in blood tests
- Recovery is possible, depending upon the extent of the infection and how soon diagnosis occurs. If the cat survives the first week of clinical disease, careful nursing care can lead to recovery, but the intestine may suffer permanent damage, seen as poor absorption of nutrients and constant diarrhoeal episodes.
- Any affected animal should be isolated.
- Vaccination provides effective immunity with a booster every year. The term 'prevention is better than cure' is highly applicable in the case of FIE.

Feline infectious peritonitis

- Feline infectious peritonitis (FIP) is a highly contagious disease caused by a feline coronavirus.

- Coronaviruses are found in a cat's surrounding environment, and the rate of infection is higher where many cats are found, such as in rescue centres, breeding catteries, or multi-cat households.
- Infected cats shed the virus in their faeces, and other cats can become infected via ingestion of the virus through eating or grooming, for example. Not all infected cats will develop FIP as the disease is only caused when the coronavirus mutates within the cat.
- Clinical signs include:
  - Lack of appetite and gradual weight loss
  - Lethargy
  - Swollen abdomen due to an accumulation of yellow fluid
  - Possible breathing difficulties dependent on amount of fluid in the abdomen
  - Diarrhoea and vomiting
- Progressive signs include:
  - Neurological signs including inability to stand, paralysis and convulsions
  - Inflammation within the structure of the eye, affecting sight
- If clinical FIP becomes established, then the disease is fatal.
- Any treatment is provided to relieve suffering and ease the signs of disease displayed. Euthanasia should be considered if the disease is suspected.
- There are two forms of FIP. One form is characterised by the formation of fluid in the abdomen, and the disease is said to be 'wet' in form (effusive). If lesions form on the organs instead of fluid building up, then the disease is said to be 'dry' in form (non-effusive).
- The form of FIP can only usually be confirmed on post-mortem examination as there is no definitive diagnostic test.
- To assist in preventing FIP, strict hygiene and disinfection are essential, particularly in multi-cat environments. Litterboxes should be kept away from food and water bowls, and in multi-cat households, there should be one litter box available for every two cats as a minimum.
- There is currently no vaccine available in the United Kingdom to prevent FIP.

Feline leukaemia virus

- Feline leukaemia virus (FeLV) is a common contagious illness in cats that affects approximately 1% of healthy pet cats in the United Kingdom.
- FeLV is caused by a *retrovirus*.
- Infection rates are higher in cats living in a multi-cat environment and where cats are in close contact as this supports transmission of the virus. Prevalence is higher in unhealthy cats.
- The disease is almost always fatal once signs of disease appear.
- FeLV is a fragile virus and is easily destroyed by disinfectants. It cannot exist for a long time in the environment without a host animal.
- Transmission is via saliva either through fighting/biting, grooming, or use of feeding bowls, water bowls, bedding, etc.
- A pregnant queen may pass the infection on to her unborn young, or the virus can also be passed to kittens through milk in a lactating queen. Infected cats may become persistently infected, but this does not happen in all cases of infection.
- Once the virus enters the body, usually via the mouth or nose, replication occurs before the virus enters the bloodstream. Once in the bloodstream, the virus targets the bone marrow specifically. Cats that can mount a suitable immune response to the virus will do so within 3 months, but if the bone marrow becomes significantly infected, then it is likely that the cat

will subsequently suffer from a persistent infection due to suppression of the immune system. Young kittens are most susceptible to the virus.

- Most cats die within 2–3 years of exposure or because of FeLV-related disease conditions, which include:
  - Anaemia (lack of red blood cells)
  - Lymphosarcoma (tumours of the lymph system)
- Evidence of the virus' presence can be obtained through testing blood samples using several diagnostic tests.
- Clinical signs of FeLV infection include:
  - High temperature (fever)
  - Lethargy
  - Poor appetite and weight loss
  - Anaemia
  - Enlargement of the spleen
- Control of FeLV disease is via:
  - Testing, particularly in multi-cat households
  - Animals testing positive being isolated from others
  - Disinfection and strict hygiene in cat areas
  - Retesting 12 weeks after positive test to ensure true result
  - Testing all new cats that join a household
- After two positive tests, the safe choice is to permanently isolate or euthanise the cat.
- Cats can be vaccinated from 9 weeks of age with a second dose being administered 2–4 weeks later followed by annual boosters to maintain immunity. Vaccination does not prevent FeLV infection, but it aims to prevent cats from becoming persistent shedders of the disease.

Feline viral respiratory diseases

Many microorganisms can be responsible for causing respiratory disease in cats. Feline viral respiratory disease can also be known as:

- Cat flu
- Feline upper respiratory disease (FURD)
- Feline viral rhinotracheitis (FVR)
- Feline viral respiratory complex

The two main viruses involved are:

1. *Feline* calicivirus
2. *Feline* herpesvirus

Cats are particularly susceptible to infections (both bacterial and viral) of the nose and throat. Due to their location, these infections are called upper respiratory infections or cat flu. While it is essential to vaccinate, the vaccine does not always protect against some strains of this disease, especially *feline calicivirus*. It depends which strains are in general circulation.

Feline calicivirus
- *Feline calicivirus* is easily destroyed outside the host by disinfectants.
- Transmission of the virus is by aerosol or direct contact. As a result of this, any grouping of cats may lead to infection, i.e. shows, boarding catteries, rescue centres, and veterinary surgeries.

- Many cats that have survived the disease become carriers, shedding the virus for several years. It is possible to have suspected carrier animals tested by a veterinary surgeon for the presence of the calicivirus.
- The incubation period is up to 10 days after exposure to high-risk situations (groups of cats) or stress caused by a change to the environment which may lower the cat's resistance to disease.
- Clinical signs of calicivirus infection include:
  - Ulcers on the tongue – may cause secondary bacterial infection
  - Inflammation of the gums
  - Unwilling to eat but producing excess saliva
  - High temperature
  - Depressed and listless
  - Loss of voice

Feline herpes virus

- *Feline herpes virus* attacks and replicates in the tissues of the respiratory tract and conjunctiva of the eye, causing viral rhinotracheitis.
- The tissues from the nose (*rhino*) to the trachea (*tracheitis*) are affected and inflamed, causing breathing difficulties, sneezing, and coughing.
- Viral rhinotracheitis is the most serious form of upper respiratory disease, often leaving recovered animals with damage to the nasal passages. This causes the affected cat to periodically sneeze, snuffle, and have a runny nose, the discharge occasionally being thick with pus.
- Recovered animals can act as carriers, shedding the virus particularly when stressed.
- Feline herpes virus can survive outside the host for up to 8 days.
- The incubation period is from 2 to 10 days following exposure to the virus.
- Clinical signs of *feline herpes virus* include:
  - High temperature
  - Discharge from the eyes and nose, later becoming thickened due to bacterial infection
  - Depressed and listless
  - Loss of appetite
  - Sneezing
  - Conjunctivitis
  - Mouth ulcers
  - Pneumonia
  - Abortion in pregnant queens
- Vaccination against this virus is available, and boosters should be given on an annual basis to maintain protection. In high-risk situations, six monthly administration is advisable.

Rabies

- Rabies is caused by a *Lyssavirus species* from the *rhabdovirus* family and is both a zoonotic and notifiable disease.
- It is a fragile virus, surviving for only a short time in the environment, and it is destroyed by most disinfectants, heat, and light.
- Transmission is via the saliva of infected animals.
- Following infection, the virus replicates in the muscle cells at the site of infection, from where it travels to the spinal cord and the brain, via the peripheral nerves. Once situated in the

central nervous tissues, neurological signs of disease are observed. The virus then travels to the salivary glands, where it is shed to infect other mammals, both human and animal.

- The incubation period following infection is from 10 days to 4 months, depending on how near to the central nervous system the virus is initially introduced into the body.
- There are three stages to the disease signs. However, not all stages will occur in all affected animals:
  1. *Preclinical stage* – generally lasts 2–3 days with increased body temperature, slow eye reflexes, and signs of irritation at the site of the original injury. In some cases, the preclinical stage can last for several months during which the virus is shed in the saliva.
  2. *Excitable stage* – lasting up to 1 week with the animal becoming irritable, aggressive, and disorientated, having difficulty standing and epileptic-type fits.
  3. *Dumb stage* – lasting 2–4 days during which the animal becomes progressively paralysed in the throat and skeletal muscles, leading to salivation, respiratory difficulties, coma, and death.
- Rabies diagnosis is confirmed post-mortem, following examination of the central nervous tissues for signs of the virus.
- Vaccination is available for dogs that live in countries where rabies is endemic or for travelling to a country with rabies in the wild or domestic animal population. The vaccine can only be given from 3 months of age, and boosters should be administered annually to maintain protection.
- If a dog, cat, or human is bitten by an animal suspected of being infected with rabies:
  - Clean the wound immediately using soap or antiseptic solutions
  - Seek medical attention straight away

Myxomatosis

- Myxomatosis is caused by the *Myxoma virus* and is often fatal for rabbits.
- The virus is carried and spread by insect vectors such as mosquitoes, fleas, flies, fur, and harvest mites.
- Infection can also occur via direct contact with affected rabbits, as well as via inhalation and through fomites.
- The incubation period is 8–21 days.
- Clinical signs include:
  - Swelling around the eyes
  - White eye discharge
  - Genital swelling
  - High temperature
  - Lethargy
  - Loss of appetite
  - Skin lesions
- Once clinical signs are seen, death usual occurs within 2 weeks.
- Prevention is via:
  - Minimisation of insects in the environment where possible (e.g. avoid stagnant water building up that attracts mosquitoes).
  - Vaccination can be given from 5 weeks of age with an annual booster to maintain immunity.
  - Flea treatments suitable for rabbits can also be given.
  - Prevent wild rabbits from coming into the environment.

Rabbit viral haemorrhagic disease

Can be referred to as VHD (viral haemorrhagic disease) or RHD (rabbit haemorrhagic disease).

- A usually fatal, highly contagious disease of rabbits caused by a *Calicivirus*.
- Two strains exist – VHD1/RHD1 & VHD2/RHD2. Strain 2 is less virulent (causes less rabbits to die).
  - The virus is hardy and difficult to get rid of once in an environment. If a rabbit has been diagnosed with VHD/RHD, then everything must be destroyed after its death, e.g. accommodation, food bowls.
- The incubation period is shorter for VHD1/RHD1 (16 hours to 3 days) than for VHD2/RHD2 (3–9 days).
- Transmission can be airborne, through direct rabbit contact, and via insects or fomites, such as bedding and clothing of handlers.
- Clinical signs include:
  - Difficulties breathing
  - Fever
  - Reduced appetite
  - Lethargy
  - Bleeding from the nose, mouth, or anus prior to death
  - Usually fatal within 2 days
- Prevention is via:
  - Minimisation of insects in the environment where possible (e.g. avoid stagnant water building up that attracts mosquitoes).
  - Vaccination can be given, but two injections are needed to ensure both strains are received. The first vaccine is a combination of VHD1/RHD1 and myxomatosis. The second vaccine is a combination of VHD1/RHD1 and VHD2/RHD2. Vaccines can be given from 5 weeks of age with an annual booster to maintain immunity.
  - Flea treatments suitable for rabbits can also be given
  - Preventing wild rabbits from coming into the environment

Ferret distemper

Ferret distemper is a highly contagious, often fatal disease of ferrets. Where ferrets visit areas that dogs frequent, then they should be vaccinated with the canine distemper vaccine as there is no ferret distemper vaccine licensed for use in the United Kingdom.

- Clinical signs may include
  - Eye discharge
  - Nasal discharge
  - Loss of appetite
  - Neurological signs
- Treatment may include:
  - Fluid therapy to replace lost fluids
  - Painkillers
  - Antiemetics
  - Euthanasia

Ferret influenza

Both zoonotic and anthropozoonotic in that the influenza virus can be passed from animal to human and from human to animal.

- Clinical signs may include:
  - Sneezing
  - Coughing
  - High temperature
  - Lethargy
  - Reduced appetite
  - Nasal discharge
  - Mild conjunctivitis
- Treatment includes hydration and rest. The virus is usually cleared from the system without further intervention being required.
- Prevention measures include human individuals with influenza should not handle or carry out husbandry for ferrets at that time. High standards of hygiene should be implemented.

Psittacine beak and feather disease

Psittacine beak and feather disease (PBFD) is a highly infectious viral infection caused by a group of viruses called *Circoviruses*.

- The virus is hardy and can survive for a long time in the environment.
- Transmission is via the oral and nasal cavities following contact with faeces, sharing of food from the crop (with nestlings), and exposure to feather dust in accommodation and on the clothes or hair of handlers.
- Incubation period can be up to 2 years following exposure to the causative pathogen.
- Young birds are more likely to be affected.
- Clinical signs usually include:
  - Dead or abnormally formed feathers (feather dystrophy)
  - Beak deformities, including overgrowth, excess flakiness, and breakage on handling.
- There is no treatment for PBFD.
- Death will usually occur up to 2 years following appearance of the disease.
- Infected birds should be separated from others.

Adenovirus infections

Adenovirus infections are commonly found in reptile species but can be found in many other species.

- There are many different strains of *adenovirus* that can cause infection.
- Transmission route is inhalation of the virus after contact with faeces of an infected animal.
- Incubation period.
- Clinical signs may include:
  - Weakness
  - Lethargy
  - Reduced appetite

- Weight loss
- Diarrhoea
- Sudden death
- Treatment
  - Fluid therapy
  - Assisted feeding
  - Isolation from other animals
- Prevention involves maintaining high standards of hygiene and regular, thorough cleaning of animal accommodation.

Fungal Diseases

There are several fungal infections that animals can be susceptible to and some of the common ones are:

Ringworm (dermatophytosis)

Ringworm is a zoonotic, contagious fungal infection of the skin that can affect several animal species.

- Fungal species responsible for causing ringworm may include:
  - *Microsporum canis* (affects cats, dogs, and to a lesser extent large animals)
  - *Trichophyton mentagrophytes* and *Trichophyton verrucosum*
  - *Microsporum gypseum* (found in the soil)
- Transmission is usually via direct contact between animals, but indirect contact, such as through contact with equipment used on infected animals, can also spread infection.
- Clinical signs may include:
  - Crusty, hairless patches of skin
  - Raised lesions (a circular shape gives the disease its name; however, lesions are not always circular in shape)
  - Itchy skin
- Ringworm is self-resolving, but treatment may be given to shorten the length of time that an animal has the signs of the disease.
- Anti-fungal drugs may be prescribed along with a topical shampoo.
- Avoiding overcrowding of enclosures can help reduce spread of the disease.
- Handlers should wear disposable gloves when dealing with infected animals.

Candidiasis

Candida infection is a yeast like fungus that can affect different species of animals but is particularly seen in birds.

- The most common species of yeast causing infection is *Candida albicans*.
- *Candida albicans* is normally present in the body of animals and can grow and cause infection when the animal is stressed or immune-compromised. It is an opportunistic pathogen and can affect the digestive system, skin, and urinary tract.
- Transmission is via ingestion of the organism.
- Diagnosis is via culture of the organism.

- Clinical signs may include:
  - Regurgitation of food
  - Reduced appetite
  - White plaques in the mouth
  - Weight loss
- Treatment is with antifungal medication.

Aspergillosis

Aspergillosis is a fungal disease of birds that affects the respiratory system in immunocompromised birds. *Aspergillus* spp. are opportunistic pathogens.

- The most common *Aspergillus* spp. that is found infecting birds is *Aspergillus fumigatus*.
- Some species of birds appear to have a predisposition for developing the infection, e.g. African grey parrots, cockatiels, and Amazon parrots.
- Transmission is through inhalation of spores through the nasal passages or ingestion into the mouth.
- Clinical signs may include:
  - Lethargy
  - Reduced appetite
  - Weight loss
  - Difficulty breathing
  - Irregular breathing
  - Tracheitis
  - Nasal discharge
- Diagnosis is based on blood tests and diagnostic imaging.
- Treatment is with antifungal drugs. More severe cases may need oxygen therapy or surgery.
- Prevention includes ensuring that bedding is regularly changed to prevent it getting mouldy, having high standards of hygiene, and ensuring adequate ventilation as warm, humid environments can increase the presence of the disease.
- Where aspergillosis is present, handlers should wear face masks.

Protozoal Diseases

Protozoa are single-celled organisms, some of which can cause disease.

Coccidiosis

Coccidia species are opportunistic pathogens that can affect cats, dogs, rabbits, and birds as well as other livestock species.

- *Eimeria* species can affect rabbits and birds. *Isospora* species can affect dogs and cats.
- Once coccidia have entered the body, the pathogen matures in the intestine and eggs called oocysts are shed in the faeces. Spread of infection is due to the coccidial oocysts being ingested by another animal.
- Clinical signs may include:
  - Diarrhoea

- Dehydration
- Weight loss
- Lethargy
- Abdominal pain
- Reduced appetite
- Coccidial infection is usually self-resolving, but some anti-coccidial medication may be given.
- Prevention includes regular cleaning and disinfection of the accommodation and removal of faeces. Overcrowding should also be avoided. Vaccines exist for some species.

Cryptosporidiosis

- *Cryptosporidium parvum* is the species that most frequently infects animals. It is zoonotic.
- Transmission is due to ingestion of oocysts that have been shed in faeces by infected animals.
- Clinical signs of infection may include:
  - Watery diarrhoea, yellow in colour
  - Dehydration
  - Abdominal pain
  - Lethargy
- Treatment includes rehydration therapy to balance electrolytes. Disposable gloves should be worn when dealing with infected animals.
- Prevention includes regular cleaning and disinfection of the accommodation and removal of faeces. Overcrowding should also be avoided.

Giardiasis

Giardia infection affects the gastrointestinal tract and can be caused by several *Giardia species*. Domestic mammals and birds can be affected as well as wild mammals.

- *Giardia muris* affects rodents, *Giardia duodenalis* affects mammals, and *Giardia psittaci* can affect birds to give examples.
- Transmission is through ingestion of *Giardia* cysts shed in the faeces of infected animals.
- Clinical signs of infection may include:
  - Watery diarrhoea (may be intermittent)
  - Weight loss
  - Dehydration
- Infection is confirmed following the results of faecal diagnostic tests.
- Treatment is for the clinical signs observed, combined with strict hygiene procedures. Reinfection can be common and so an extended period of treatment may be required.
- Prevention includes regular cleaning and disinfection of the accommodation and removal of faeces. Overcrowding should also be avoided.

Prion Disease

Prion diseases are rare but can affect both humans and animals. Prions are proteins that have misfolded and become abnormal. Once a prion protein has been formed, it causes other proteins to misfold. When the number of prions has increased, they cause disease. They are smaller than viruses and do not contain any genetic material.

- Prion diseases affect the nervous tissue particularly in the brain and they cause tiny bubbles in the brain cells, which makes it look like a sponge under the microscope. Affected cells will die.
- Transmissible Spongiform Encephalopathy (TSE) diseases are caused by prions.
- Transmission of disease occurs when an animal:
  - Eats an infected animal
  - Encounters an infected animal's body fluids or waste
  - Encounters soil contaminated by infected animals
  - Is housed with infected animals
- Farm livestock are particularly affected by TSE diseases, but they also exist in cats and mink.
- There is no treatment for TSE diseases and they are inevitably fatal.

Vaccinations for dogs

Diseases that dogs should be vaccinated against in the United Kingdom include:

- Canine distemper
- Canine viral hepatitis
- Canine leptospirosis
- Canine parvovirus

Diseases that dogs may be vaccinated against include:

- Kennel cough
- Rabies
- Canine herpes virus in breeding bitches

Vaccinations for cats

Diseases that cats should be vaccinated against in the United Kingdom include:

- FIE (feline panleukopenia)
- Feline viral respiratory diseases (cat flu):
  - Feline herpesvirus
  - Feline calicivirus
- Chlamydiosis or feline pneumonitis
- Feline infectious anaemia (FIA)
- Feline infectious peritonitis (FIP)

Diseases that cats may be vaccinated against include:

- Feline leukaemia virus (FeLV)
- Feline immunodeficiency virus (FIV)
- Rabies

Vaccinations for rabbits

It is advised that rabbits in the United Kingdom are vaccinated against

- Myxomatosis
- Viral haemorrhagic disease

Annual boosters are required following the primary course of vaccination.

Vaccinations for ferrets

It is advised that ferrets in the United Kingdom are vaccinated against rabies if they are travelling abroad.

If ferrets are walked or taken to areas where dogs visit regularly, then it is advised that they receive a canine distemper vaccination. There is no ferret distemper vaccine licensed for use in the United Kingdom.

Summary of Diseases

There are many diseases that animals can be infected with, and it is the responsibility of the owner/carer/keeper to ensure that strict hygiene routines are followed to prevent the build-up of pathogens in the environment and limit a potential disease outbreak.

Owners/carers/keepers should be aware of the normal indicators of health for the species and be able to detect when something is unusual for that animal so that closer monitoring can take place. This may include veterinary consultation for the diagnosis of disease.

14

Zoonotic Diseases

Learning goals

In this chapter, the learning goals are:

- To define the term zoonoses
- To define the term anthropoonoses
- To define the term notifiable disease
- To be able to name examples of zoonotic, anthroponotic, and notifiable diseases from a range of species
- To identify methods for preventing zoonotic and anthroponotic diseases

Definition of Terms

Zoonoses

- These are diseases that are transmissible from animals to humans.
- Most domestic animals can transmit zoonotic disease.
- Examples are listed in Tables 14.1–14.3:

Prevention of zoonotic diseases

To minimise the risk to people from diseases that can be transmitted from animals, the following simple but effective hygiene precautions must be taken:

- Wash hands after handling any animal
- Control fleas and worms
- Vaccinate animals
- Do not allow pets to lick children's faces
- Do not feed pets from household plates or dishes
- Use separate utensils for food preparation of human and animal food
- Daily collection and safe disposal of faeces, wearing disposable gloves
- Always wear gloves when handling body discharges
- Investigate any signs of unexpected illness after contact with animals

Animal Biology and Care, Fourth Edition. Emily Jewell.
© 2026 John Wiley & Sons Ltd. Published 2026 by John Wiley & Sons Ltd.
Companion Website: https://www.wiley.com/go/animal/biology4e/jewell

Table 14.1 Examples of zoonotic diseases transmitted from dogs.

Dog infection	Effects in humans
Leptospirosis	Weil's disease
Toxocariasis	Visceral larva migrans
Echinococcosis	Hydatid disease
Sarcoptic mange	Skin rash and bites causing scabies
Cheyletiella mites	Skin rash and bites
Ringworm	Skin lesions and hair loss
Salmonellosis	Diarrhoea/vomiting
Campylobacter	Diarrhoea/vomiting
Rabies	Rabies (hydrophobia)

Table 14.2 Examples of zoonotic disease transmitted from cats.

Cat infection	Effects in humans
Pasteurellosis	Bites or scratches become infected
Bartonella henselae infection	Cat Scratch Fever – high temperature, flu-like signs, and rash
Ringworm	Raised, circular, inflamed skin lesion
Toxoplasmosis	Abortion of foetus
Rabies	Fever, itching at original bite area, behaviour changes, paralysis, and death

Table 14.3 Examples of zoonotic diseases transmitted from other species.

Human disease	Causal microorganism	Originating species
Avian influenza	Virus	Birds
Brucellosis	Bacteria	Cattle
Campylobacter	Bacteria	Hamsters
Psittacosis	Bacteria	Birds
Salmonellosis	Bacteria	Mice, rats, and guinea pigs
Tetanus	Bacteria	Horses and other herbivores

Anthropoonoses

- These are diseases that are transmissible from humans to animals.
- May also be called *reverse zoonosis* or *zooanthroponosis*.
- Examples include:
  - SARS-Cov-2 virus
  - Influenza viruses
  - *Giardia* infection

- Paramyxovirus, e.g. mumps
- Ringworm
- MRSA (Methicillin-resistant *Staphylococcus aureus*)

Prevention of anthroponotic diseases

To minimise the risk to animals from diseases that can be transmitted from humans, the following simple but effective hygiene precautions must be taken:

- Wash hands before handling any animal
- Ensure face masks are worn when suffering with cold/flu viruses
- Ensure disposable gloves are worn when suffering with skin conditions
- In some cases, vaccination of humans and animals may be needed

Notifiable Diseases in Animals

Under Section 88 of the Animal Health Act 1981, a notifiable disease in animals is one that must be reported to the Animal and Plant Health Agency (APHA) in the United Kingdom, whether suspected or diagnosed. Notifiable diseases may also be zoonotic. The UK Government also work with the European Union to monitor diseases under the EU's Animal Health Regulation of 2021.

Notifiable disease of animals in the United Kingdom can be classed as being endemic or exotic.

- Endemic – already present in the United Kingdom
- Exotic – not usually present in the United Kingdom

Notifiable diseases are usually categorised as such because they can have a significant impact on animal health, public health, and the country's economy. They must be reported by law and officials from the APHA, and the Department for Environment, Food and Rural Affairs (DEFRA) will step in to prevent the spread and control any outbreaks of disease. Alerts will be issued to veterinary professionals, livestock keepers, and the public to be aware of the spread of the disease, e.g. Avian Influenza.

The APHA are the key body responsible for coordinating the information reported with regard to watching out for, discovering, and controlling notifiable diseases in the United Kingdom.

Control measures that may be put in place to control an outbreak of a notifiable disease and stop it spreading further include:

- Movement restrictions between areas and premises
- Culling of affected animals
- Strict disinfection procedures
- Strict biosecurity measures
- Vaccination in some cases

Examples of notifiable animal disease in the United Kingdom

- Avian Influenza (Bird Flu) (all birds)
- African Horse Sickness (horses)
- Blue Tongue (Ruminants & camelids)
- Foot & Mouth Disease (Ruminants)

- Peste des petits ruminants (sheep and goats)
- Paramyxovirus (pigeons)
- Rabies (all mammals including humans)

Please note that this is not an exhaustive list. It is the responsibility of animal owners to keep themselves up to date with current legislation and notifications from APHA, DEFRA, and the UK Government.

Summary of Zoonotic Diseases

There are many different diseases that can affect animals, some of which may be spread to humans and some that may be transmitted to them from humans. Some of these diseases can have a significant impact on the national economy, animal, or public health, and so legislation requires that they are reported. It is the responsibility of animal owners to keep themselves up to date with current legislation.

15

Parasitology

Learning goals

In this chapter, the learning goals are:

- To define the term parasite
- To name and describe the effects of key external parasites for a range of species of animals
- To name and describe the effects of key internal parasites for a range of species of animals

What Is Parasitology?

Parasitology is the study of parasitic organisms.

A *parasite* is an organism that lives in or on another living body known as the *host*. The parasite benefits by taking nourishment from the host. Parasites can either be host-specific or they can have a range of hosts. Parasites may live on the inside or outside of the animal's body. An *endoparasite* lives on the inside of the body, and an *ectoparasite* lives on the external surface of the host's body.

The parasite feeds on the host but has no intention to kill it, as this would destroy its food source. Unfortunately, some hosts may die because of the parasite's feeding activities or from toxins released by it.

To prevent disease or death of the host species, prophylactic control of parasites is important (see Chapter 8). Routine control in equine and large animals is necessary to keep parasite numbers down. Control in small animals (dogs, cats, rabbits, etc.) aims to completely remove all parasites, whether internal or external. There are many easy-to-use and effective products for removing external parasites such as fleas and lice, with a residue effect which will last for varying periods of time. The products supplied for eliminating internal parasites are collectively called *anthelmintics* or *wormers*. Some worms are zoonotic, and so, their elimination from the animal is extremely important.

Parasitology Terms

- *Transport host* – transports the parasite to the next host. No development takes place in the parasite.
- *Paratenic host* – same as transport host but the parasite must be eaten, to be excreted and passed on to the next host.

Animal Biology and Care, Fourth Edition. Emily Jewell.
© 2026 John Wiley & Sons Ltd. Published 2026 by John Wiley & Sons Ltd.
Companion Website: https://www.wiley.com/go/animal/biology4e/jewell

- *Intermediate host* – some parasites must spend time on/in this host to develop to their next life cycle stage.
- *Final host* – host in which the parasite completes its development.
- *Permanent parasite* – develops through all life stages and lives on one host.
- *Temporary parasite* – moves from host to host.
- *Endoparasite* – lives inside the host's body.
- *Ectoparasite* – lives on the surface of the host's body.

External Parasites

Fleas

Flea infestations are one of the most common problems occurring in dogs and cats. It can be almost guaranteed that every cat and dog will have a flea infestation during their life. Fleas can cause severe problems on their own, or they can act as vectors for other organisms. It is adult fleas that cause the clinical problems seen in animals and these can include:

- Severe skin irritation
- Eczema
- Anaemia
- Flea allergy dermatitis

Fleas may act as vectors for:

- *Yersinia pestis* – causes plague
- *Rickettsia*
- *Tapeworms*

Common flea species
- Human flea – *Pulex irritans* (may also affect dogs, cats, and horses)
- Dog flea – *Ctenocephalides canis* (may also affect humans and cats)
- Cat flea – *Ctenocephalides felis* (may also affect humans and dogs)
- Chicken flea – *Echidnophaga gallinacea* (may also affect dogs, cats, humans, cattle, and horses)

Ctenocephalides species (Figure 15.1)

- Adult fleas can live for 2 years without feeding
- Flea eggs hatch in 1–2 days
- Flea larvae feed for 4–8 days (in carpets or bedding)
- Larvae spin cocoons and adults emerge in 5 days or less
- Adult flea cycle may take only 3 weeks, but if the environment is unsuitable, the larval stage can last for months before becoming an adult.

Diagnosing fleas
Fleas are often hard to detect due to their size. In heavy infestations, fleas may be seen in the coat, especially in light-coloured animals, or they may collect around the base of the tail, in the ears, or in the groin/armpits.

Figure 15.1   Flea – *Ctenocephalides* spp.

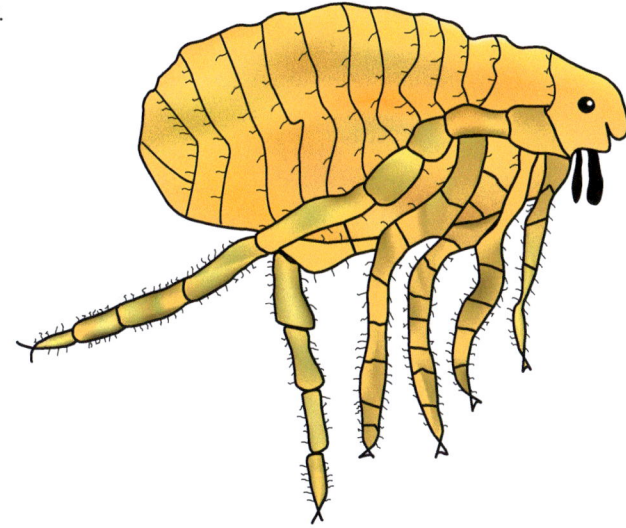

The best and easiest way to check for fleas is to look for 'flea dirt'. Flea dirt is dried pieces of blood excreted by the flea.

- Comb the animal's coat over a piece of damp white paper or cotton wool. If the specks that fall onto the coat dissolve and turn red/brown, then the animal is likely to have fleas.
- If the animal does have fleas, then as well as treating the animal, it is essential that the environment in which it lives is also treated. A few sprays to do this are available, and advice on their use can be obtained from the veterinary practice or the retailer.

Prevention and treatment of fleas

There are a wide range of products available for the control of fleas. It is important, however, to treat the environment as well as the animal. Thoroughly disinfect the environment and replace any bedding with fresh, clean bedding. The animal may need to be washed in an insecticidal shampoo. Products bought under veterinary prescription are usually more effective than those bought from the pet shop:

- Sprays
- Powders
- Spot-on preparations
- Shampoo
- Pills
- Collars
- Liquid in the food

All products have their advantages and disadvantages – if you are unsure, seek help from your veterinary practice.

Ticks

Ticks are temporary parasites that spend short periods of time on the host, as they need more than one host to complete their life cycle.

- Ticks live on the surface of the animal's skin.
- Ticks feed on the blood of the animal.
- Ticks may produce toxins to aid with digestion.
- Ticks may act as vectors for microorganisms or endoparasites.
- When engorged with blood, ticks are easily spotted on the animal.
- Ticks may cause severe irritation or *alopecia*.

Common species of ticks

There are three common types of ticks seen in animals and all are *Ixodes* species:

- *Ixodes ricinus* – sheep tick – very common and affect various species.
- *Ixodes hexagonus* – hedgehog tick – common and affect various species.
- *Ixodes canisuga* – dog tick – affects various species. Can be a problem in kennels as it can survive in crevices in floors and walls.

Ixodes species (Figure 15.2)

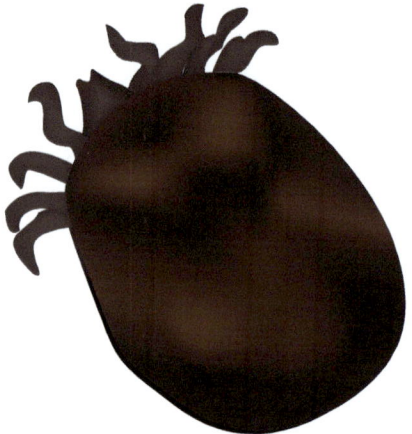

Figure 15.2   Tick – *Ixodes* spp.

- An adult tick can live for 2 years without feeding.
- An engorged female can lay 1000–3000 eggs.
- Larva hatches in 30 days.
- Nymphs emerge from moulted larva.
- Adult tick emerges after 12 days.
- Feeding is required between each stage of development.

Diseases can be transmitted by ticks in their saliva to other host animals. These diseases include:

- **Lyme disease** – a bacterial tick-borne infection caused by *Borrelia burgdorferi*. The bacteria may cause skin discolouration along with cardiac and joint disease in an infected animal. It is endemic in several states of the USA and in Europe by ticks of wildlife hosts, such as rodents and deer.
    Signs of Lyme disease are:
  - Sudden onset lameness with arthritic pain in one or more joints (i.e. carpal or wrist joint), which may last only a few days but recurs intermittently.
  - High temperature with enlarged surface lymph nodes.

- **Ehrlichiosis** – caused by a tick-borne bacterium, which lives inside monocytic white cells. It is transmitted by ticks when they feed on the host animal's blood. It is found in the Mediterranean countries of Europe. The severity of infection and recovery of the host animal depend on its immune status. Certain breeds of dog appear to be particularly susceptible to infection, e.g. German shepherds. *Babesiosis* may also be present, having been passed by the tick at the same time.

  Signs of ehrlichiosis are:
  - High temperature and inappetence
  - Lymph nodes enlarged
  - Bleeding from the nose and under the skin
  - Anaemia

- **Babesiosis** – caused by a protozoan that develops and multiplies in the salivary glands of the tick, from where it is transmitted to the host animal during feeding and infects red blood cells. It is endemic across much of Europe. The severity of the disease varies, depending on the species and strain of Babesia and the health status of the animal.

  Signs of babesiosis are:
  - Pale mucous membranes
  - Anaemia
  - Breathing problems and collapse

Treatment of ticks

- To remove a tick, dab with an *acaricide* and remove with a specialist device. Surgical spirit may also be used but it is not always effective.
- Do not pull live ticks off the host as their mouthparts can be left embedded in the skin and cause a secondary infection.
- Injections containing the active ingredient *ivermectin* may also be given in animals where there is repeated and heavy tick infestation.

Lice

Lice are host-specific parasites. This means that they only live on one species, i.e. each animal species has its own type of louse. Lice can affect cats, dogs, rabbits, guinea pigs, rodents, birds, and humans.

- Lice can be classified as *biting* or *sucking lice* depending on their feeding technique.
- Lice are transmitted by direct contact or by transfer of eggs collected and passed on during grooming.
- Lice can cause severe problems on their own, or they can also act as vectors for other organisms such as *rickettsia*.

Problems that may be caused directly by lice include:

- Severe irritation and *pruritus*
- Loss of condition
- Alopecia
- Depression
- Anaemia in severe sucking louse infestations
- Excessive scratching due to lice can cause tissue damage and secondary infection

Common species of lice
- *Trichodectes canis* – canine-biting louse
- *Trichodectes equi* – equine-biting louse
- *Linognathus setosus* – canine-sucking louse

The louse's life cycle
Lice complete their whole life cycle on the host by:

- Laying and cementing their eggs to the hair shafts. Louse eggs are commonly known as *nits*.
- Once hatched, the immature lice are identical to the adults except for their size and are known as *nymphs*.
- After several moults, the immature lice become adults.
- The whole life cycle takes approximately 2–3 weeks.

Diagnosis and treatment of a louse infestation
Lice are often easily spotted due to their size.

A range of products are available for the control of lice. It is important to treat the environment as well as the animal. Thoroughly disinfect the environment and replace any bedding with fresh, clean bedding. The animal may need to be washed in an insecticidal shampoo. If seen by a vet, the animal is likely to be given an ivermectin injection.

Mites

Mites can live on the surface of an animal's skin, or they can burrow just under the skin and so are classified as *burrowing mites* or *surface mites*. Mites are very small in size and can only just be seen by the naked eye.

Common species of mites
There are five common species of mites that affect animals:

- *Sarcoptes* – burrows into skin
- *Psoroptes* – live on the surface
- *Demodectes* – burrows into skin
- *Otodectes* – live on the surface
- *Cheyletiella* – live on the surface

The mite's life cycle
Mites complete their whole life cycle on the host:

1. Females lay their eggs.
2. Eggs hatch into larvae.
3. Larvae undergo several moults to become adults.

A mite's life cycle can be as short as 13 days in some species.

Treatment of mites
- Clean the infected area and use an acaricide to kill the mites.
- Repeat treatments at regular intervals to ensure all life cycle stages are eliminated.
- Ivermectin injections may also be given.

Sarcoptes mites, *e.g. Sarcoptes scabiei*

- Burrow into skin surface
- Collects where there is little hair growth, i.e. around ears, face, muzzle, and elbows
- Presence of mites+intense scratching=soreness and damaged skin tissue with hair loss and possible secondary infection
- May get pustule formation
- Causes sarcoptic mange

Psoroptes mites

- Live on skin surface
- Cause localised lesions
- Live in the scabs formed by lesions from their bites
- Can cause sheep scab, body mange, and ear mange
- e.g. *Psoroptes cuniculi* causes ear canker in rabbits

Demodectes mites

- Burrowing mites
- Found in dogs – *Demodex canis*
- Causes a non-itchy alopecia and skin thickening
- May spread to cause demodectic mange which may be dry or may allow secondary bacterial infection to establish
- A similar mite is found in guinea pigs – *Trixacarus caviae*

Otodectes mites

- Surface mites living in the external ear canal
- Causes irritation and can lead to intense head shaking and *aural haematomas*
- Causes *otitis*
- The most common type is *Otodectes cynotis.*

Cheyletiella mites – *fur mites*

- Found all over the body surface.
- Live off the dead skin and carry it around the skin surface and so referred to as 'walking dandruff'.
- Cause an itchy dermatitis which is characterized by small red spots from the bites.
- There are three main species of *Cheyletiella* mite seen in small animals:
  - *Cheyletiella yasguri* – canine species
  - *Cheyletiella blakei* – feline species
  - *Cheyletiella parasitovorax* – rabbits and guinea pigs
- Cheyletiella life cycle

  1. Eggs are laid and cemented to coat hairs, similarly to lice.
  2. Eggs hatch into six-legged larvae.
  3. Moult into eight-legged larvae.
  4. Adult stage is reached.
  5. *Cheyletiella* mites are treatable with insecticidal shampoos.
  6. *Cheyletiella* mites are zoonotic and highly contagious. They can burrow through clothing and cause intense itching in humans.
  7. Adopt barrier-nursing techniques when dealing with infected animals.

Flies

- Flies can be parasitic to animals.
- Flies are attracted to soiled areas whether in the housing or on the animal itself. They lay their eggs, and once the maggots have hatched, they burrow into the skin of the animal, causing a condition known as *fly strike*.
- Prevention of fly strike is particularly important in longer-haired animals, e.g. Angora rabbits, and in livestock such as sheep.
- During hot, summer months, it is best to clip the rear end of species prone to fly strike to make detection of any soreness that may be caused by flies and maggots easier.

Ectoparasites in Birds

Ectoparasites that can be seen in captive birds are described in this section.

Mites

- *Cnemidocoptes* – mainly seen in budgies and canaries – causes scaly beak and feet. In pigeons, this species of mite causes feather disintegration.
- *Dermanyssus* – red feather mite – seen in raptors, pigeons, and parrots. This mite lives in the crevices of the housing and attacks the birds when they are roosting at night. As they suck the blood, this mite can cause anaemia.
- *Ornithonyssus* – the northern fowl mite – this mite sucks the host's blood and lives on the host continuously, and so, it is easier to detect and treat.
- *Sarcoptes* mites are not usually seen in birds but there have been recorded incidences in macaws.

Lice

- All lice found on birds belong to the order *Mallophaga* and cause damage by chewing the feathers.
- Lice are more common in birds housed outdoors due to transmission from wild bird species.

Flies

- Many different families of flies can affect birds, e.g. blue, black, and green bottles.
- Flies are attracted to birds with diarrhoea, they lay their eggs, and the maggots eat into the bird and can cause a great deal of soreness in the rear area.

Ticks

- Tick infestations can be rapidly fatal in birds due to a toxin in the saliva of the tick.
- Can be seen in hunting raptors and birds kept in aviaries under trees.

Ectoparasites in Reptiles

Ectoparasites that can be seen in reptiles are described in this section.

Mites

Ophionyssus natricis

- Most common mite found in snakes
- Appears as red-dark pinhead mites living under the overlapping edges of scales
- Mites may be seen in water dishes after bathing
- Mites can cause severe irritation and trauma as well as anaemia and *dysecdysis* (problems with skin shedding).
- May also transmit *Aeromonas* spp. of bacteria and this can cause septicaemia in the animal.

Flies

Tortoises can suffer from fly infestations in the summer months if housed outdoors. The maggots can burrow into the tortoise within 2 hours and cause severe trauma, infection, shock and even death.

Ticks

Wild-caught reptiles often suffer from ticks but so may garden-kept tortoises. The ticks commonly seen in the UK are *Ixodes ricinus* and *Ixodes hexagonus*. These ticks may transmit the bacteria *Staphylococcus aureus* and *Borrelia burgdorferi* that cause Lyme disease.

Internal Parasites

Endoparasites for small animals are divided into two groups

- Roundworms
- Tapeworms

Animals with internal parasites do not always show signs of infestation. The signs only start to appear if the infestation becomes overwhelming to the health of the host animal.

Clinical signs may include:

- Scooting on bottom (anal irritation)
- Constantly hungry and eating (polyphagia)
- Weight loss
- Vomiting and diarrhoea seen in heavy infestation
- Unhealthy, dull coat
- Enlarged abdomen

Roundworms

Nematodes (Figure 15.3):

- Are unsegmented
- Have a body cavity
- Have an alimentary tract throughout

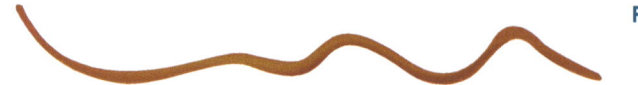

Figure 15.3 Roundworm.

- Roundworms can be divided into six groups:

1. Ascarids
2. Hookworms
3. Lungworms
4. Whipworms
5. Heartworms
6. Bladder/liver worms

Roundworms in the United Kingdom

1. *Toxocara canis*
   Toxocara canis is a roundworm of dogs and is zoonotic. It migrates in human tissues and causes *visceral larval migrans and toxocariasis* in humans, which can cause blindness in children.
   - Infective eggs or larval forms of the roundworm are eaten by the dog.
   - The eggs/larvae migrate to the body tissues, often migrating to developing foetuses.
   - They develop locally in the intestines, moving to the unborn foetus before the end of pregnancy or infecting neonates through the mother's milk after birth.
   - The larvae are now mature, passing eggs in the puppies' faeces.
   - These eggs are swallowed by other puppies, the mother, or paratenic hosts, and the cycle repeats unless the dogs are treated. Puppies should be wormed monthly from 3 weeks of age.
2. *Toxocara cati*
   Toxocara cati is responsible for infections in cats and kittens. It is also zoonotic and can cause *visceral larval migrans* and *toxocariasis* in humans.
   - Kittens become infected with tapeworm larvae either from their mother's milk or from ingestion of eggs in the environment.
   - Adult cats are infected through ingestion of eggs or paratenic hosts in the environment.
   - Heavy infections lead to stunted growth and potbellied kittens. Kittens should be regularly wormed (monthly) from 3 weeks of age.

Preventing toxocariasis

- Worm animals regularly.
- Clean up and dispose of faeces immediately.
- Disinfect where faeces have been.
- Always wash hands thoroughly.
- Teach children to wash hands after playing in grass and soil.
- Teach children to wash hands before eating food.
- Wash animals' bowls separately from human utensils.
- Do not let the animal lick your face.
- Keep the animal's anal area clean.

- Examine faeces regularly for signs of worms.
- Keep animals away from children's play areas and sports pitches.

Lungworms

Lungworms are short, slender worms that live in the heart chambers and the pulmonary artery of the animals that they infect.

Prevalence has increased in the United Kingdom, and this has been attributed to climate change and movement of infected animals. It is recommended that dog owners routinely worm their pets for lungworm as lungworm is now considered to be endemic.

- *Angiostrongylus vasorum* – dog lungworm
  - Dogs become infected when they eat slugs and snails containing the infective larvae (or encounter their slime).
  - Clinical signs of infection include irregular breathing and coughing and weight loss.
  - Treatment is with anthelmintics fenbendazole...
- *Aelurostrongylus abstrusus* – cat lungworm
  - Cats become infected when they eat slugs and snails containing the infective larvae.
  - *Aelurostrongylus abstrusus* can also live in birds and mice and so cats are at risk of infection when they hunt these other animals.
  - The adult worm lives in the cat's lung tissue.
  - Clinical signs include coughing, breathing problems, nasal discharge, and anorexia.
  - Treatment is with anthelmintic products.

Hookworms

Hookworms have a short, stout appearance with hooked heads. Two species may be found, and they differ in the appearance of their head:

- *Uncinaria stenocephala* – plates in mouth – tends to affect greyhounds and dogs in hunt kennels and is found in the small intestine of dogs.
- *Ancylostoma caninum* – large teeth – found in the small intestine of dogs.

As their name suggests, hookworms attach to the small intestine with their mouthparts and use their teeth to damage the surface and then digest the damaged tissue. They can cause weight loss and anaemia. Their eggs are passed into the environment in faeces.

Whipworms

Whipworms, as their name suggests, have a whip-like appearance. The worms burrow into the large intestine to feed. The eggs are characteristic of the worm and are protected by a thick shell that makes them resistant to damage in the environment. They can survive in the ground for several years. Whipworms are rarely seen in the United Kingdom, but an example is *Trichuris vulpis* – whipworm of the dog.

Heartworms

An example of heartworm is *Dirofilaria immitis*, heartworm of the dog – tends not to occur in the United Kingdom at the current time but may be seen in dogs imported from warmer countries.

Bladder/liver worms (*Capillaria* species)

Bladder/liver worms are not found in the United Kingdom at the current time.

Tapeworms

Cestodes (Figure 15.4):

- are segmented
- each segment is independent
- have a complete alimentary tract in each segment

Tapeworms in the United Kingdom

1. *Dipylidium caninum*

   This tapeworm affects both dogs and cats and uses the flea as an intermediate host.
   - Animal passes egg-filled tapeworm segments in its faeces (Figure 15.5).
   - The segments burst, releasing individual eggs that are eaten by the flea larvae.
   - During grooming, the animal swallows the tapeworm-carrying flea larvae.
   - The tapeworm matures in the animal host.

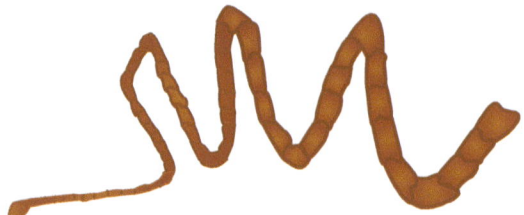

Figure 15.4   Tapeworm.

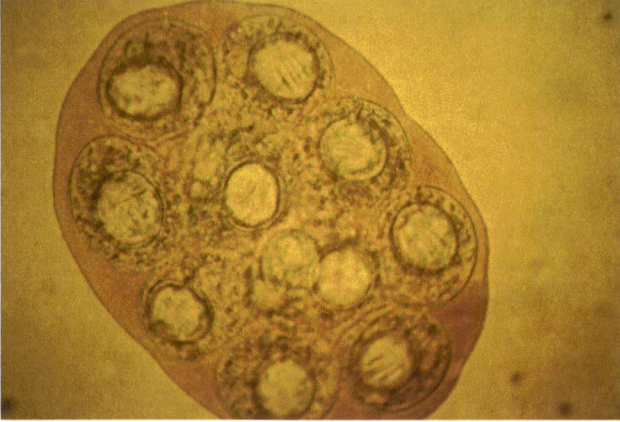

Figure 15.5   *Dipylidium caninum* worm egg.

- The adult tapeworm releases mature, egg-filled segments.
- If the host is not treated with anthelmintic drugs, the cycle begins again and will continue to repeat to increase the level of infection.

2. *Echinococcus granulosus*
   - *Echinococcus granulosus* is an important zoonotic parasite in the United Kingdom.
   - Found more commonly in rural areas as it has a dog-to-sheep life cycle.
   - Adults are approximately 6 mm in length, and there can be thousands in one animal's intestines.
   - Treatment includes preventing access to sheep carcasses.
   - If humans ingest an egg or a segment from their dog, then a *hydatid cyst* may develop in their liver or lungs in much the same way as it does in the sheep.
   - Infected people are treated using an anthelmintic before drainage of the cyst. Surgical removal of the wall of the cyst is necessary.
     Echinococcus granulosus equinus
   - This species has a dog-to-horse life cycle and is common in hounds fed on horse offal.
   - This species is not believed to be zoonotic.

3. *Taenia species*
   - There are three common *Taenia* species in the United Kingdom:
     - *Taenia hydatigena (dogs)*
       - A large tapeworm that can grow up to 5 m long.
       - Lives in the small intestines of dogs, foxes, and other wildlife species
       - Sheep are a common intermediate host
     - *Taenia solium (pigs)*
       - Humans can suffer from *taeniasis* if infected from eating raw or undercooked pork
     - *Taenia saginata (humans and cattle)*
       - *Taenia saginata* is transmitted by humans to cattle through faeces. The cattle suffer with a disease called *cysticercosis* and if people eat undercooked beef, they can become infected with the tapeworm.
       - Infected cattle show no signs of infection. The infection is diagnosed *post-mortem*.
       - Infected humans may have abdominal pain, mild diarrhoea, weight loss, and anal irritation.

Tapeworms in other animals

- Other species that may be infected with tapeworms include birds, rabbits, mice, rats, and hamsters.
- All tapeworms are specific to a species and the intermediate hosts tend to be mites or beetles.

Treatment of tapeworms

- Adult tapeworms are much easier to destroy than immature tapeworms.
- Treatment includes the use of an anthelmintic that has specific activity against a tapeworm (cestocidal).
- The product used may also have activity against roundworms and so may be called a broad-spectrum anthelmintic.
- More than one dose may be required if the infestation is heavy.

Summary of Parasites

There are many different parasites that can affect animals.

Keeping animals up to date with routine preventative treatment for both internal and external parasites is key in reducing their occurrence.

Many insurance companies require this for insurance policies to remain valid.

16

First Aid Care

Learning goals

In this chapter, the learning goals are:

- To identify the aims and objectives of first aid for animals
- To classify a first aid situation according to its severity
- To describe the initial management of a first aid situation
- To identify the correct method of transporting an injured animal
- To explain the term ABC, describe the recovery position for an animal, and describe a body scan for an animal
- To describe the life-saving techniques of artificial respiration and cardiac compression for animals
- To describe action to be taken in a range of situations requiring first aid for animals

First Aid

First aid is the first emergency care and treatment an animal receives following sudden illness or injury. First aid takes place before any veterinary medical or surgical care takes place. The main objectives of first aid are to:

1. Keep the animal alive
2. Make it comfortable
3. Assist in pain control
4. Prevent its condition from getting worse

Different first aid situations need different approaches. Some situations will allow plenty of time to attend to injuries or problems and will never be life-threatening. Other situations are so severe that the animal will die if urgent and skilled emergency care is not available.

First aid treatment is limited in its approach. It does not involve diagnosis or medical treatment of injuries but is designed to preserve life and temporarily prevent a condition from getting worse. It should allow time to get the animal to a veterinary surgeon who can diagnose the full extent of the condition, which is not always obvious at first.

First aid kits are available for animals, but unless the animal is at home, a person providing first aid for an animal is unlikely to be able to lay their hands on a kit immediately.

Animal Biology and Care, Fourth Edition. Emily Jewell.
© 2026 John Wiley & Sons Ltd. Published 2026 by John Wiley & Sons Ltd.
Companion Website: https://www.wiley.com/go/animal/biology4e/jewell

Classifying First Aid Situations

Very Severe Immediate action	Severe 1 hour for action	Serious 4–5 hours for action	Major 24 hours for action

Very severe

Very severe situations that *need immediate action* or the animal will die:

- The heart has stopped (cardiopulmonary arrest)
- Breathing is obstructed due to an object in the air passages
- Breathing has stopped
- Bleeding from a main artery or vein
- Acute allergic reaction to an insect sting or other substance

Severe

These are situations where first aid must be *provided within 1 hour* or the animal may die:

- Deep cuts and considerable blood loss
- Established shock
- Head injuries
- Breathing difficulties

Serious

These are situations where *first aid action must be taken within 4–5 hours* or more serious problems will develop that could be life threatening:

- Bone fractures that puncture through the skin (*compound fractures*)
- Spinal injuries
- Early stages of shock
- Difficulties in giving birth (*dystocia*)

Major

In these situations, *first aid action must occur within 24 hours* to prevent further damage:

- Fractures with no skin injury (*simple fractures*)
- Prolonged vomiting and diarrhoea
- Foreign bodies in the eyes or ears

Initial Management of First Aid Situations

1. *Assess the situation and keep calm* – briefly examine the animal and note any obvious injuries.
2. *Contact the veterinary practice* – for advice and to let them know you are coming.

3. *Ensure your own and the animal's safety* – make sure the animal is properly restrained before handling and lifting, so that no one is bitten, and the animal is not injured further.
   - Stop and cover any obvious bleeding – use sterile dressings, if possible, to prevent further contamination.
4. *Make sure the animal can breathe* – clear the airway if it is obstructed.
5. *Treat for shock* – keep the animal warm by maintaining the body temperature.

Recovery Position for an Animal

In animal first aid, as in human first aid, there is a recovery position in which to place the animal to ensure breathing is assisted and the heart is exposed for emergency procedures, if required (Figure 16.1).

- Lie the animal on its right side
- Straighten the head and neck
- The tongue is pulled forwards and behind the canine tooth (to one side of the mouth)
- Remove any collar or harness
- Check the heart and pulse regularly

Initial Assessment

DRABC checks

These checks should be carried out prior to a more thorough body scan taking place:

- *Danger* – is there any surrounding danger around the incident that needs to be removed before providing any first aid?
- *Response* level – check if the animal is responding to any stimuli such as noise, movement, calling its name, or responding to touch. This is an indicator of its level of consciousness.
- *Airway* – check that the airway is not obstructed; if it is, then clear it if safe to do so.
- *Breathing* – check the animal's breathing and if needed, assist with artificial respiration.
- *Circulation* – check the pulse and heart – check the beat, its rate and strength, and record the information. If the heart has stopped, then proceed with heart massage.

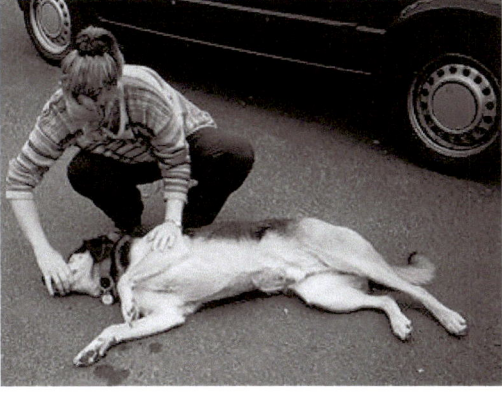

Figure 16.1   Recovery position for an injured animal, keeping the airway straight.

Body scan

Following DRABC checks, carry out a body scan to assess the animal further:

- Check mucous membranes (Figure 16.2) or the eyes and gums:
  - *Pale* – indicating shock or serious bleeding (internal or external).
  - *Blue* – also referred to as *cyanotic*, indicates lack of oxygen to the tissue cells.
  - *Yellow* – also referred to as *jaundice*, can be caused by an excess of bile pigment in the bloodstream and usually involves the liver in some way.
  - *Red/congested* – indicates over-oxygenation after exercise, in heat stroke cases or fever conditions.
- Check capillary refill time (Figure 16.3):
  - Lift the upper lip and press the gum over the top canine tooth with a little pressure. This squeezes the blood out of the surface capillaries, causing the area to go temporarily white. The refill time is the time it takes for the gum to become the normal pink colour again as the capillaries refill, usually 1–1½ seconds. Any time longer than that is considered 'slow' and may indicate a degree of shock.

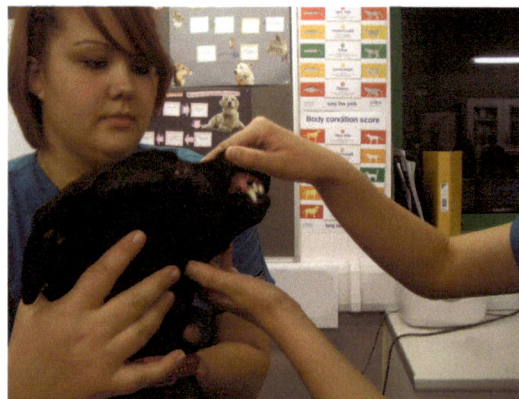

Figure 16.2   Checking mucous membrane colour.

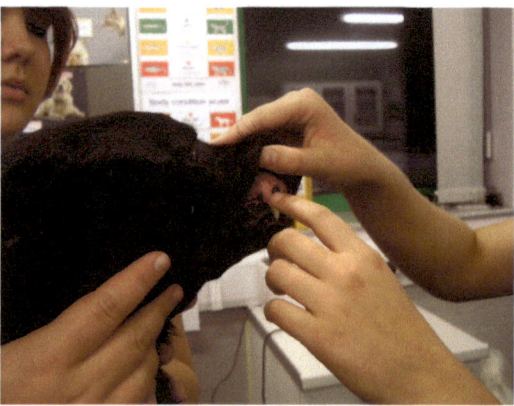

Figure 16.3   Checking capillary refill time.

- Check the rate and quality of the pulse:
  - Assess using the *femoral artery* located in the groin area of the hind leg. This artery is exposed over the femur bone at this point, allowing the pulse to be taken. If the animal is unconscious, the *sublingual artery* under the tongue can be used.
    - The rate refers to the speed of the pulse, which reflects the heartbeat.
    - The quality of the pulse refers to whether it is strong, thready, weak, or normal. To describe this accurately, the handler must have some experience of pulse taking.
    - The pulse should be taken for a full minute for a true recording.
- Check the breathing rate:
  - Record observations as normal, slow, fast, or shallow.
  - Assess for a full minute for a true recording.
- Assess body temperature through feeling the extremities of the animals, such as the feet and tail end. If the temperature is lower than it should be, the handler will feel this, because the normal body temperature of most animals (mammals and birds) is higher than that of humans.
- Check for any unusual odour from the animal's body, whether it comes from the animal's mouth, anus, or coat.
- Check for signs of bleeding from the animal's surface or from a body opening, such as the mouth, rectum, vulva, prepuce, or ears.
- Check limbs for any unnatural posture that may indicate dislocation or fracture.

Life-saving Techniques

Life-saving techniques will be needed in two situations that may occur following sudden illness, injury, or trauma:

- *Cardiac arrest* – the heart has stopped
- *Respiratory arrest* – breathing has stopped
- If both the heart and breathing have stopped, this is called *cardiopulmonary arrest*

In all cases, the animal will need to have resuscitation to restore heart and lung function and keep oxygen circulating around the body to prevent irreversible brain and/or cell damage, which can be caused from oxygen deprivation.

This is referred to as *cardiopulmonary resuscitation (CPR)*.

Cardiac compressions (heart massage)

The aim of cardiac compressions is to keep blood moving through the body, thereby providing the oxygen that may be left in the blood to the tissues. The amount of pressure and rate of compressions will depend on the size of the animal.

1. Small dogs, cats, or other small animals
   - Place in recovery position (on its right side, head and neck extended and tongue pulled forwards).
   - Hold the animal's chest between the thumb and fingers of the same hand, over the heart, and just behind the elbows.
   - Support the body of the animal with the other hand on the lumbar spine area.

- At all times, keep the head and neck in a straight line to assist breathing.
- Squeeze the thumb and fingers of the hand over the heart together; this will compress the chest wall and the heart, which is squeezed between the ribs.
- Repeat this action approximately 120 times per minute.
- Check every two minute to assess heartbeat/pulse – stop if the heart has restarted or continue compressions until further help arrives.

2. Medium-sized dogs and other species
   - Place in the recovery position.
   - Put the heel of one hand on the top of the chest, just behind the elbow and over the heart (Figures 16.4 and 16.5).
   - Place the other hand either on top of the first hand or under the animal to support the heart as it is compressed.
   - Press down onto the chest with firm, sharp movements.
   - Repeat this action about 80–100 times per minute.
   - Check every 2 minutes to assess heartbeat/pulse – stop if the heart has restarted or continue compressions until further help arrives.

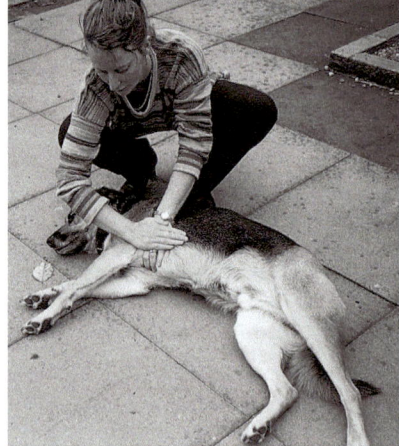

Figure 16.4   Position of hands when doing cardiac massage.

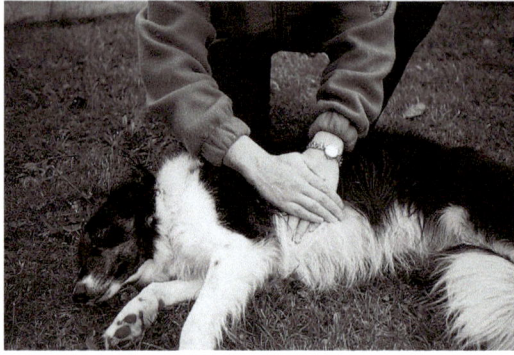

Figure 16.5   Same hand position, behind the elbow and over the heart.

3. Large, barrel-chested or fat dogs and other species
    - Place on its back, with head slightly lower than its body, if possible.
        - ○ Put the heel of one hand on the abdominal end of the sternum (breastbone).
    - Place the other hand on top of the first.
    - Press firmly onto the chest, pushing the hands forwards towards the head of the animal.
    - Press down in this way 80–100 times per minute.
    - Aim to always keep the head and neck straight during the procedure.
    - Check every 2 minutes to assess heartbeat/pulse – stop if the heart has restarted or continue compressions until further help arrives.

Respiratory arrest

If the breathing has stopped, then it must be restarted urgently. There are two first aid methods that can be used for restarting breathing:

- Artificial respiration – manual method
- Mouth-to-nose technique

Artificial respiration

- Place in recovery position.
- Clear the airway of any blocking material.
- Place a hand over the ribs, behind the shoulder bone (Figure 16.6).
- Compress the chest with a sharp, downward movement.
- Allow the chest to expand and then repeat the downward movement.
- Repeat approximately every 3–5 seconds, until breathing restarts.
- Always keep head and neck straight to maintain the animal's airway.

Mouth-to-nose technique

- Place in recovery position.
- Clear the airway.

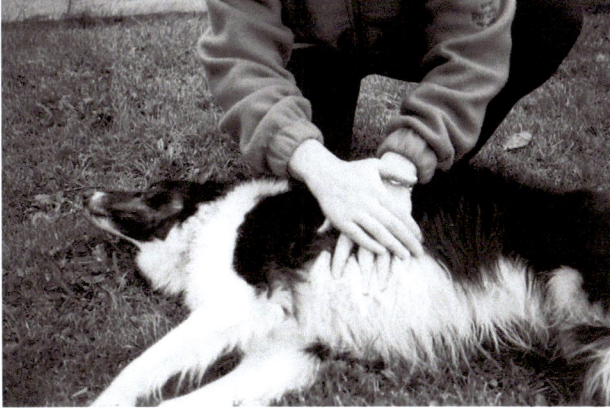

Figure 16.6   For artificial respiration compression, hands are placed over the chest.

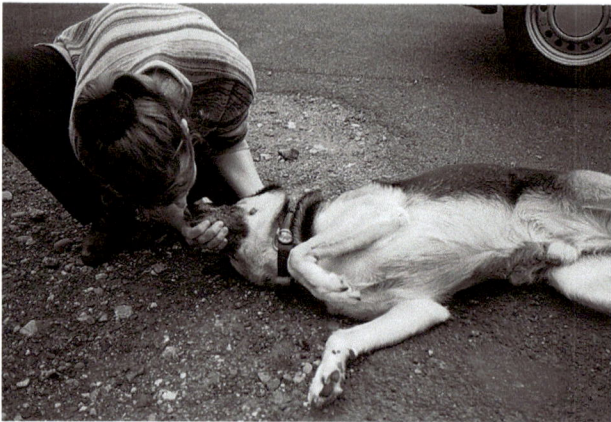

Figure 16.7   Mouth-to-nose resuscitation with the airway kept straight and mouth held shut. The operator breathes down the nose.

- Place a tissue or thin cloth over the animal's nose (for personal hygiene).
  - Always hold the animal's neck straight.
- Keep its mouth closed by holding upper and lower jaws together.
- Breathe down its nose to inflate the lungs (Figure 16.7).
- Repeat this inflation of the lungs at 3–5 second intervals.
- Check for independent breathing after each cycle of artificial breaths.

This technique provides the animal with the unused oxygen in the handler's breath and their exhaled carbon dioxide, which helps to stimulate the breathing or gasp reflex in the animal.

Movement of an Animal Requiring First Aid

If the animal's life is in danger, then it must be moved. Injured animals are usually in pain, shocked and frightened and may attack anyone who tries to approach or handle them. To protect both the handler and the animal from further harm or injury, great care is needed:

- Make slow, deliberate movements
- Use a calm, soothing voice
- Handle the animal as little as possible
- Muzzle if necessary and only if the animal has no breathing difficulties
- Transport to the surgery

Before moving the animal, quickly assess the condition. This is referred to as initial assessment, and the sooner this is done, the more improved the chances of survival are. The initial assessment and any help provided must be reported to veterinary staff on arrival at the surgery.

Species consideration is important when considering handling. The method for moving an injured dog or cat will vary from the method used for rodents, horses, reptiles, or birds, for example.

Small dogs, cats, rabbits, and smaller pets

Use a pet carrier or cat-sized basket, making sure there are plenty of breathing holes and space for the animal (Figure 16.8). Alternatively, and depending on the injury, the animal can be held in the owner's arms although this is not recommended (Figure 16.9).

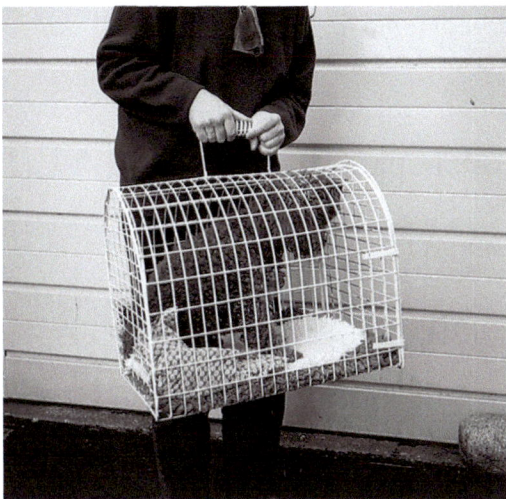

Figure 16.8   Carrier cage for a small dog, cat, or other animal.

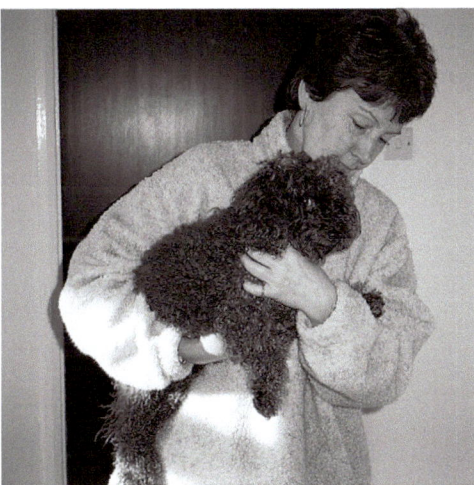

Figure 16.9   Small dog held in arms.

Medium-sized dogs or other animals

If the animal only has minor injuries, encourage them to walk slowly. If they are not able to walk, then pick them up with one arm around the front of the forelegs and one around the hind legs (providing this does not make any injuries worse), lift and hold against your body, with the legs hanging downwards (Figure 16.10).

Large breeds of dog or similar sized animals

This size of animal (20 kg+) should *always* be lifted by more than one person, one supporting the head and chest and another supporting the abdomen and hindquarters (Figure 16.11). If the dog is too large for lifting, then with two or more handlers, use a stretcher or blanket lift (Figure 16.12).

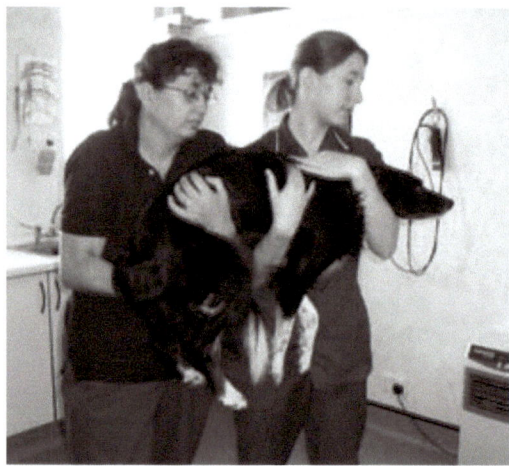

Figure 16.10   Medium dog lift.

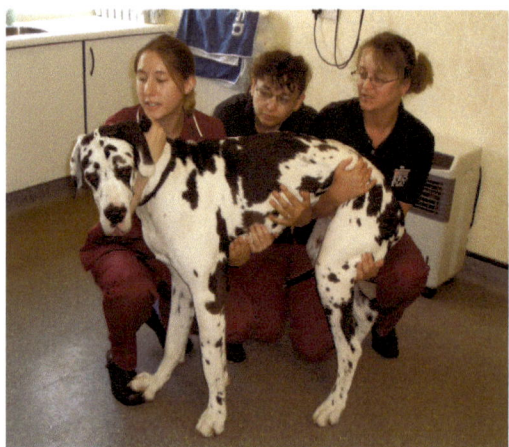

Figure 16.11   Giant breed lift.

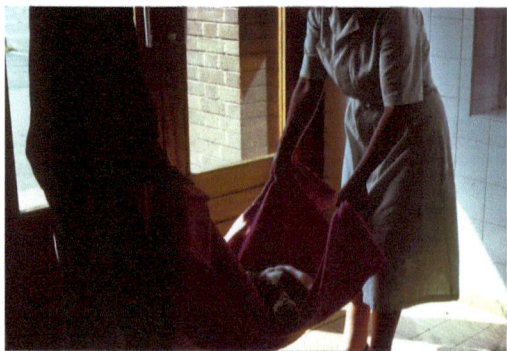

Figure 16.12   Blanket lift requires two or more people for a large animal.

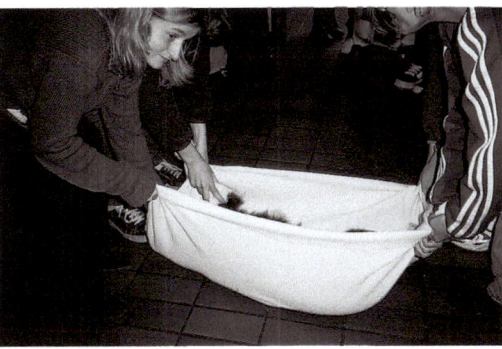

Figure 16.13   Blanket lift for a smaller dog with spinal injuries.

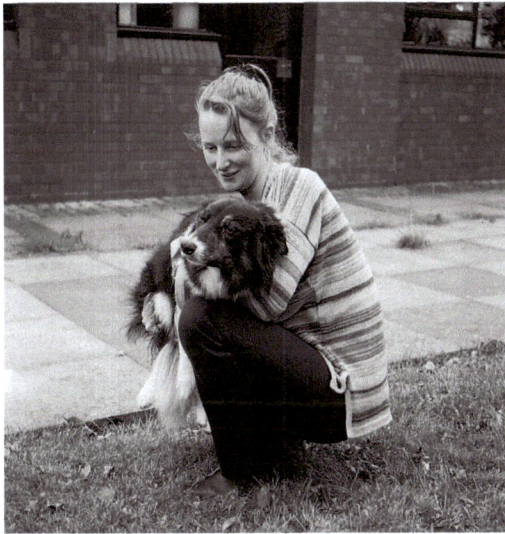

Figure 16.14   Lift with straight back and bent knees to prevent back strain injury of the handler.

Pull the animal onto the blanket, lying on its side, and lift using the corners of the blanket or, if not enough handlers are available, simply drag the blanket, provided the surface is smooth. This blanket technique is also used for smaller animals with spinal injuries (Figure 16.13).

Whatever the size of the injured animal, always lift in the correct manner; bend your knees before lifting rather than bending from the waist (Figure 16.14). This reduces the risk of back injury for the handler. If you are in doubt, get more help.

Transporting injured birds and reptiles

Due to their fragile bones, transport of injured reptiles and birds requires safe, careful handling and minimisation of stress.

- Ensure handler safety using gloves and eye protection where possible.
- Cover birds with a towel or clothing and place in a well-ventilated cardboard box and close the box as a darkened environment helps to reduce stress.

- For lizards, a similar procedure as that for birds can be used but a covered heat pack is useful to place in the bottom of the box.
- Snakes may need a hook or tongs to be lifted. They can be transported in a cardboard box or in a pillowcase secured at the top to prevent escape.

Situations Requiring First Aid for Animals

Many factors can contribute to an animal requiring first aid and some of the most common factors are:

- Poisons
- Insect stings
- Injuries causing bleeding
- Burns and scalds
- Eye injuries

Poisons

A poison or toxin is any substance which, on entry to the body in sufficient amounts, has a harmful effect on the individual. Poisons can gain entry to the body by various means:

- By mouth
- Via the lungs
- Absorbed through the skin surface or directly through a cut/wound

Animals can be poisoned by a multitude of potentially toxic substances, many of which are ordinary household products. The source may be poisonous plants, garden products, or toxic chemicals used or stored near the animal in the household or garden environment. Such poisons would include:

- Pesticides for the garden, such as slug bait and weedkillers
- Toxic plants or bulbs, e.g. daffodils, lilies, and rhododendrons
- Rodent killers, such as warfarin poison
- Paint and cleaning solutions for paint brushes
- Cleaning products such as bleach, toilet cleaners, and washing powder pods
- Drugs such as aspirin, ibuprofen, blood pressure tablets, and sleeping tablets
- Human food, e.g. raisins, onion, chocolate, grapes, and xylitol

Signs of poisoning

Very few poisons produce distinctive signs. Most cause non-specific signs, such as:

- Becoming aggressive, excited, or depressed
- Unsteady on its feet
- Salivating, vomiting, and/or having diarrhoea
- Abdominal pain and fitting-type episodes
- Pale, with lowered body temperature
- Slow capillary refill time

The owner/carer/keeper knows best what is normal and what is unusual in their animal, so record all information and contact the veterinary practice as soon as possible for advice on the next steps. If the owner knows the chemical involved and has the container or packet, take that to the veterinary surgeon too. Unless instructed to make the animal sick, do not attempt to do so as this may cause more harm.

Immediate first aid includes:

- Place in recovery position
- Support for any breathing problems
- Keep warm to reduce shock
- Record pulse and heart rate
- Comfort and do not leave unattended
- Get to the veterinary surgery as quickly as possible

Insect stings

Insect stings usually cause more pain than harm. However, it is possible that an animal may have an allergic reaction to the insect venom, or if the sting is near to the airway, any subsequent swelling could obstruct breathing.

If the venom sac from an insect sting is embedded in the skin, never squeeze it, as this may inject more venom into the animal. Leave the venom sac to be removed by veterinary staff.

- *Wasp stings* (Figure 16.15) *are alkaline*. Treatment is therefore with an acid solution, such as household vinegar in the form of a pad or compress.
- *Bee stings are acidic*. Treatment is therefore with an alkali such as bicarbonate of soda mixed with water and soaked into a pad or compress.

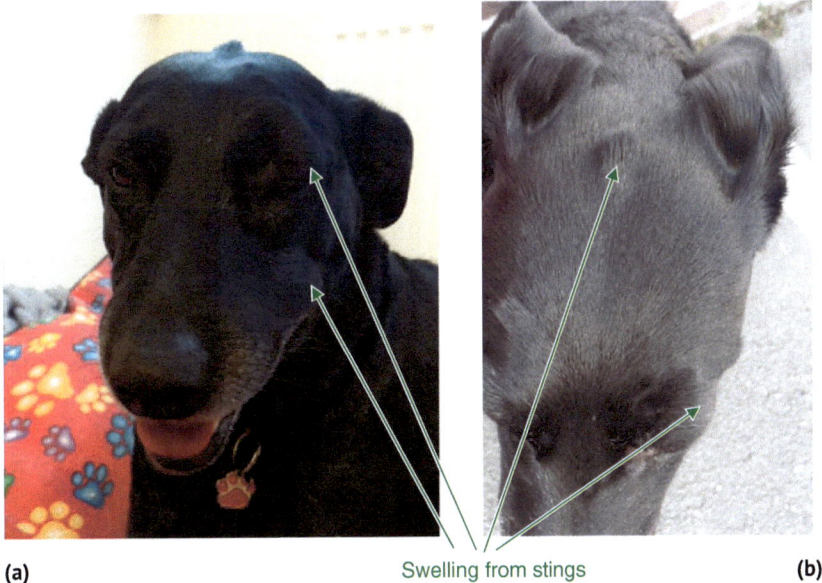

(a) Swelling from stings (b)

Figure 16.15 Dog with wasp stings to face (a) before and (b) after treatment.

Wasp = V
Bee = B

Treatment for insect stings aims to neutralise them. Unless someone has seen it bite or sting, it is not always possible to know which insect is involved. If this is the case, then apply a cold compress or face flannel filled with ice cubes to the area to reduce the swelling and give some pain control.

Bleeding

Bleeding or *haemorrhaging* is the escape of blood from damaged blood vessels and can cause serious problems. Blood loss often leads to the development of shock due to the reduction in circulating volume of blood.

Bleeding may be external (obviously seen) or internal (not always obvious). Internal bleeding should be suspected after incidents such as road traffic accidents, heavy falls, or crush injuries, and so, it is important that the following signs are watched for:

- Mucous membrane colour is pale and getting paler
- Behaviour is dull or listless
- Animal appears thirsty
- The pulse and breathing rate are fast and appear weak
- Feet and tail are cold to the touch
- Body temperature is subnormal
- Capillary refill time is slow

If blood loss is severe, then signs include those of blood loss to vital organs, such as the following:

- The animal becomes restless and will not settle
- Breathing difficulties
- Fitting-type episode
- The animal is unable to stand and becomes unconscious

For reporting purposes, the following information is useful to the veterinary surgeon:

- The type of blood vessel damaged
- Location of injury on the body
- When the bleeding started
- Whether the bleeding is internal or on the surface
- Treatments carried out so far

What type of blood vessel is damaged?

- *Artery* – blood is bright red (oxygenated) in colour and comes out as spurts that are synchronised with the heartbeat
- *Vein* – blood is dark red (deoxygenated) in colour and is a steady flow
- *Capillary* – is bright red and seen as a steady ooze

Heavy bleeding can reduce the circulating blood volume enough to cause shock. Bleeding that is less heavy may still cause the tissue cells to be deprived of oxygen, which could be permanently damaging. Even small losses of blood can delay wound healing and contribute to development of an infection. Therefore, any type of blood loss puts the animal at risk of further complication.

Stopping bleeding

The following methods are temporary solutions to use in first aid incidents until veterinary attention is available:

- *Direct pressure*
  - Use on surface wounds by pressing a sterile or clean pad of absorbent material on the injured area to control the blood loss (unless there is a foreign body such as metal, glass, or material fibres in the wound as pressing directly on this could push it deeper, where it would be harder to locate or may cause damage to internal structures). The direct pressure method could be adapted to aim to press either side of the foreign body if possible.
  - This method can be used for about 5–15 minutes before tissues beyond the injury must receive a reviving flow. Then, pressure can be re-established.
- *Pressure points*
  - Pressure points are located where major arteries of the body are located near the surface of the body. Where they cross a bone, pressure can slow, or even stop, the supply reaching an area beyond. If the wound is on the extremity, these points can be used as a temporary measure:
    - Forelimbs – the pressure is put on the inside or medial elbow area, to slow the *brachial artery* flow
    - Hindlimbs – the pressure is put on the same site used for pulse taking, in the groin area on the femur, to slow the *femoral artery* flow
    - Tail – the pressure is applied to the ventral or underside of the base of the tail, to slow the *coccygeal artery* flow
  - Pressure points can only be used for about 5–10 minutes or damage to tissues can occur.
- *Pressure bandages*
  Pressure bandages may be used initially or after the previous methods have been used to establish the extent of the injury.
  - Pressure bandages can only be applied to extremities, such as limbs and tail. They are applied tightly to constrict and slow the surface vessels supplying the area, thus limiting blood loss.
  - Plenty of padding material is applied over the dressing on the wound and is then tightly bandaged in place. If blood seeps through, then more padding is applied and bandaged in place.
  - This is a temporary measure to be used for the maximum of an hour before veterinary attention is obtained.

Shock

Shock is a very complex and potentially fatal clinical syndrome involving insufficient blood supply to the tissues, resulting in a lack of oxygen to the cells. Lack of oxygen to the cells is called *tissue hypoxia*, and this can be fatal if not corrected.

When blood is lost from the body, the body tries to compensate by redistributing blood to vital structures like the brain and heart, at the expense of other organs like kidneys, skin, intestines, and muscles. Organs can be severely damaged by the resulting lack of oxygen.

The causes of shock vary, but some examples are:

- Blood loss from damaged vessels
- Trauma injuries to tissues from a road traffic accident

- Pain due to injury or surgical procedures
- Heart problems that interfere with its normal pumping action
- Infections that cause blood to 'pool out' in the capillary beds, by affecting the walls of the blood vessels

Shock takes three forms:

- *Impending* – it is expected to happen, bearing in mind the events or injuries.
- *Established* – it is in place and the animal must have urgent medical treatment involving whole-blood transfusions or use of plasma expanders.
- *Irreversible* – treatment is unlikely to save the animal's life as systems are too damaged.

Signs of shock include:

- Pale colour
- Cold extremities
- Weak or slipping into an unconscious state
- Increase in the heart rate and breathing
- Slow capillary refill time of longer than 2 seconds

Preventing shock:

- Maintain body temperature using blankets, towels, or foil blankets (Figure 16.16). This is probably the single most useful thing that can be done. If blood flow is maintained to the peripheral vessels in the limbs and tail, shock will be at least delayed and possibly even prevented.
- Stimulate peripheral blood flow by rubbing or massaging extremities.
- Position the head slightly lower than the body to encourage the blood flow to the brain.
- Assist the animal to breathe by placing in the recovery position, and give artificial respiration if breathing stops.
- Keep the animal calm and still to prevent further injury.
- Ensure good ventilation but avoid draughts.
- Regular monitoring and recording of pulse, breathing, and mucous membrane assessments.
- Do not give food or drink until assessed by veterinary staff.
- Do not give any medications unless advised to by veterinary staff.
- Get to the veterinary surgery as quickly as possible.

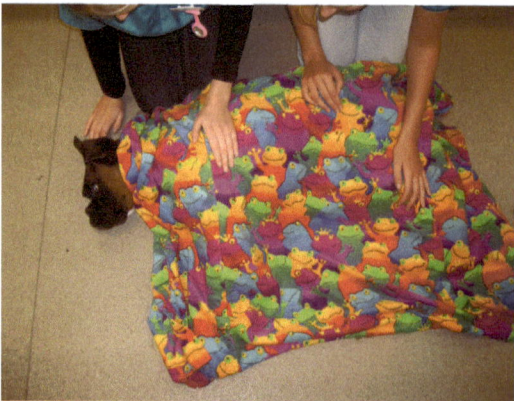

Figure 16.16   Maintaining body temperature.

Heat stroke (hyperthermia)

Heat stroke results from an excessive rise in body temperature caused by high environmental temperatures. Dogs and cats do not lose body temperature through the skin due to their dense coats and lack of sweat glands. Therefore, to eliminate excessive body heat, they use the respiratory system, inhaling cool air through the nose and exhaling hot air from the body through the mouth. The faster this exchange occurs, the faster their body will cool down, which is why dogs pant after exercise. Heat stroke is rarely seen in cats, and in dogs, it usually occurs because the animal has been confined, on a hot day, with no access to shade, or in a small area without sufficient ventilation.

Small mammals can be affected by heat stroke if they have no shade area when environmental temperatures are high. If hutches have inadequate ventilation or are placed in direct sunlight for most of the day, the animal occupants can be affected by heat stroke. Ferrets are particularly susceptible to heat stroke and placing cool packs or frozen water bottles in their accommodation covered by blankets can be useful to try and cool them down.

It is important to note that on a hot day, the temperature in a car soon becomes higher than the environmental temperature, even if windows are left open. Do not leave dogs in cars on a hot day even if parked in the 'shade'.

When the environmental temperature exceeds the animal's body temperature, it ultimately becomes impossible to maintain body temperature within normal limits for that animal.

Heat stroke affects all dogs, but those most at risk, if exposed to excess heat, are:

- Those with thick dense coats
- Overweight animals
- Short-nosed breeds
- Animals with heart conditions
- Elderly animals
- Animals with medical conditions that affect the breathing

Panting becomes ineffective and the body temperature will rise rapidly; death follows quickly if the body temperature is not immediately reduced.

Signs of heat stroke include:

- Excess panting and salivation
- Bright red mucous membranes (check the gums)
- Vomiting
- Excitement/anxiety
- Disoriented
- Collapsed/unable to stand
- Body temperature high (41–43 °C)

It is essential to reduce body temperature urgently but not too quickly as this may cause additional issues:

- Remove the animal from the hot environment.
- Cool the animal using:
  - A pack of frozen vegetables held on the neck area.
  - Wrap in towel/blanket soaked with cold water and continue to hose water over the soaked wrapping, keeping clear of the face.

- Monitor the animal's body temperature.
- If collapsed, put into the recovery position to assist breathing.
- If conscious, encourage to drink restricted amounts of water frequently (if unrestricted, the animal may swallow too much water too quickly and cause vomiting).
- With small animals, syringe feeding the water is a useful method of rehydrating them.

Hypothermia

Hypothermia is commonly seen in young or small animals, due to an inability to control body temperature within normal limits. This may be caused by illness or accident, leaving the animal unable to restore temperature loss unless assisted. Working animals such as gundogs are susceptible to hypothermia as they spend long periods of time outside in damp undergrowth.

Signs of hypothermia include:

- The animal appears sleepy or lethargic
- Its movement becomes weaker
- It is unconscious

Treatment of hypothermia includes:

- If the animal is wet, dry it by rubbing vigorously with a towel
- Wrap, using a lightweight covering, to preserve heat
- Increase the environmental temperature but do not overheat
- Monitor constantly by taking temperature and do not leave unattended
- Honey can be given to increase blood sugar and give an easily digestible source of energy to produce internal warmth

Bone fractures

A fracture refers to an incomplete or complete break in a bone's structure. Breaks in the bone are usually obvious but may not always be, and so, the objectives of first aid for fractures are to prevent the situation from getting worse and make the animal comfortable for transportation to the veterinary surgery.

The causes of bone fracture can include:

- Road traffic accidents
- The animal landing badly after jumping
- Muscles contracting to break small bones, particularly in the legs of racing dogs or horses
- Bone disease that has weakened the bone structure

Types of fracture
Fractures are classified according to the type of break and associated damage:

- *Simple* – the bone is completely broken but there is no connecting skin injury (Figure 16.17)
- *Compound* – the bone is completely broken, and there is a wound connecting to the skin, or the bone is protruding through the skin. A badly handled simple fracture can become a compound fracture.
- *Greenstick* – the break in the bone is incomplete. This type of break is often seen in young animals as their bones are softer than adult animals and so appear to bend like a young twig on a tree.

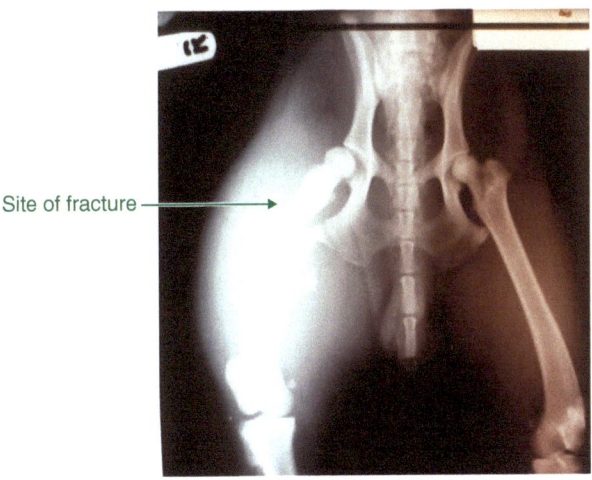

Site of fracture

Figure 16.17   X-ray shows fractured right femur and extent of tissue swelling.

Signs of a fracture may include:

- Loss of use of the affected limb (animal will not bear weight)
- Pain on handling or will not allow handling
- Unusual position or shape to the limb – usually obvious to see
- Swelling and bruising
- Unusual movement of the limb

Some fractures are also complicated by damage to surrounding tissues, such as blood vessels, nerves or organs.

Depending on the type of fracture, first aid aims to:

- Stop any bleeding.
- Clean and cover any wounds.
- Immobilise the fracture site if the joints above and below the site can be immobilised by a splint. If splinting is possible, always apply the splint to the limb in the position in which it is found. For example, if the foot and carpals of the foreleg are now positioned sideways instead of facing front, do not correct the position – splint it.
  - Materials that can be used for splinting include:
    - Rolled-up magazine or newspaper
    - A ruler or piece of wood
    - Cardboard
    - A matchstick
  - Areas of the body that can be splinted are:
    - Forelimbs
    - Hindlimbs
    - Tail
- If a splint is not possible, then:
  - Restrict movement of the animal.
  - Make comfortable on plenty of bedding.
  - Reassure animal and do not leave them unattended.

- Treat for shock.
- Transport to the veterinary surgery as quickly as possible.

Wounds

A wound is damage to body tissue that usually involves a break in the surface of the skin or a mucosal surface.

Wounds can be caused by a range of factors and may be minor or severe depending on if they involve additional tissues such as muscles, nerves, or bones.

In a first aid situation, common causes of wounds are:

- *Trauma*: Accidents, falls, crushes, tears, etc.
- *Burns*: Exposure to heat, chemicals, or radiation.

Types of wounds

Wounds are described as being *open* or *closed*.

- *Closed* wounds do not penetrate the whole thickness of the skin as a structure and include bruises or blood blisters (*haematoma*), or pockets of blood from a small, damaged blood vessel.
- Treatment involves the use of a cold compress, such as ice cubes held in a face flannel, immediately after injury, to reduce the swelling of local tissues and help control pain. This treatment is only useful immediately after injury.
- *Open* wounds are those where damage to surface tissue is also sustained and some bleeding occurs. Open wounds are named according to how the wound occurred and whether tissue is missing (Table 16.1):

Table 16.1 Types of open wound.

Type of wound	Characteristics of wound	Possible causes of wound
Abrasions	• Torn, ragged edges of skin • Embedded contaminants • Surface layer damage • Little bleeding	• Glancing blows • Dragging • Road traffic accidents
Incised	• Clean cut wound • Painful due to nerve ending damage • Bleed freely	• Sharp edged materials e.g. glass, metal, knife blades
Lacerated	• Jagged flaps of skin • May have tissue missing (*avulsed*) • Less painful due to torn, stretched skin • Less bleeding	• Bite injuries • Barbed wire • Road traffic accidents
Puncture	• Long narrow deep tracks into tissue • Small entry wound into skin covered by a scab • Prone to infection as scab holds microbes in the wound • Painful abscesses may form	• Sharp pointed objects • Teeth • Nails • Thorns

Stages of wound healing

The healing process consists of several stages until it is complete.

1. *First-intention healing*

   This takes place in wounds that:
   - Are not contaminated with grit, soil or micro-organisms.
   - Have clean-cut edges that can be held together.
   - Have been cleaned within one hour of injury.

   In this type of healing, the edges should have rejoined within 10 days following injury.

2. *Second-intention healing or granulation*

   This takes place in wounds that:
   - Are contaminated with grit, soil, and microorganisms.
   - Have jagged edges and possibly sections of skin missing.
   - Have not been cleaned within 2 hours of injury.
   - Have edges that gape open.
   - Become infected.

   This type of healing can take weeks to months.

Wound care

The sooner an open wound is cleaned using a water-based antiseptic solution, the more chance there is that infection will not develop. At a first aid situation, the solutions used for wound cleaning must not cause any further inflammation or damage to the wound and therefore should not contain any detergent.

If microorganisms in the wound are prevented from multiplying, it could mean the difference between the wound healing within 10 days (first intention) and the delayed healing of the second-intention or granulation method.

Water is the best liquid to use for cleaning a wound in the first instance and once at the veterinary surgery, an antiseptic product, e.g. Chlorhexidine, can be used to clean the wound further.

Once cleaned, the wound should be covered to prevent contamination and further aggravation of the area by the animal.

Burns and scalds

Burns can be caused by direct heat, e.g. a fire, electrical, or chemicals

  Scalds are caused by hot liquids.

Burns and scalds can be minor or severe. All burns and scalds should be reviewed by a veterinary surgeon. Any burn or scald that covers more than 10% of the body's surface area is a large injury.

Burns and scalds may be deeper than they look and damage the deeper layers of the skin and other tissues.

First aid treatment involves:

- Safely remove the item causing the burn.
- If the burn is chemical in nature, wear gloves if possible.
- Cooling the area immediately – this is of the utmost importance.
- Ideally use cool running water for 5–10 minutes, but in the absence of running water, immerse in cool water. Avoid ice cold water as this can cause further tissue damage.
- Ensure any coverings are clean and non-stick to avoid contamination of the wound.

- Avoid applying creams, etc. as they can hold the heat in, doing further damage to the under-lying tissues.
- Treat for shock.
- Get veterinary attention immediately.

Eye injuries

Any animal with an eye injury will have their vision affected and be in pain and consequently this may cause substantial changes in the animal's behaviour. It is very important to approach the animal slowly and talk gently to the animal so that it is warned of your approach. Once you have reassured the animal, examine the eye carefully (Figure 16.18).

Types of eye injury that may be seen include the following:

Chemicals

- These can cause serious injury to the eye structures.
- Always wash the eye out as soon as possible, using cool (not cold) tap water to remove any chemical.
- Do not leave the animal unattended.
- Get veterinary help immediately.

Prolapsed eyeball

This means the eye is now in front of the eyelids and the optic nerve is being stretched as the lids swell. Never touch the eyeball. The important point to remember is that the eye must not be allowed to dry out.

Give the following first aid treatment:

- Keep the eye moist at all costs. Use tap water soaked into a pad, squeeze out, and apply to the eye area.
- Once moistened, soak the pad again in tap water and place gently over the eye.
- Hold or bandage in position.
- Do not leave unattended and stop any self-mutilation.
- Keep warm, quiet, and comfortable.
- Seek veterinary assistance urgently.

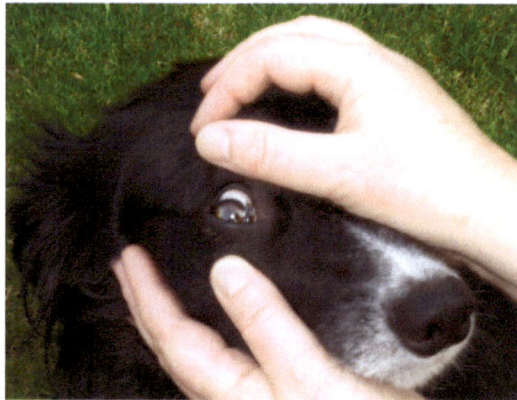

Figure 16.18 Examine the eye carefully, touching the lids only.

Some breeds of dog, such as Pugs, Pekingese, and Boxers, are prone to eye prolapse due to their shortened faces; therefore, always use extra care when handling these breeds.

Perforating injury

A perforating eye injury occurs when a sharp object becomes embedded in the structure of the eye.

Never pull the foreign body out of the eye, even if it is large enough to grasp. If it is removed non-surgically, the front chamber of the eye would leak fluid (*aqueous humour*), causing the back chamber to prolapse forwards, thereby destroying the eye structure.

Treatment is to keep the eye moist, prevent self-mutilation, and get to the veterinary surgery quickly.

Summary of First Aid Care

First aid is the first emergency care and treatment an animal receives following sudden illness or injury. There are many situations when first aid may be required for an animal and the key objectives are to:

1. Keep the animal alive
2. Make it comfortable
3. Prevent its condition getting worse

First aid provision allows the first aider to identify the severity of the situation using DRABC and a body scan so that information can be recorded for handover to the veterinary staff upon arrival at the surgery.

17

Basic Bandaging

Learning goals

In this chapter, the learning goals are:

- To identify the reasons for bandaging
- To identify the aims of bandaging
- To describe how to apply a bandage
- To describe the precautions that should be observed when bandaging an animal

Bandaging is one of the most important skills that can be learnt by an owner/carer/keeper of an animal in order that they can monitor a bandage that has been applied after injury or surgery.

Reasons for Bandaging

There are several reasons that bandaging may need to be applied:

- Protect a wound
- Prevent self-mutilation and interference
- Support soft tissues (muscle or ligament) in sprains and strains
- Stop bleeding (pressure bandage)
- Prevent contamination of a wound
- Reduce swelling (cold bandage or pack)
- Hold a dressing in place

A clinically applied bandage has three different layers for maximum effect. The layers of a bandage are:

1. *Primary or contact layer*
   Dressings are placed on the surface of the skin against the wound to assist healing. The type of dressing is dependent on the type of wound:
   a. *Adherent dressings*, i.e. gauze swab, tend to stick to the wound and may be difficult to remove without damaging a layer of new tissue.
   b. *Non-adherent dressings*, i.e. Melolin, absorb wound fluids into the cotton wool-type backing. They do not stick to wounds or cause so much damage on removal.
   c. *Moist dressings*, i.e. Intrasite gel to encourage healing.
   d. *Impregnated dressings*, e.g. silver or iodine based, to promote rapid healing.

Animal Biology and Care, Fourth Edition. Emily Jewell.
© 2026 John Wiley & Sons Ltd. Published 2026 by John Wiley & Sons Ltd.
Companion Website: https://www.wiley.com/go/animal/biology4e/jewell

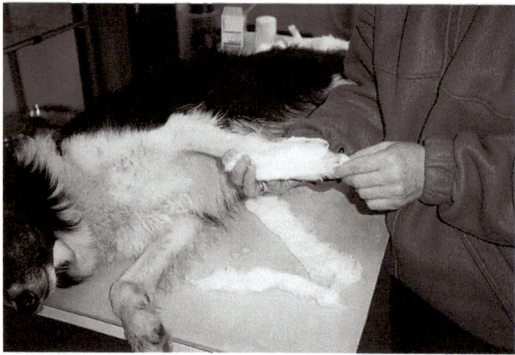

Figure 17.1 The area to be bandaged is protected with a padding material, between the toes and dewclaw.

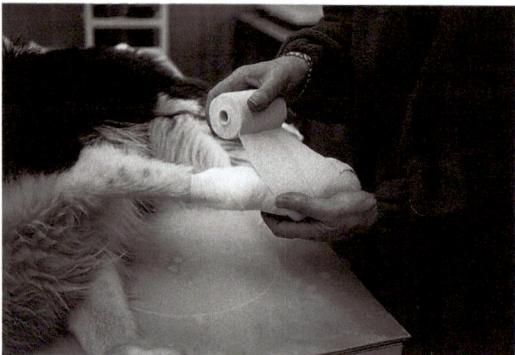

Figure 17.2 A protective layer covers the bandage.

2. *Secondary layer*
   a. This provides the absorption and padding, which promotes comfort for the animal.
   b. Suitable materials that can be used as a secondary layer in bandaging are cotton wool (Figure 17.1), foam, and synthetic padding.
3. *Top layer*
   a. The top layer is known as the *conforming layer*.
   b. The top layer secures the primary and secondary layers and protects from the environment and the patient. This is either an adhesive or a self-adherent material, i.e. Elastoplast or VetWrap (Figure 17.2).
   c. Examples include open weave bandages, tubular bandages, and conforming bandages.

Aims of Bandaging

- The bandage must be comfortable for the animal.
- If the bandage is too loose, the animal will remove it.

- If the bandage is too tight, the animal will try to remove the bandage, and the surface tissues may be damaged by the animal's constant licking.

The aims of bandaging are to:

- Prevent the animal interfering with the area affected under the bandage
- Limit movement in the case of broken bones or tissue damage and therefore limit pain
- Stay on for the required amount of time
- Look neat but will do the job until professional help is reached

Once the bandage has been applied, then it is necessary to watch out for any of the following:

- Smell coming from the bandage
- Obvious discharge or wound leakage
- Discomfort
- Interference or self-mutilation to try and remove the bandage
- Over-exercising
- Bandage getting wet or dirty
- Any signs of ill health

If any of the signs listed previously are seen in an animal with a bandage, seek advice from a veterinary surgeon straight away.

Rules for Bandaging

- Wash hands before starting to prevent introducing infection.
- Get all the materials together before restraining the animal.
- Never stick adhesive tapes onto the animal's coat or hair as it is hard to remove.
- Do not use safety pins or elastic bands to secure the ends of any bandage. Use narrow adhesive tape on the bandage surface.
- In the case of a leg bandage, include the foot; otherwise, it will swell.
- Have the animal restrained in the correct position for application of the bandage.
- If unsure of temperament, always muzzle for safety.
- Apply the bandage in a spiral fashion to prevent the development of pressure rings.
- Bandage limbs from the distal end to the proximal end in a figure of eight spiral pattern.

A tight bandage can cause fluid to build up in the tissues and prevent its proper flow. To make sure a bandage is not applied too tightly, it should be possible to easily slip two fingers under the edge of the bandage.

On limb bandages, only the tips of the toes should be left visible. If exercising an animal outside with a bandaged limb, then several products are commercially available to prevent the bandage from being soiled, e.g. booties.

If an animal is paying too much attention to the bandaged area, then initially check that the bandage is suitably applied and use distraction techniques with treats or toys before considering the use of a bitter-tasting spray or an Elizabethan collar to prevent access to the area.

Figures 17.3–17.8 demonstrate bandaging technique.

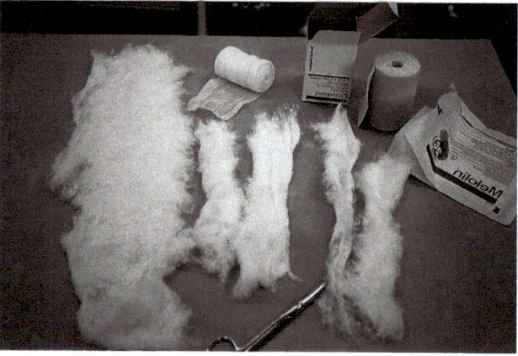

Figure 17.3 Prepare all materials prior to restraint of the animal.

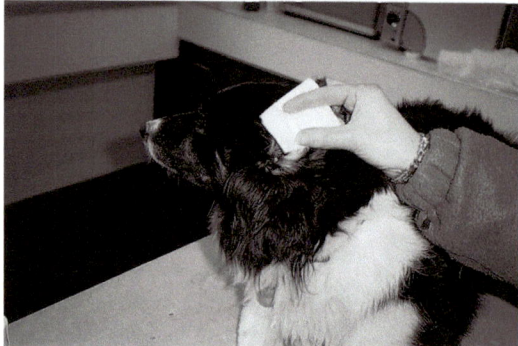

Figure 17.4 Ear bandage. First, protect the wound with a dressing.

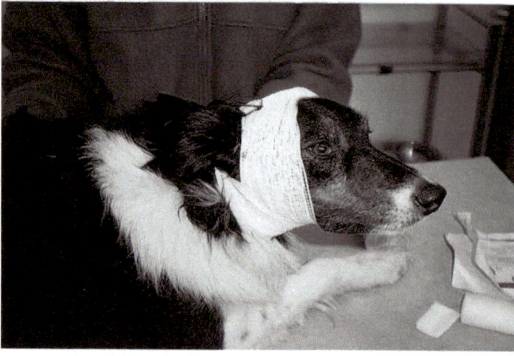

Figure 17.5 Hold dressing in place with the injured ear flap bandaged against the top of the head.

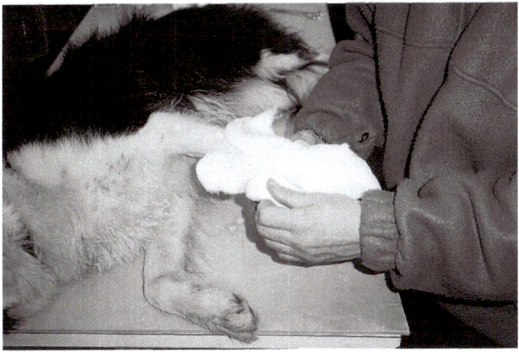

Figure 17.6 The padding.

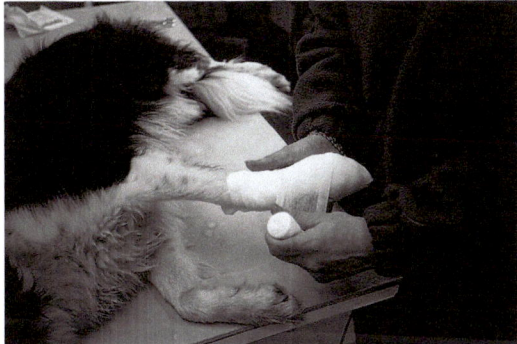

Figure 17.7 The bandage in figure of eight from distal to proximal.

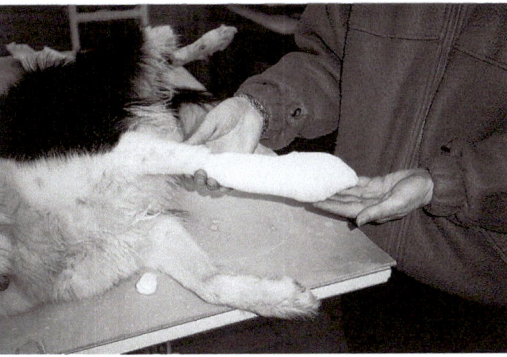

Figure 17.8 The top protective layer.

Summary of Basic Bandaging

There are several reasons for bandaging to be carried out on an animal with the key reason being to protect a wound from deteriorating further and becoming infected.

Bandages should have a primary and secondary layer to protect the wound, along with a top layer to secure the other layers. Once a bandage has been applied, the limb should be monitored to ensure the bandage is not too tight or that infection is not developing under the bandage.

If an animal pays too much attention to a bandaged area, commercial products are available to prevent the animal from interfering and therefore allow the area to recover and heal as quickly as possible.

18

Isolation and Quarantine

Learning goals

In this chapter, the learning goals are:

- To identify the difference between isolation and quarantine
- To describe the processes of isolation and quarantine
- To identify basic guidelines for quarantine of animals in the United Kingdom

The terms isolation and quarantine are often mistakenly interchanged, but it is important to remember that they occur at two very different times and so are separate processes.

Isolation

Isolation is required when an animal has or is suspected of having a contagious disease (Table 18.1). Susceptible animals, such as unvaccinated young, may be subject to *protective isolation* to keep them away from any disease until they have received their primary vaccinations. The home setting becomes the controlled environment.

In many veterinary establishments, there is a purpose-built isolation unit where contagious animals can be housed and nursed. In other animal establishments, an isolation facility may have to be created, as the necessity dictates. This may be a separate room, or it may involve the use of a foldaway cage or cage box in a non-animal area of the unit that can be carefully controlled.

An infected animal should be housed in an area that prevents other animals from being in contact with the disease-producing organisms it will be shedding. Microorganisms can be shed via:

- Urine
- Faeces
- Blood
- Discharges from eyes, ears, nose, mouth, prepuce, vulva, or a wound
- Respiratory tract via sneezing or coughing
- Vomit

Following consideration of the transmission routes for contagious diseases, animals in isolation should be managed as followed:

- Allocate one member of staff to the isolation area
- Wear protective clothing that is only used in that area

Animal Biology and Care, Fourth Edition. Emily Jewell.
© 2026 John Wiley & Sons Ltd. Published 2026 by John Wiley & Sons Ltd.
Companion Website: https://www.wiley.com/go/animal/biology4e/jewell

Table 18.1 Examples of contagious diseases of animals needing isolation.

Dog	Cat	Other species
Canine Distemper	Feline Calicivirus	Avian Influenza (birds)
Canine Infectious Hepatitis	Feline Infectious Peritonitis	Influenza (ferrets)
Canine Influenza	Feline Leukaemia Virus	Pasteurellosis (rabbits)
Canine Parvovirus	Feline Panleukopenia	Psittacosis (birds)
Leptospirosis	Rabies	Salmonella infections (reptiles and birds)
Kennel cough	Ringworm	
Rabies		
Ringworm		
Sarcoptic mange		

- Wear protective footwear or set up a footbath containing disinfectant
- Use gloves and masks as additional protection
- The unit must contain:
  - all required food preparation equipment and food bowls
  - all cleaning equipment and products
  - all instruments that may need to be used
  - medical supplies that may be needed
  - a sink so that all equipment can be cleaned within the unit
  - an area for safe examination of the animal(s)
  - an area for safe disposal of soiled bedding, faeces, urine, vomit, blood, and saliva, which may contain infectious microorganisms

An isolation facility must be suitable for the species it is housing with a separate, effective ventilation system. There should be rest areas and exercise areas appropriate to the species. Any treatments required by the animals must take place within this area. All cleaning equipment and feeding supplies for patients must be for use in isolation only. Hygiene is essential to assist the full recovery of the patient. Thorough cleaning of all surfaces, feeding equipment and bedding materials will reduce the number of microorganisms present.

It is essential never to put healthy animals or humans at risk by careless behaviour. There is also the possibility that the disease may transmit from animals to human owners/carers/keepers (*zoonotic disease*).

Quarantine

Quarantine refers to the process of detaining animals coming into the United Kingdom for a set time of 4 months, in isolation from other animals to screen for disease, specifically rabies.

Quarantine legislation in the United Kingdom applies to pet cats, dogs, ferrets, rabbits, and rodents that are brought into the country.

Legislation that applies to quarantine in the United Kingdom is:

- The Non-Commercial Movement of Pet Animals Order 2011
- Rabies (Importation of Dogs, Cats and Other Mammals) Order 1974

Quarantine applies to:

- Pet cats, dogs, and ferrets that are travelling to the United Kingdom that do not meet the pet travel rules (see Chapter 6)
- Rabbits and rodents travelling from outside the European Union
- Rabbits and rodents travelling from European Union who have not been living there for more than 4 months

Quarantine does not apply to:

- Animals travelling within the United Kingdom
- Animals travelling between the United Kingdom and the Channel Islands or the Isle of Man
- Animals that meet the pet travel rules (see Chapter 6)
- Rabbits and rodents that have been living in Europe for 4 months before entry to the United Kingdom
- Animals that enter and leave within 48 hours and stay in the holding facility at the licensed entry point (port/airport)

Animals coming into the United Kingdom for quarantine processes should only arrive at specifically licensed ports or airports. If your pet needs to go through a Border Control Post, then the animal is limited to arrival at three airports only. This situation applies when pets are arriving directly from a non-European Union country and not travelling with you or is being transported for a commercial purpose.

Animals must only be transported from the entry point to the quarantine premises by a licensed carrier, not by the owners.

All animals are given appropriate accommodation according to size and species. There are recommended minimum internal measurements for individual units, which also state sleeping area and adjoining exercise area size.

Guidelines are in place for the general standards of hygiene and materials used for surfaces in quarantine kennels (e.g. non-slip floors). Also stated are the feeding and management routines, the need for visual stimuli and fresh air access, and the condition and minimum temperature of the sleeping area.

The animal's owner is allowed reasonable access for visiting during the quarantine period. If any signs of ill health arise during the quarantine, the attending veterinary surgeon is consulted, and the owner of the animal is informed immediately.

Release from quarantine can only happen when:

- The animal has been in quarantine for 4 months
- The animal is going back to the country it came from

It is down to the veterinary surgeon responsible for the quarantine premises to decide whether the animal may leave the premises.

Quarantine may be extended if there is an outbreak of rabies at the premises or if the animal is in shared accommodation (only if from same household) and one of the animals dies and rabies cannot be ruled out as the cause of death.

Animal owners are responsible for any costs associated with travel, entry to the United Kingdom, and the quarantine period.

Up to date quarantine rules can be found on the United Kingdom's Government's website www.gov.uk.

Some animal collections operate shorter periods of quarantine (around 30 days) when an animal is brought into the collection to again prevent disease from entering the main collection of animals.

Summary of Isolation and Quarantine

Although the terms isolation and quarantine are often used interchangeably, there are differences between them.

Isolation occurs when an animal has or is suspected of having a contagious disease to prevent it from passing the disease onto other animals.

Quarantine occurs when an animal is brought into the United Kingdom that does not meet the Pet Travel rules.

Similarities in the two processes occur in terms of management of the animals, PPE, and husbandry procedures, ensuring that disease transfer risk is minimised. Any equipment allocated to a specific animal must only be used for that animal and should be cleaned within the facility.

19

Care of the Hospitalised Patient

Learning goals

In this chapter, the learning goals are:

- To identify reasons that an animal may be hospitalised
- To be able to describe the hospital environment for animals
- To be able to describe husbandry and monitoring processes relating to the hospitalised patient
- To describe a nursing care plan
- To describe the importance of isolation and barrier nursing
- To describe the importance of hygiene and cleaning processes in the veterinary hospital

Animals may be hospitalised for several reasons:

- Observation prior to diagnosis
- A surgical operation
- Medical treatment
- Collection of samples or to run diagnostic tests
- Nursing care

When an unwell animal is admitted to the veterinary hospital, it is vital that everything is done to support its recovery. To ensure a high standard of care, there must be adequate facilities, equipment, and trained staff.

Four key concepts that will aid recovery include:

- High standards of hygiene
- Observation of each animal
- High animal welfare standards
- Accurate and diligent record keeping

Hygiene

Within the veterinary hospital environment, high standards of hygiene must be of the utmost importance to protect vulnerable patients. The hospital environment may contain high concentrations of *pathogenic* microorganisms. Injured or diseased patients are at risk due to decreased resistance to infection. Every effort must be made to decrease the microbe population in the hospital environment to safeguard patients.

Animal Biology and Care, Fourth Edition. Emily Jewell.
© 2026 John Wiley & Sons Ltd. Published 2026 by John Wiley & Sons Ltd.
Companion Website: https://www.wiley.com/go/animal/biology4e/jewell

To protect the patient:

- Use disinfectants and antiseptics to control the source of the disease.
- Prevent the transmission of disease – ventilation, isolation of suspect animals, and use of disposable protective clothing.

If mops are used for washing the floor, the following rules should be followed:

- Move the mop around in the disinfectant solution, wring out, and proceed to clean.
- Move the mop from left to right across the body; never push back and forwards in front of the operator.
- Start with the area furthest from the door and move across towards the door methodically to ensure the whole floor is mopped.
- Do not allow anyone to walk on the floor until it is dry.
- Use yellow wet floor signs to indicate that the floor is wet.
- Change the disinfectant solution between rooms.
- Separate mop heads should be used for sterile areas of the hospital.
- Mop heads should be washed in the washing machine and dried daily.
- If used more than once daily, soak 30 minutes in a bucket of disinfectant.
- Never leave in soaking solution for more than 30 minutes.
- Wring out thoroughly before using on the floors.

Regular checks must be made throughout the day to make sure no animal is in soiled housing (Figure 19.1). If the kennel is soiled by body excretions, samples may need to be collected for investigation once the animal has been removed to clean accommodation. Incontinence pads may be used to soakaway any urine.

Basic room cleaning procedure

The basic room cleaning procedure applies to all rooms in the veterinary hospital, but there may be additional elements in rooms such as the surgical theatre, triage room, consultation area, and recovery area.

- Ensure appropriate PPE is worn
- Consider the timing of any cleaning procedures to minimise disruption to patients and clients
- Vacuum or sweep the floor to remove any material and animal hair

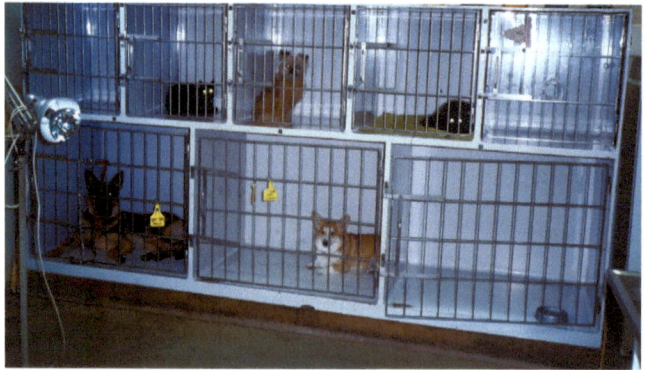

Figure 19.1   Hospital kennels allow easy monitoring of animals.

- Prepare an appropriate disinfectant at the right dilution rate
- Remove waste from all bins and replace plastic liner
- Spot clean surfaces, examination tables, cupboard doors, room doors, light fixtures, and equipment routinely kept in this area
- Clean and disinfect walls
- Check and restock any disposable equipment
- Clean and disinfect the sinks
- Mop the floor with disinfectant
- Regularly empty the vacuum cleaner and change the bag/filter (weekly or more often if required)
- Clean, disinfect, and store cleaning equipment

Adjustments for the consultation room (Figure 19.2a,b)

- Equipment may need to be washed and sterilised
- Clinical waste needs to be disposed of in yellow bags
- Disinfect the room at the end of every consultation period
- Hand drying should be via paper or disposable cloth towels

Adjustments for the triage area (Figure 19.3)

- Removal of all coat clippings
- Equipment may need to be washed and sterilised, including cleaning and lubrication of clippers
- Clinical waste needs to be disposed of in yellow bags
- Spot-clean the room after every patient
- Restock supplies
- Hand drying should be via paper or disposable cloth towels
- Take any samples for analysis to the laboratory or to the office for posting to a distant laboratory

The triage area is where samples may be taken during consultations and where pre-operative procedures are carried out. Pre-operation preparation may include anaesthetising and

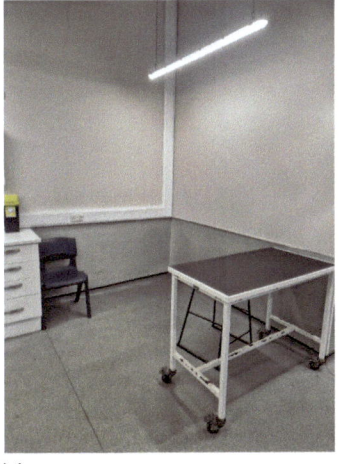 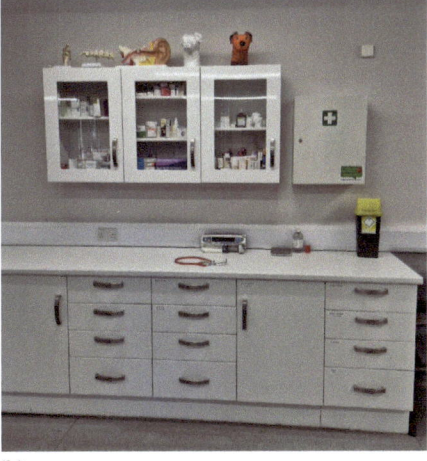

(a)   (b)

Figure 19.2   (a and b) Consultation area.

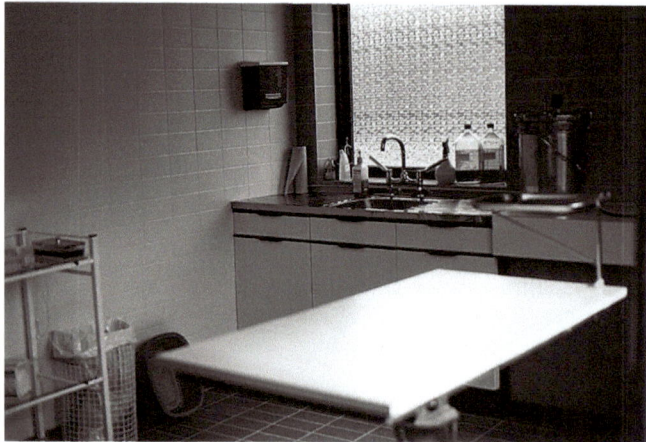

Figure 19.3   Triage area.

clipping the site of surgery in triage, which means no cross-contamination of patients takes place because of high standards of maintenance. In the triage area, there will usually be piped oxygen or a mobile oxygen delivery cylinder, plus emergency treatment drugs, and materials for first aid.

The triage area is always located near to the surgical theatre and sterilising areas for the packing and cleaning of surgical instruments.

Adjustments for sterile areas

- High levels of sterility need to exist in the theatre, the scrubs area, and the equipment preparation areas.
- Personal hygiene needs to be high.
- Surgical wounds can become infected from:
  - The environment
  - The staff
  - Surgical instruments
  - The patient's own microorganisms
- Infected wounds will cause a delay in the healing process.
- Ensure equipment is washed, sterilised, labelled, dated, and stored away for its next use (Figure 19.4).
- Ensure equipment is stored in an organised manner so that all members of the team know where everything is and that it is to hand as necessary.
- Ventilation in the theatre should replace the theatre air with clean air approximately 10 times per hour in order to prevent airborne contamination.

Hygiene terms reminder:

- *Sterilisation* – the removal or destruction of all living microorganisms including bacterial spores.
- *Disinfectants* – will kill pathogenic microorganisms.
- *Antiseptics* – prevent microorganisms from multiplying and therefore infection fails to develop.
- *Asepsis* – is a state of being free from microorganisms.

See Chapter 11 for further information on hygiene.

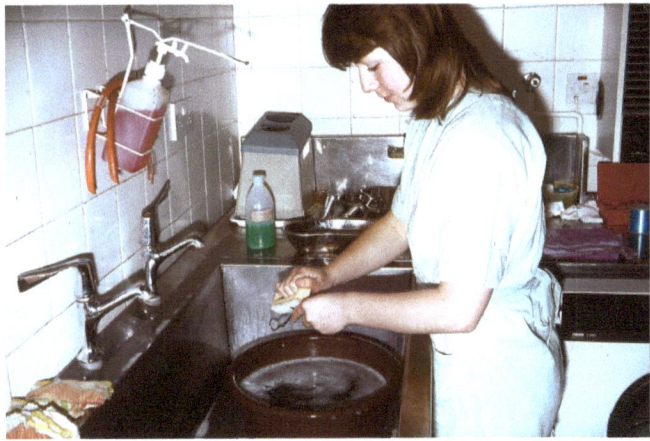

Figure 19.4   Instruments in cold water/detergent ready for sterilisation.

Observation

There should always be staff within the veterinary hospital who are monitoring the animals throughout their shift. The veterinary surgeon should examine an animal at least twice daily to assess progress.

Nursing or veterinary care assistant staff are responsible for the animal's cleanliness, feeding, watering, and medication at correct times and reports on any changes to its condition.

The observation process should monitor the following:

- The patient's behaviour along with any behavioural changes
- Signs of pain or discomfort
- The appetite of the animal
- The ease of feeding, quantity of food eaten, and any favourite foods
- Amount of water consumed
- Urine output, characteristics, and ease of passing
- Faecal output, characteristics, and ease of passing
- Breathing rate and characteristics, e.g. does the animal cough after waking up, as this could be indicative of heart issues
- TPR assessments recorded as often as is necessary
- Mobility of the animal
- Self-grooming
- Sleep/rest periods

Animal welfare

In line with the five animal needs (Chapter 6), animal welfare should be of a high standard in the veterinary environment and incorporated into a *nursing care plan*. Hospitalised animals are dependent upon their carers to meet all their needs.

1. *Health*:
    a. Admittance to the hospital is to reduce any effects of disease, injury, or illness. Pain relief will be provided as necessary and medication and surgical treatment will be administered as required according to the results of diagnostic procedures undertaken.

  b. Check medications for:
  - **i.** Timing
  - **ii.** Dosage per day
  - **iii.** Form of medication, e.g. tablets, injection, ointment
  - **iv.** Whether assistance is required for successful administration

2. ***Behaviour*:**
   - **a.** It is more than likely that behaviour will deviate from normal for the animal whilst it is hospitalised, as it will be trying to cope with an unfamiliar environment and any illness or surgical procedure.
   - **b.** Some animals may not cope well with the change of environment and require different care to others
   - **c.** When an animal starts to show normal behaviour again, it indicates that the animal is on its way to recovering.

3. ***Companionship*:**
   - **a.** Social species are unlikely to be housed with other animals of the same species during long stays in the veterinary hospital. Day cases may allow a companion to be admitted for company, depending on the procedure being undertaken. In most cases of hospitalised animals, human contact that is gentle and reassuring is calming for the animal.

4. ***Diet*:**
   - **a.** A suitable diet should be available for the animal. In some cases, the owner will bring the usual diet from home to prevent digestive upset from a change of diet.
   - **b.** Fresh water should always be available unless the animal is on a restricted water intake or having its urine output specifically measured (Figure 19.5).
   - **c.** Feeding bowls and equipment should be washed and disinfected daily.
   - **d.** Feeding bowls should not be able to be tipped over and therefore leave the animal in a wet environment.
   - **e.** If an animal is not to be fed or watered, then a sign should be placed on the housing (Figure 19.6). This may be due to:
     - **i.** The animal having surgery scheduled
     - **ii.** Medical conditions
     - **iii.** The animal is or has been recently vomiting
     - **iv.** Recovering from surgery to the gastrointestinal tract

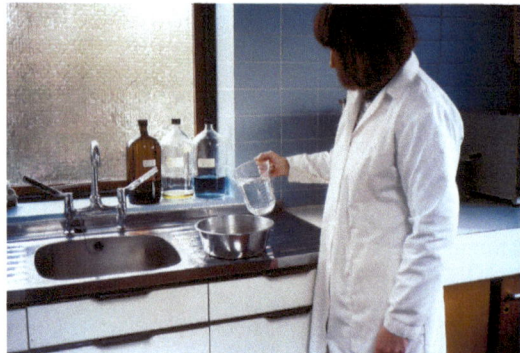

Figure 19.5   Measure the required amount and record on the observation chart.

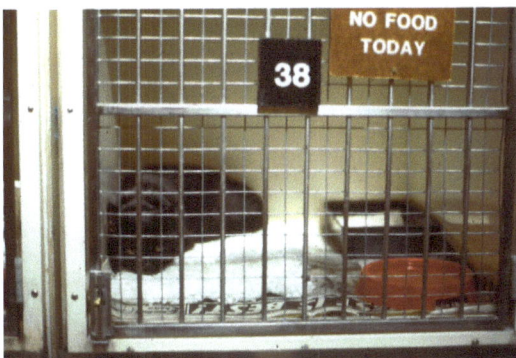

Figure 19.6   Identify kennels where restrictions are in place.

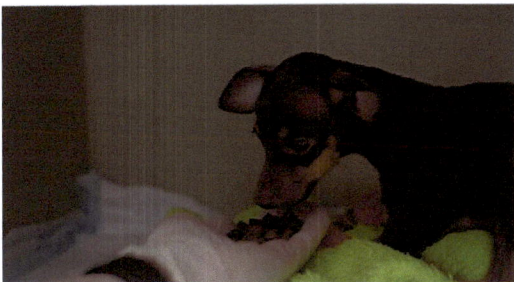

Figure 19.7   Post-operatively, patients may need encouragement to feed. *Source*: Hand feeding a dog recovering from surgery stock photos, royalty-free images, vectors, video.

        v. The animal requires blood tests

        vi. The animal has diarrhoea

    f. Feeding routine in a veterinary hospital is usually twice daily to:

        i. assess appetite in the morning and evening

        ii. assist with administration of medication

    g. Handfeeding may be required for post-operative patients to encourage eating (Figure 19.7).

5. *Environment*:

A hospitalised animal has been taken from its normal environment and routine and has been admitted into an environment where the scents, sounds, and people are different. Combined with any ill health or surgical procedures, the animal will feel vulnerable.

    a. The environment should be as suitable as possible for the animal but hygienic enough to prevent any contamination of surgical wounds.

    b. Exercise may be possible, depending on whether the animal is able to walk comfortably.

    c. The environment must be kept at a suitable temperature and have adequate ventilation (no draughts) with bedding provided where possible (often in the form of Vetbed – Figure 19.8) that is easy to remove, wash, and dry.

    d. *Temperature control*

        i. Most mammals and birds regulate their own body temperature through homeostatic processes. When conscious and healthy, temperature control is usually good, but when ill, injured, pre- or post-operative, then patients may need help to regain lost body heat and prevent the development of shock.

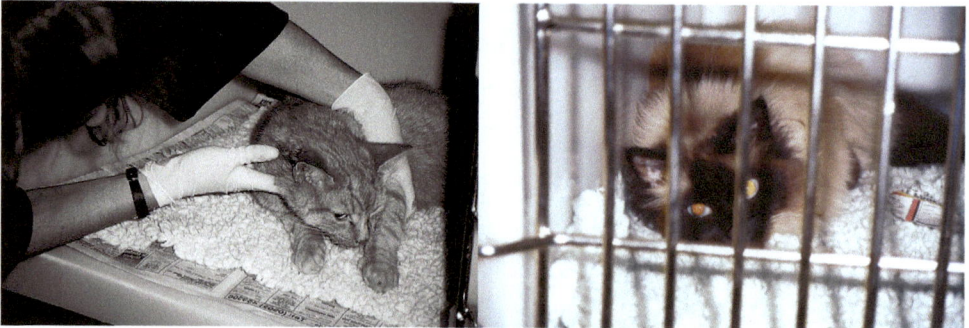

Figure 19.8 Bedding will support body temperature post-operatively.

    ii. Conditions causing a raised body temperature include:
- Heat stroke
- Infection
- Stress
- Exercise
- Poisons

    iii. Conditions causing a lowered body temperature are:
- Very young/old
- Serious haemorrhage
- Shock
- Recovery from anaesthesia
- Poisons

    iv. It is important not to overheat an animal but simply support the reestablishment of their own thermoregulatory processes within normal range for the species.

    v. External heat can be provided via:
- Environmental thermostat controls
- Kennels with underfloor heating
- Heat pads
- Incubator for small or newborn animals
- Bubble wrap
- Lightweight blankets
- Space blankets
- Vet beds
- Bean bags

    vi. Using external heat lamps can be harmful if the animal is unable to move away as the animal could overheat and potentially suffer burns to the skin if the lamp is too close. Always keep the lamp a minimum of 1m from the body of the animal to avoid any overheating or burns.

    vii. Reptiles will require an external source of heat due to being ectothermic. Ensure that the heat source is appropriate for the species.

e. *Environmental enrichment*

    i. Most of the enrichment for hospitalised patients will come via human contact, such as assisting with eating and drinking, grooming, and TLC time spent reassuring the animal (Figure 19.9).

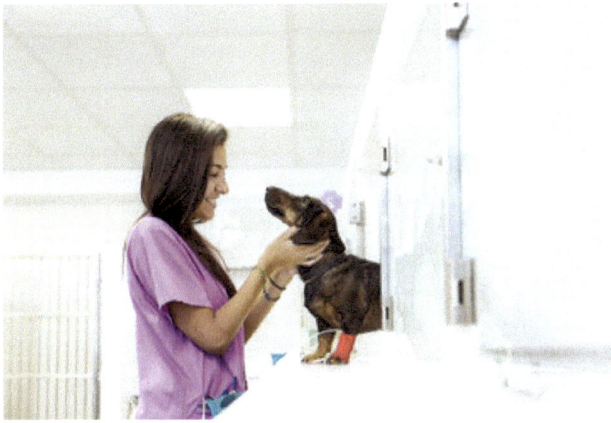

Figure 19.9 TLC to promote recovery. *Source*: Veterinary nursing stock photos, royalty-free images, vectors, video.

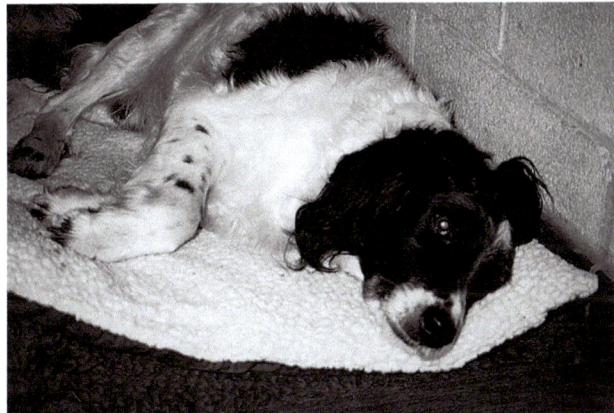

Figure 19.10 Plenty of bedding for recumbent patients.

    ii. Additional enrichment can be provided by feeding favourite foods and providing toys once the animal is able to interact with them, providing they do not become too excited.

    iii. Calming music can be beneficial

    iv. Pheromone plug ins may also be of use

Recumbent patients

In the veterinary context, a *recumbent patient* is an animal that is unable to stand or move on its own. It often stays lying down for a long time. Recumbent patients often need more individualised care to promote recovery.

    Measures that can be implemented include:

- Using deep bedding to prevent pressure on any bony areas (Figure 19.10). Bedding should be comfortable and supportive to prevent pressure sores developing

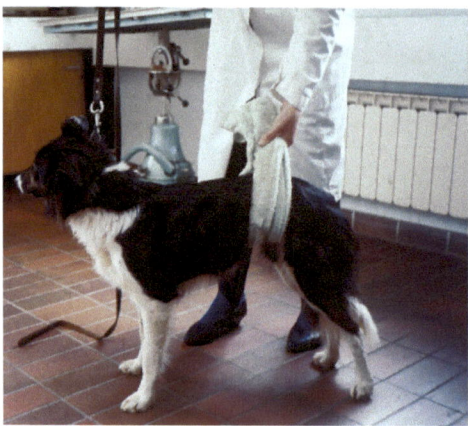

Figure 19.11   Assisting a dog to stand using a sling to support hindquarters.

- Regular hygiene checks to ensure the animal does not stay in a soiled kennel. Consider using incontinence pads to help soak up any urine
- Assist drinking to prevent dehydration
- Assist eating, giving small meals often
- Groom and clean away any food on the coat after feeding
- Encourage limb movements to stimulate circulation (Figure 19.11) unless the veterinary surgeon has advised against this
- Provide the relevant medication on a timely basis
- Turn the animal every 1–2 hours to prevent fluid pooling in the chest due to shallow breathing
- Rub and stroke the body to stimulate surface circulation, generating heat and fluid movement within the tissues
- Spend time playing with the animal
- Assist the animal to urinate or check any inserted urinary catheter

Nursing care plans

Nursing care plans are dynamic plans that should be developed following an initial assessment of the physical, psychological, and environmental needs of an animal as identified on the list for observation. Talking to the owner can help in establishing the usual behaviour and routines of the animal.

The initial assessment can identify potential problems as well as actual problems, and from this information, the goals of the nursing team for the individual care of the animal are created.

The care plan includes any interventions that are needed, such as medical treatment, surgery required, dietary adjustment, and environmental modifications. It should be implemented by the nursing team and constantly evaluated during the time of hospitalisation for the animal.

If the animal is not recovering as expected or deteriorates in any way, the plan should be adjusted by the veterinary surgeon and the nursing team.

Animals should be seen as holistic beings, and any treatment should be designed accordingly.

Handling hospitalised patients

Handling should be carried out as part of routine husbandry procedures such as grooming/coat care along with health checking. Wiping any discharges from the nose, eye, or ears and keeping the area around the mouth moistened using damp cotton wool will help to simulate the animal's own grooming routines. This contributes to a feeling of well-being for the animal, familiarises them with the nursing team, and promotes recovery.

Any handling for diagnostic or surgical procedures should be gentle and considerate of the animal's condition.

Isolation and barrier nursing

If the patient has a suspected contagious or zoonotic disease, it must be moved to the isolation area. Barrier nursing follows strict rules to prevent cross infection between routine patients or staff members.

Barrier nursing provision involves:

- Wearing protective clothing – disposable apron, intact gloves, and mask if necessary
- Change of footwear
- Required drugs and medical equipment for patient care
- Cleaning equipment for unit use only
- Feeding materials and cleaning of bowls in the unit
- One member of the staff to work in isolation only and not handle any other patients

Recordkeeping

1. Accurate records must be kept for each animal. At the time of writing, records are often kept digitally in which case access to them must be secure to maintain confidentiality. Paper records may be attached to the front of the hospital cage for ease of access during daily monitoring.
2. Hospital kennels should be numbered to ensure the right records are kept for the right animal (Figure 19.12)
3. Records should contain pet details and other information which is vital to the veterinary surgeon who must assess the patient's progress (Figure 19.13):

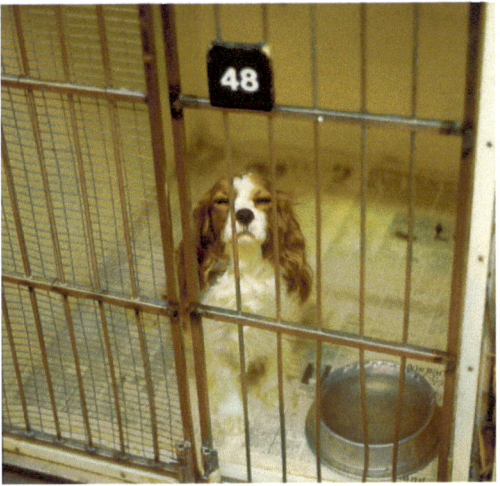

Figure 19.12 Numbering of kennels for ID purposes.

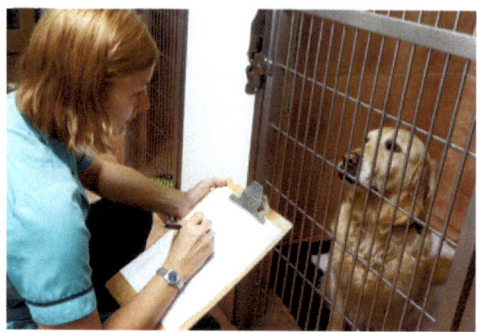

Figure 19.13 Recording information on patient. *Source*: Veterinary nurse stock photos, royalty-free images, vectors, video.

Summary of Care of the Hospitalised Patient

There are many reasons why an animal may be admitted to a veterinary hospital, but for all reasons, it is important that the animal has a positive experience.

Ensuring that the animal is well cared for and that it is not subject to any additional health concerns contributes to that experience.

Maintenance of high standards of hygiene in all areas of the veterinary practice, close observation of individual animals, implementation of high animal welfare standards, and accurate, diligent record keeping all help to promote recovery of the animal.

20

Medication for Animals

Learning goals

In this chapter, the learning goals are:

- To define the term pharmacology
- To identify the possible routes of administration of medication in animals
- To describe the handling and dispensing of pharmacological products
- To identify and describe relevant legislation relating to veterinary medicines including:
  - Veterinary Medicines (Amendment, etc.) Regulations 2024
  - Misuse of Drugs Regulations 2001
  - Misuse of Drugs and Misuse of Drugs (Designation) (England and Wales and Scotland) (Amendment) (No. 2) Regulations 2024
  - Small Animal Exemption Scheme (SAES)

Pharmacology is the branch of science concerned with the study of drugs. It covers the following aspects in relation to any drug administered to the body:

- The way in which the drug affects the body
- Absorption of the drug into the body
- Metabolism of the drug by the body
- The process of excretion of the drug from the body

The process of giving out drugs to the person responsible for an animal is known as *dispensing*. Drugs can either be dispensed by the veterinary practice at which the owner is registered or by taking a prescription to a dispensing pharmacist. There are licensed online providers who dispense veterinary medications once a prescription has been received from the consulting veterinary surgeon. Clients must pay for the prescription to be dispensed, but the cost of the medication from the online provider may be less than the veterinary practice.

Animal Biology and Care, Fourth Edition. Emily Jewell.
© 2026 John Wiley & Sons Ltd. Published 2026 by John Wiley & Sons Ltd.
Companion Website: https://www.wiley.com/go/animal/biology4e/jewell

Routes of Administration

Administering medication

Drugs can be administered in various ways to the animal's body. The method in which the drug is administered to the body is known as the *route of administration*. The route of administration often depends on:

- the part of the body that is the target of the drug,
- how quickly the effect of the drug is required,
- the ability of the owner to give the drug.

1. ***Oral administration***
   - *Oral administration* is the most frequently used route for drugs because the owner can treat at home. The products are supplied in various forms, e.g. tablet, powder, paste, and liquid (Figure 20.1).
   - Many tablets have an outer coating and therefore should never be broken up or crushed in case the action of the drug is reduced. Reasons for coating tablets include:
     - Protection of the drug from moisture
     - To hide an unpleasant taste
     - To assist in identification
     - To protect the drug from hydrochloric acid in the stomach (enteric coated)
     - Protection of the stomach from the irritant effect of a drug
   - Oral administration can have disadvantages:
     - If the animal is vomiting
     - Absorption can be slow and some of the drug may not be absorbed at all
     - The presence of food may reduce the drug's effect
     - The animal may refuse to swallow the drug
     - The owner is unable to give the drug to the animal

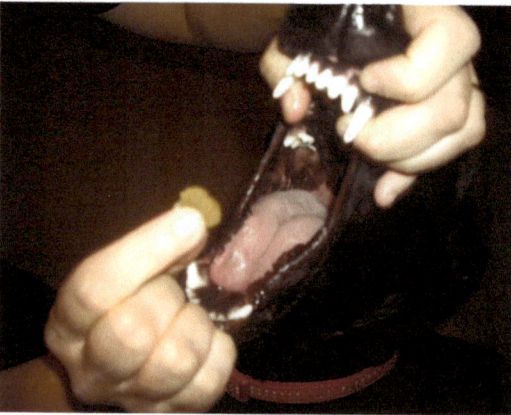

Figure 20.1 The mouth is opened wide so that the tablet can then be placed at the back of the throat for swallowing. Once the mouth is closed, the throat should be rubbed to encourage swallowing of the tablet.

2. *Parenteral administration*

- The *parenteral administration* route is any other administration route into the body than the mouth. It usually refers to or is taken to mean 'by injection'. Any drug administered by this method must be sterile, and the method involves cleaning of the skin site and personal hygiene. The most frequently used injection methods are:
  - *Subcutaneous* – into the connective tissues below the skin (below the hypodermis). This method is for non-irritant drugs, and absorption of the drug is slow.
  - *Intramuscular* – directly into a muscle body (hind leg or back). This method is used for small volumes of drug only and can be painful, but the drug is more rapidly absorbed than by the subcutaneous route.
  - *Intravenous* – into a surface vein (foreleg, hind leg, or neck vein). This method places the drug directly into the bloodstream and has very rapid action.
  - Other injection routes used less frequently are:
    - *Epidural* – into the vertebral canal to give spinal pain control (analgesia)
    - *Intra-articular* – directly into a joint
    - *Intradermal* – into the skin structure

3. *Topical administration*

- Drugs administered via the *topical route* are applied to a surface tissue of the body like the skin, eyes, or ears (Figure 20.2).
- They are either absorbed just into the surface of the skin or mucous membranes or deeper into the structure of the skin, depending on the material used to carry the drug.
- Some topical drugs may be able to move into body systems, and that is why the operator must immediately wash off any drug that contacts their skin.
- Types of carriers used include:
  - Water to place wettable powder against the skin
  - Petroleum jelly an ointment that melts with body heat
  - Oil and water together as a cream, which will penetrate the skin layers
  - Detergent-based products as medicated shampoos to cover the skin surface before rinsing off

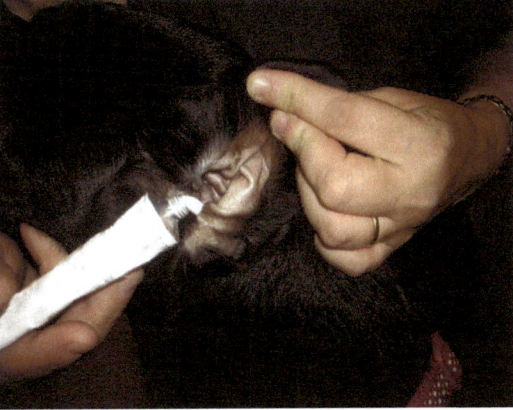

Figure 20.2   The cream is applied to the ear flap.

Pharmacology and Dispensing of Drugs

Drug administration

For safe drug administration, be sure that the following are checked and confirmed before medication is given:

1. Is it the right:
   a. drug?
   b. patient?
   c. dosage?
   d. route for the drug?
   e. time interval?
2. Administering the right drug:
   a. Check label
   b. Check against the animal's medical record, if available
   c. If the writing is illegible on the medical record, get it clarified
   d. Understand the difference between trade names and generic names
3. Administering the right drug to the right patient:
   a. Check the ID on the animal
   b. Check the ID on the kennel
   c. Check any medical records
4. Administering the right dose:
   a. Read instructions
   b. Check with supervising member of staff
5. Administer the drug by the correct route:
   a. Know the meaning of abbreviations:
      i. *i.m.* – intramuscular
      ii. *p.o.* – by mouth *(per os)*
      iii. *i.v.* – intravenous
      iv. *s.c.* – subcutaneous
   b. Do not crush 'delayed action' capsules/tablets to mix with food.
   c. Some drugs must be given *i.m.* for absorption as they may be irritant given *s.c.*, so always check the instructions on the container or product leaflet.
6. Administering the drug at the right time:
   a. Know the abbreviations:
      i. *b.i.d.* or *b.d.* – twice daily or every 12 hours
      ii. *t.i.d.* or *t.d.* – three times daily or every 8 hours
      iii. *q.i.d.* or *q.d.* – four times daily or every 6 hours
   b. Ensure the drug intervals are adhered to for best therapeutic levels.

Any drugs given to an animal should be documented on the animal's records:

- The drug, dose, route, site of administration, date, and time
- If there is no recording, assume the drug has not been given
- Record after drug is given, not before, in case of problems
- Be aware of drug/food or drug/drug interactions
- Some drugs must be given with food, like aspirin
- Some drugs must be given on an empty stomach, like the antibiotic ampicillin

- Drug interactions when treating for heart disease, arthritis, and epilepsy
- Record any adverse effects seen

Labels for drug containers

For legal requirements, the essential information on a container label is:

a. Veterinary practice name and address
b. Date of dispensing
c. Owner's name and address
d. Animal's name
e. Product name and strength, e.g. Metacam 1.5 mg/ml
f. Total quantity supplied
g. Dose rate, e.g. 1 tablet
h. Directions for use, e.g. twice daily
i. Any specific precautions (e.g. store in the fridge)
j. The words KEEP OUT OF REACH OF CHILDREN
k. The words FOR ANIMAL TREATMENT ONLY
l. If applicable, the words FOR EXTERNAL USE ONLY
m. Expiry date if relevant
n. Withdrawal period if relevant (usually applies to animals in the food chain)

Warnings should also be attached to certain drugs such as aspirin in full-strength form (150 mg). Labels should read 'Unsuitable for cats'. This drug can be used in humans and dogs, but in cats, its effect lasts a lot longer. If a second dose is given by the owner too soon, then the cat will be overdosed. Clearance time for aspirin is:

- Humans – 4 hours
- Dogs – 8 hours
- Cats – 30 hours

Handling and dispensing of drugs

Legal aspects

Drugs used in the treatment of animals are classified under the Veterinary Medicines (Amendment, etc.) Regulations (VMR) 2024 into four groups. VMR control the following aspects relating to veterinary medicines in use in the United Kingdom – manufacture, advertising, marketing, supply, and administration.

Current information relating to the categorisation of medicines can be located on the Veterinary Medicine Directorate website:

- **POM-V** – these are *prescription-only medicines – veterinarian*; dispensing of these medicines can only occur once they have been prescribed by a veterinary surgeon. The veterinary surgeon must make a clinical assessment of the animal or relevant information in order to prescribe drugs in the POM-V category. POM-V drugs must be dispensed by the veterinary surgeon or a pharmacist. Examples include antimicrobials, controlled drugs (CD), and vaccinations. Some medicated feedstuffs fall into this category.
- **POM-VPS** – these are *prescription-only medicines – veterinary surgeons, pharmacists* and *suitably qualified persons (SQP)*; these medicines must be prescribed and supplied by a veterinary

surgeon, pharmacist, or SQP and dispensed from registered premises. A clinical assessment of the animal or relevant information is not essential to prescribe these drugs. Clients may request prescriptions to obtain the drugs elsewhere for this category of medicine. Examples of POM-VPS drugs include spot-on medications, anthelmintics, and some vaccinations in farm livestock. Some medicated feedstuffs also fall into this category.

- **NFA-VPA** – these are *non-food animal medicines – veterinary surgeons, pharmacists and SQP*; medicines in this category are only for companion animals but not horses. These drugs must be supplied from registered premises by either a veterinary surgeon, pharmacist, or SQP. A clinical assessment is not required to supply these drugs, and they do not require a prescription. Examples of these drugs include anthelmintics for companion animals.
- **AVM-GSL** – these are *authorised veterinary medicines – general sales list*; these drugs can be supplied by any retailer such as pet stores and supermarkets. Drugs in this category usually have a wide margin of safety in their usage. Prescriptions are not required. Examples include vitamins and minerals.

The classification group to which the medicine belongs is found on the drug container label and any outer packaging. For medicines in the POM-VPS and NFA-VPS categories, users must be advised of the safe and effective use of the medicine.

A special category of drugs, those that could be abused by humans, is known as *CD*. The legislation applicable is the Misuse of Drugs Regulations (MDR) 2001, which are supported by The Misuse of Drugs and Misuse of Drugs (Designation) (England and Wales and Scotland) (Amendment) (No. 2) Regulations 2024.

The MDR 2001 is divided into five schedules. These schedules are set out in decreasing order of the need to control the drug:

a. *Schedule 1* – These are drugs with no recognised medical use and which have high potential for abuse. They include drugs like methylenedioxymethamphetamine (MDMA; ecstasy) and hallucinogenic drugs such as lysergic acid diethylamide (LSD) and are not legally held in veterinary practice for the purpose of treating animals. They can only be used by research premises with a Home Office Licence. Schedule 1 drugs have the strictest control measures.

b. *Schedule 2* – These are drugs recognised for medicinal use but a high potential for abuse. They include the opiate analgesics (pain control) like cocaine, morphine, pethidine, and etorphine (very strong anaesthetic agent) along with cannabis. These drugs are POM-V, and records are kept on their ordering, supply, safe storage and, if out of date or not required, their destruction.

c. *Schedule 3* – These are drugs recognised for medicinal use with less potential for abuse than those in schedule 2. Such drugs include barbiturates (used for anaesthesia, control of epilepsy, and euthanasia), some minor stimulant drugs, and some analgesics (pain control). These drugs are POM-V and must have safe storage and purchase records.

d. *Schedule 4* – includes the benzodiazepine drugs such as Valium (diazepam) (used to reduce stress). When these drugs are given to patients within the veterinary practice (e.g. in injectable form only), they are exempt from restrictions.

e. *Schedule 5* – are drugs for medicinal use with the lowest potential for abuse. These drugs contain preparations with only traces of otherwise CD, such as codeine (cough mixture) and morphine (kaolin and morphine for diarrhoea treatment). The levels of drug are so small that they are exempt from restrictions.

Some drugs carry special risks. Harmful products may produce an acute effect immediately after contact, whereas others may accumulate over time and constant exposure will be necessary before their effect on the operator or nurse is seen.

High-risk products include:

- Certain hormone products, like those used to postpone oestrus
- Cytotoxic drugs – those used in the treatment of cancers
- Gaseous anaesthetic agents like halothane
- Certain antibiotics
- Antifungal powders – those used to treat ringworm
- Insecticides

Small Animal Exemption Scheme

The SAES allows certain veterinary medicines that fall into this category to be licensed for use in certain small pet species by the Secretary of State who has reviewed the active ingredient contained in the drug and declared that it is not required to be under veterinary control. The medicine may then be marketed under the SAES. Pets covered include aquarium fish, caged birds, homing pigeons, ferrets, rabbits, small rodents, reptiles, and amphibians. Although these drugs must be manufactured under stringent conditions and vigilantly monitored as to adverse effects and efficacy, they do not have a legal distribution category but can be similarly classed as AVM-GSL drugs. SAES drugs must not contain antibiotic, narcotic, or psychotropic substances. They can only be administered orally, topically, or in water (for fish). The medicines can only be sold in single-course pack sizes and must be labelled correctly.

Drug Resistance

Since the mid-1960s, it has been identified that some pathogens can be resistant to drug treatment, and this causes problems in the animal. Such pathogens include:

a. **Methicillin-Resistant *Staphylococcus aureus* – MRSA**
In normal circumstances, *Staphylococcus aureus* is a bacterium found on the skin surface and in the oral cavity and nasal passages of animals. In hospitalised patients, *S. aureus* can multiply and invade the body itself, causing food poisoning, skin infections, and post-operative wound infections, which can lead to septicaemia. *Staphylococcus aureus* is a pathogen of concern as outbreaks are known to cause death. Antibiotics that are commonly used to treat this bacterial infection are ineffective in some cases due to the development of resistance within the bacteria. This resistance includes the drug methicillin, hence the term MRSA. If an outbreak is caused by MRSA, then early diagnosis and alternative antibiotic treatment is required. *Staphylococcus pseudintermedius* found in dogs has also shown resistance similar to MRSA.

b. ***Clostridium difficile* – *C. difficile***
Clostridium difficile is a bacterium that can be found throughout the environment in soil, water, faeces, and processed food products. Humans, mammals, some birds, and reptiles naturally carry this bacterial strain in their intestines without any effects. *Clostridium difficile* can be transmitted through faeces and accidental ingestion from contaminated surfaces. The bacterium can produce spores that can exist in the environment for weeks/months. In normal circumstances, if the bacterium is ingested, it is prevented from multiplying in the body by the healthy bacterial population found in the intestines. However, if an animal's healthy intestinal bacterial population is compromised due to disease or treatment with antibiotics such as *penicillin* and *cephalosporins*, then *C. difficile* takes the opportunity to multiply rapidly and cause

problems by producing a toxin that attacks the lining of the intestines, leading to digestive problems and watery diarrhoea. Research has shown that some *C. difficile* strains are zoonotic, e.g. *C. difficile RT078*, can spread between farm animals and humans.

c. **Salmonella species**

Some strains of Salmonella have shown resistance to commonly used antibiotics e.g. *Salmonella infantis* in poultry and *S. typhimurium* in reptiles, birds, and rodents.

d. **Escherichia coli (E. coli):**

Certain strains of *E. coli* are resistant to many antibiotics and can cause severe infections. Examples include *Extended-Spectrum Beta-Lactamase (ESBL)-producing E. coli* found in dogs, cats, farm livestock, and wildlife.

Drugs Glossary

Group	Definition
Anabolic	Promotes growth of body tissue
Anaesthesia	Causes a temporary loss of sensation for surgical procedures
Analgesic	Relieves or prevents pain
Anthelmintic	Kills internal parasitic worms
Antibiotic	Disrupts or destroys bacteria
Anticoagulant	Prevents blood from clotting
Antidiuretic	Hormone which reduces urine output
Antiseizure	Prevent epilepsy seizures
Barbiturate	Sedative and sleep-inducing drugs
Corticosteroids	Suppress inflammation
Cytotoxic	Toxic to living cells, used in chemotherapy for cancer treatment
Diuretic	Increases urine production
Emetic	Causes vomiting
Narcotic	Relieve pain, dull the senses and induce drowsiness
Sedative	Reduces awareness of surroundings
Vaccine	Stimulates the production of antibodies

Summary of Medications

Veterinary drug prescription, administration, storage, and usage are tightly controlled by legislation in the United Kingdom to keep animals and humans safe.

Prescribed drugs must be labelled accurately and only given to the animal for which they were intended.

Drugs must be handled carefully and administered in the correct way to the animal, taking account of the amount of drug to be provided and the frequency at which it must be given.

Misuse of veterinary drugs can be dangerous and cause complications in the treatment of animals.

Section 3

Animal Husbandry

21

Animal Handling and Restraint

Learning goals

In this chapter, the learning goals are:

- To identify the reasons for handling and restraining animals
- To identify the correct approaches when handling and restraining animals
- To describe suitable examples of animal handling and restraint procedures for a range of species
- To identify restraint equipment that may be used with a range of animals

Why Do We Handle Animals?

Most domestic species of animals will need handling at some point during their life. They may need to be handled for a health check, if they are injured or unwell or just for their overall safety.

For safe, effective, and sensitive handling to take place, it is important to appreciate the behavioural differences between species. Body language can be quite complex in some species and must be considered before approaching the animal.

Handling may give rise to fear and stress in the animal, which could be due to a learnt response following a bad handling experience. Any knowledge of the individual's temperament or behaviour in given situations is helpful information.

Animals should be accustomed to handling from an early age. Teaching the animal to tolerate sensitive areas like ears, feet, mouth, and teeth being examined will make life less stressful for the animal and handler in later life.

Reasons for handling animals may include:

- Daily, weekly, monthly health checks
- Grooming
- Transportation
- First aid situations
- Examination after injury
- Receiving medication

Animal Biology and Care, Fourth Edition. Emily Jewell.
© 2026 John Wiley & Sons Ltd. Published 2026 by John Wiley & Sons Ltd.
Companion Website: https://www.wiley.com/go/animal/biology4e/jewell

Why Do We Need to Restrain Animals?

We may need to restrain animals for their safety and the handler's safety.
Situations where an animal may need to be restrained may include:

- Medical procedures, e.g. injections, prophylactic treatments, administering medication, and vaccination
- Collection of diagnostic samples, such as blood, urine, and saliva
- For therapeutic purposes, such as physiotherapy and hydrotherapy

Restraint may be:

- Physical – can be manual or with the use of equipment, such as nets and muzzles
- Chemical – e.g. for surgery or diagnostic procedures
- Environmental – traps, cages, kennels, etc.

Approaching an Animal for Handling

- Assess the animal's behaviour and body language
- Be quiet but confident to establish control of the situation
- Talk in a reassuring manner
- Never corner the animal; always leave supposed escape options
- Reach out to introduce yourself to the animal with a loosely clenched fist, palm facing the floor
- Stroke the animal and accustom it to your voice and scent but be aware that some animals may be head shy
- Only lift the animal if the approach has been accepted
- Handle with minimum restraint, especially cats
- If the animal becomes or is aggressive, then a firm method of restraint is required for the safety of handlers

Examples of Behaviour Seen When Animals Are Unwilling to Be Handled

- Cats – hiss, adopt defensive posture, growl, strike with front claws, and flatten their ears to the skull and dilation of the pupils
- Dogs – hackles raised, growling, lips in snarl position, ears forward, barking, and attempting to bite
- Ferrets – may hiss or screech, fluffed up tail, and unusual biting
- Guinea pigs – squealing, teeth chattering, freezing, and hiding
- Rabbits – biting, scratching using hind legs, thumping hind legs on floor, and, if terrified, squealing
- Small rodents, e.g. rats, hamsters, and gerbils – biting, scratching
- Birds – screeching, wing flapping, biting, and hiding

- Lizards – hissing, tail flicking, making themselves look bigger, biting, and colour changes in some species, e.g. chameleon
- Snakes – hissing, striking, increase in tongue flicking, and hiding

Handling Procedures

It must be remembered that there are different handling techniques available, and these may be used within the animal industry. The information provided are examples of effective, safe, suitable methods that do not compromise the welfare of the animal being handled or the safety of the handler.

Before handling any animal, always check the reason that it is being handled as well as the behaviour and temperament of the animal.

Cats

- Use calm, confident movements
- Speak gently and quietly
- Make contact with the cat by stroking the head gently and progress along the cat's back. When the cat responds, pick the cat up by placing one hand under the cat's chest and the other hand under the cat's hindquarters. Hold the cat to the body to help it feel secure (Figure 21.1).

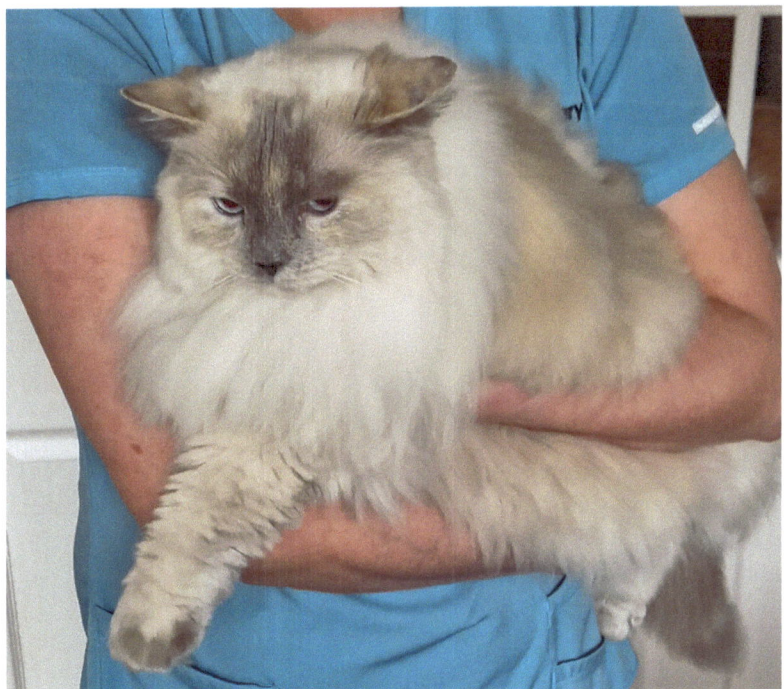

Figure 21.1   Handling technique for a cat.

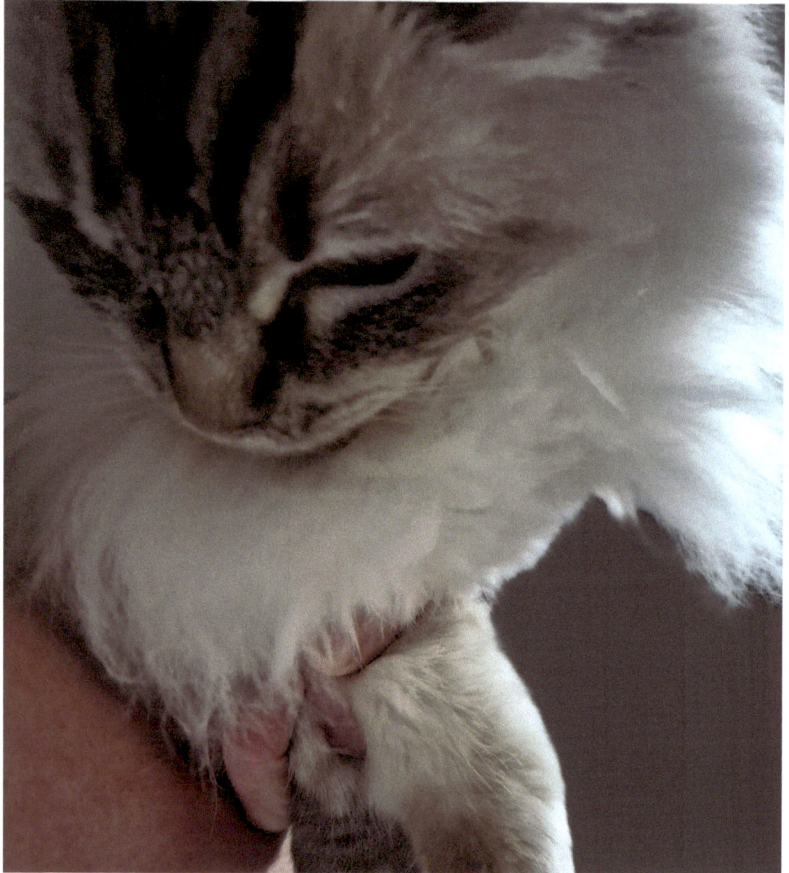

Figure 21.2   Secure hold of the forelegs of a cat.

The front legs of the cat need to be securely held between the fingers of the arm that is across the body of the cat (Figures 21.2 and 21.3).

Dogs

Before handling, always check the following:

- Their collar is securely fitted and will not slip off if held.
- Position of additional restraint device if required, e.g. Halti® or other head collars, nylon or cage muzzle or body harnesses (correct size/correct fit).
- If there is no muzzle available, a bandage muzzle can be created for the dog if required.

To apply a bandage muzzle to a dog:
Two handlers are required, one to hold the dog and one to apply the muzzle.

Dog handler:

- Stands facing the same way as the dog and to one side (alongside the shoulder).
- Have control of the scruff and collar (if worn) with both hands.

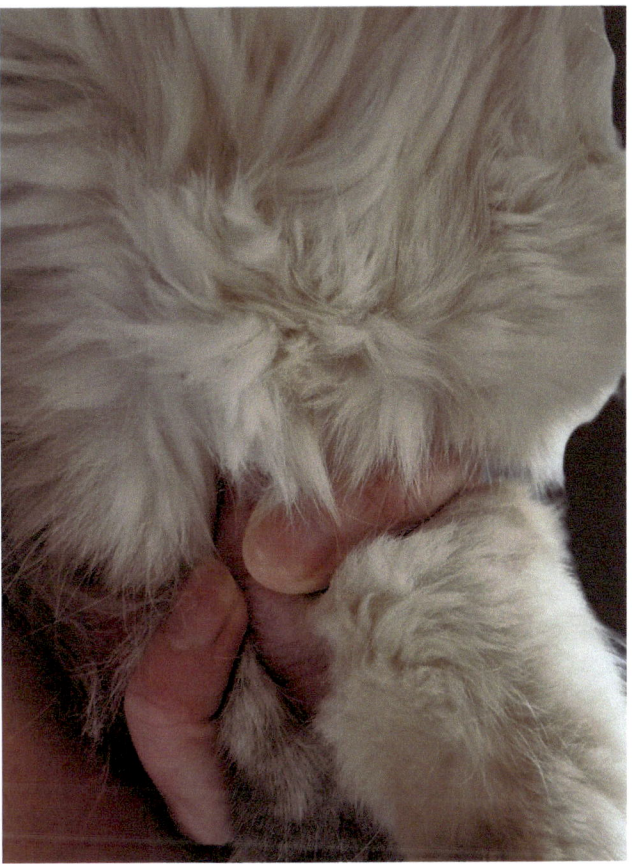

Figure 21.3 Close up of secure hold of the forelegs of a cat.

Figure 21.4 Making a loop with the bandage.

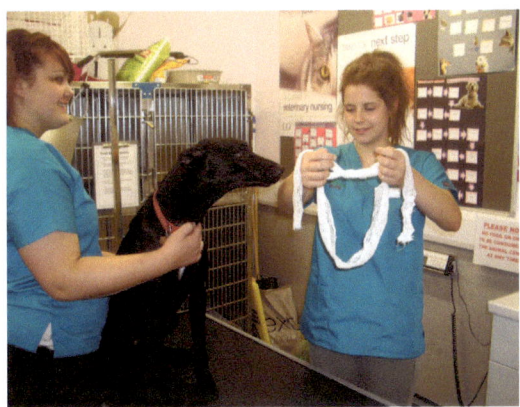

Person applying tape muzzle:

- Use a bandage that will not stretch.
- Cut a long length of bandage in excess to requirements.
- Make a loop with a double-throw knot (Figure 21.4).

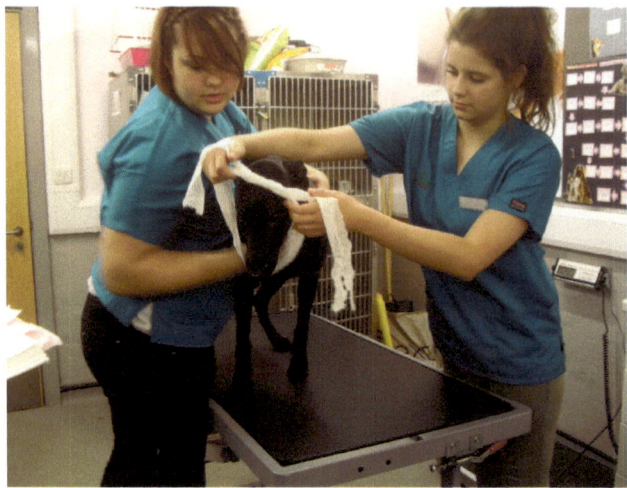

Figure 21.5 From the side, drop the loop over the dog's mouth and nose.

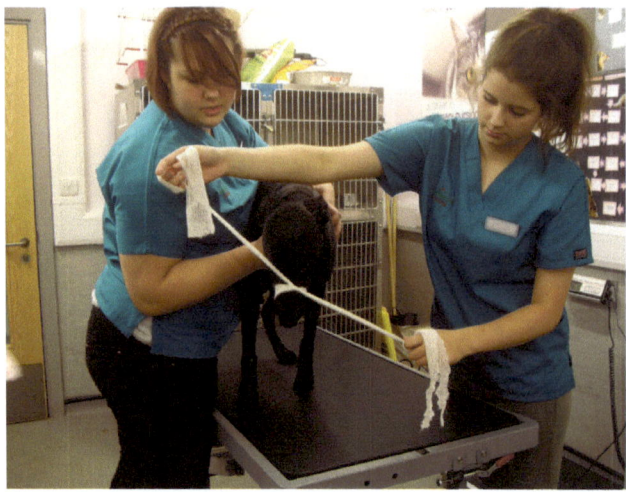

Figure 21.6 Tighten the loop over the muzzle of the dog.

- Keeping the loop open, approach from one side of the dog.
- Drop the loop over the dog's mouth and nose and tighten the loop quickly (Figures 21.5 and 21.6).
- Cross the muzzle ties under the jaw.
- Knot the ends behind the dog's ears and tie into a bow for quick release (Figure 21.7a–c).

Ferrets

Ferrets vary in size and can be nippy which may deter some handlers. The easiest way to handle a ferret is to place one hand under or around the ferret's chest and then support the hind legs with the other hand (Figure 21.8). The ferret should be held close to the handler's body so that it feels safe. Ferrets should not be held near to the handler's face.

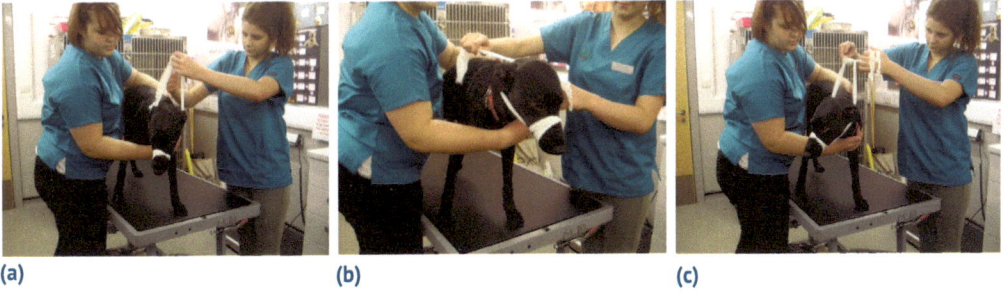

(a) (b) (c)

Figure 21.7 (a–c) Knot the ends behind the ears and tie a bow for quick release.

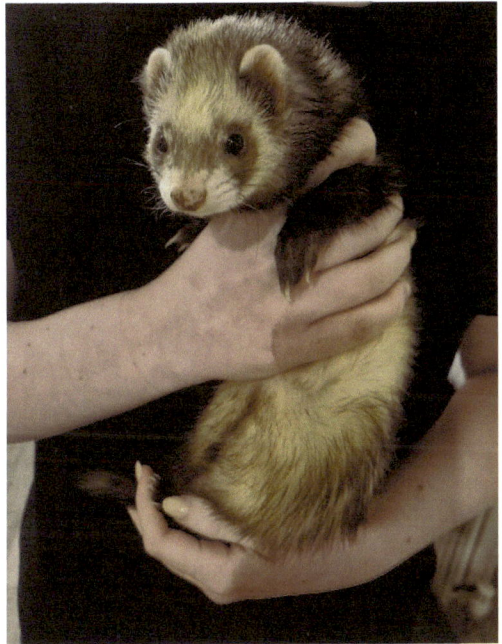

Figure 21.8 Holding a ferret.

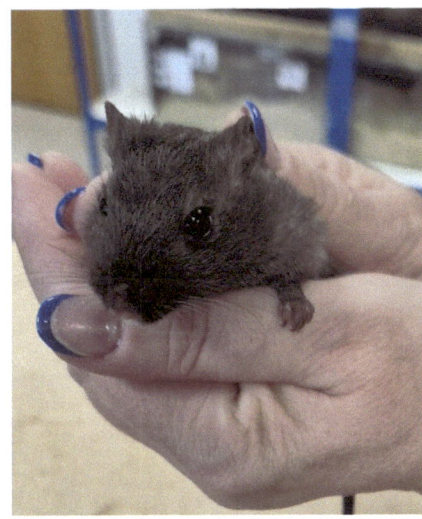

Figure 21.9 Holding a gerbil.

Gerbils

Never lift a gerbil by the middle or end of the tail. The gerbil should be picked up using an over-shoulder grip or in a small container. Cup the gerbil in your hands to prevent escape (Figure 21.9). To restrain the gerbil, either grasp the tail firmly at its base, supporting the gerbil on either side of your hand or ensure that the head is held firmly between the first and middle fingers and the body cradled in the palm of the hand (Figures 21.10a,b).

Guinea pigs

Grasp under the trunk with one hand while supporting the hindquarters with the other hand (Figure 21.11). Bring towards you and rest on your chest to promote a feeling of safety for the animal – keep one hand over the shoulders and one hand under the hindquarters.

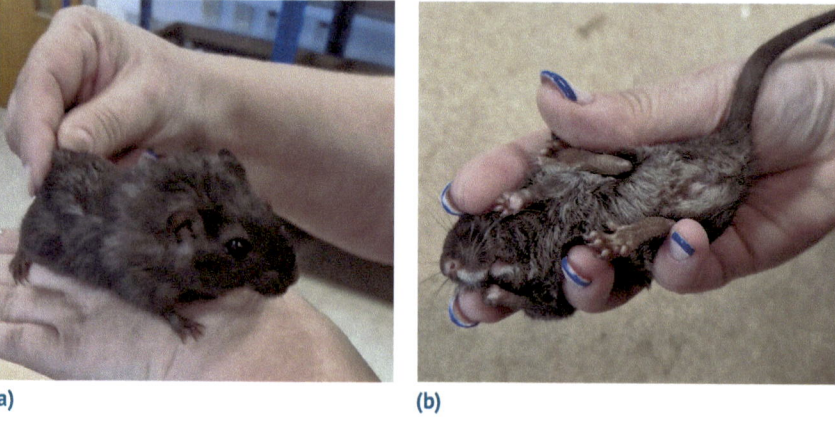

(a)   (b)

Figure 21.10   (a and b) Restraint for a gerbil.

Hamsters

Never grab a sleeping hamster. Once woken by disturbing the bedding or gently blowing on the hamster, it should be picked up using an over-shoulder grip or in a small container. Cup the hamster in your hands to prevent escape (Figure 21.12). To restrain the hamster, ensure that the head is held firmly between the first and middle fingers and the body cradled in the palm of the hand (Figure 21.13).

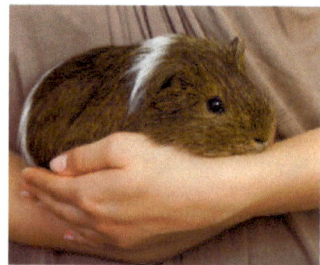

Figure 21.11   Holding technique for a guinea pig.

Rabbits

Never ever lift a rabbit using only the ears. Place one hand on the shoulder of the animal and slide the hand down the shoulder and underneath so that the first finger is positioned between the front legs of the rabbit. The thumb and middle finger can then close over the forelegs of the rabbit, and the handler's other hand can be used to lift the hindquarters. The rabbit can then be lifted and either placed in a carrier, on a handling table for examination or cradled against the handler's chest or along their arm (Figure 21.14). Rabbits need to feel secure; otherwise, they will struggle to escape. When handling on a surface, ensure hands are kept on the rabbit to prevent it escaping.

   Note: Never lift a rabbit to the point where it can try an escape over the shoulder of the handler; otherwise, severe scratching can occur to the handler and the rabbit risks injuring itself.

Rats

Place hand firmly over the back and rib cage and restrain head with the thumb and forefinger immediately behind the lower jaw (Figures 21.15 and 21.16).

Reptiles

Reptiles need to be handled very carefully as their bones are more fragile than a mammal's bones.

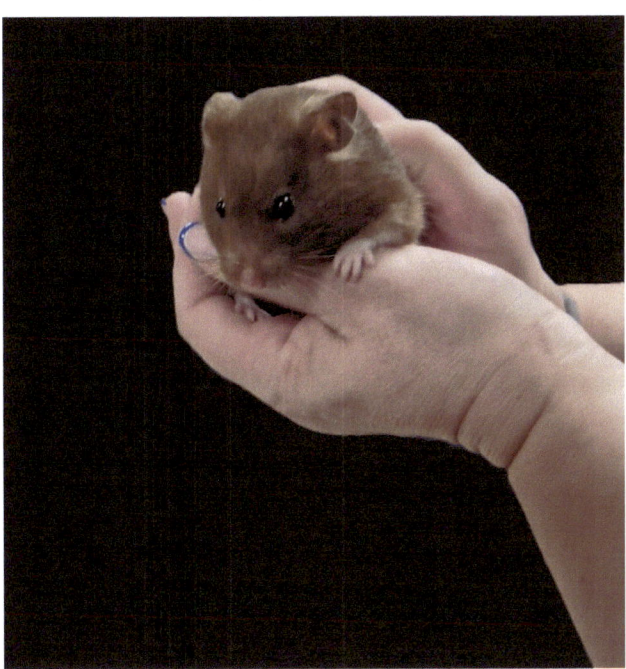

Figure 21.12 Holding technique for a hamster.

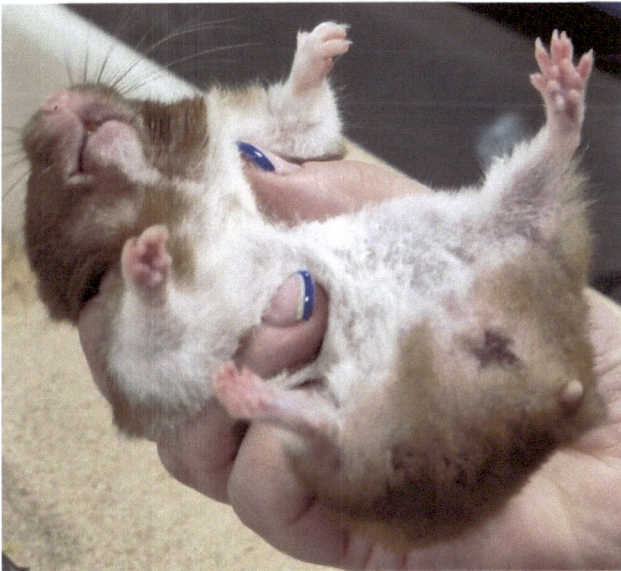

Figure 21.13 Restraint of a hamster.

Lizards

Where possible, handle the lizard on a surface then they feel they have something to grip onto. Where this is not possible, hold the lizard gently along your arm (Figure 21.17a). Avoid grabbing

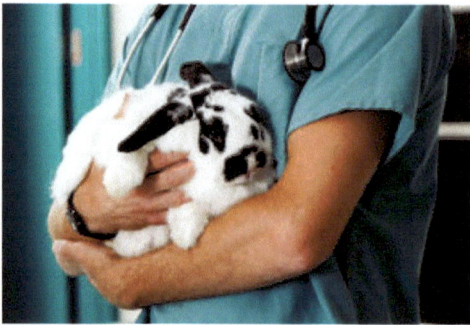

Figure 21.14 Handling technique for rabbits.

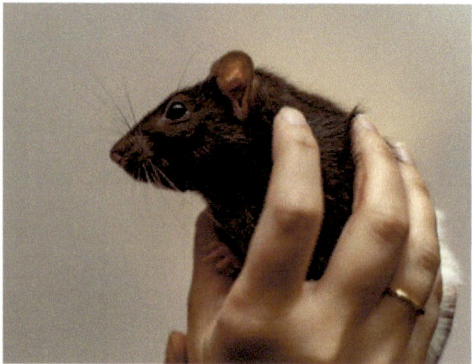

Figure 21.15 Holding technique for a rat.

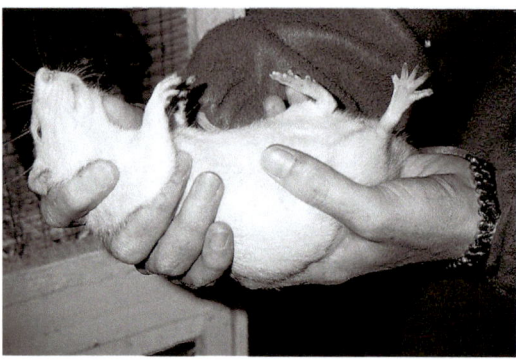

Figure 21.16 Holding technique to expose the abdomen and chest.

the tails of smaller lizards as some lizards shed their tails in a protective process called *autotomy*, e.g. geckos. For larger lizards, such as Green Iguanas, the base of the tail can be used as another supportive handling point if required. Lizards can be restrained by ensuring the head is held still on either side of the back of the skull (Figure 21.17b).

Snakes

A snake should not be put around the neck for handling purposes, especially snakes that constrict their prey.

Snakes should be handled carefully and adjustments made for the size of the individual. Smaller or more agile snakes, such as the Sinaloan milk snake, tend to move more quickly than larger snakes and so a holding tube can be of use for handling and examination purposes (Figure 21.18).

Larger snakes such as Royal Pythons or Boa Constrictors should be supported with both hands and allowed to move freely unless they need to be examined in the head area. If this is the case, then snakes can be restrained by ensuring the head is held still on either side of the back of the skull and one finger on the top of its head. Snake hooks may be used for handling snakes (Figure 21.19). For very large snakes, more than one person may be required for handling.

Restraining the Dog and Cat

For general examinations

To examine a dog, the head must be controlled (Figures 21.20 and 21.21).

Handling to examine limbs, chest, and abdomen (lateral position)

Place the animal on its side and place a hand gently on the thorax to maintain contact with the animal (Figure 21.22).

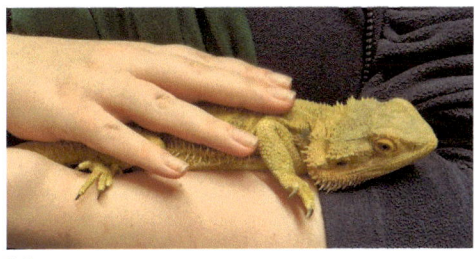

(a)

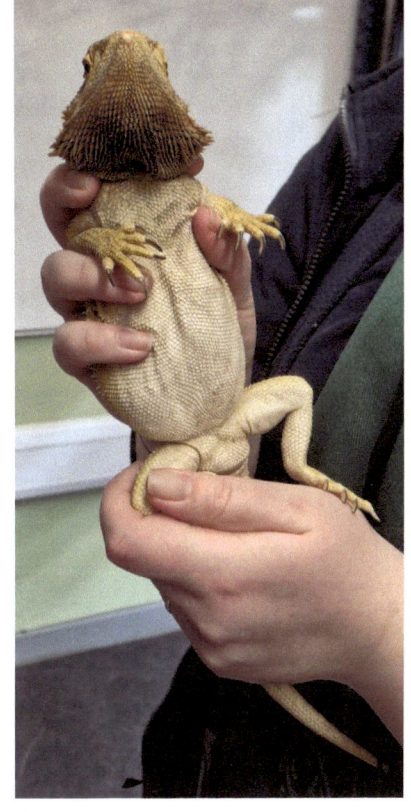

(b)

Figure 21.17 (a) Handling a bearded dragon and (b) restraining a bearded dragon.

Handling for subcutaneous injections

Use the scruff area on the back of the neck (Figures 21.23 and 21.24).

Handling for intramuscular injection

Use the muscle on the front of the hind leg. Never use the muscle at the back (*caudal aspect*) of the hind leg, to prevent damage to the main nerve supply (*sciatic nerve*). Two handlers are required, one to control the head and one to give the injection (Figure 21.25).

Handling for intravenous injection

Presenting one of the forelegs for procedures such as an injection into the vein or taking a blood sample (Figures 21.26a,b and 21.27).

Transferring an animal from basket to examination surface

There are many different animal carriers on the commercial market (Figure 21.28). The advice provided is for a top opening basket (Figure 21.29).

- Place one hand under the chest of the animal and support the hindquarters with the other hand before lifting carefully.
- Hold under one arm, hand still under the chest, and transfer the other hand to support and control the animal's head.
- Never overrestrain an animal unless necessary.

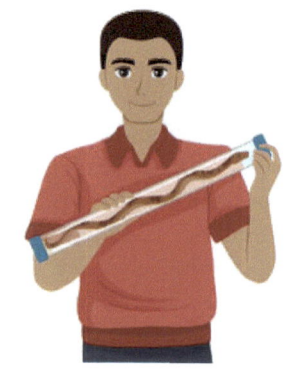

Figure 21.18 A holding tube for a snake.

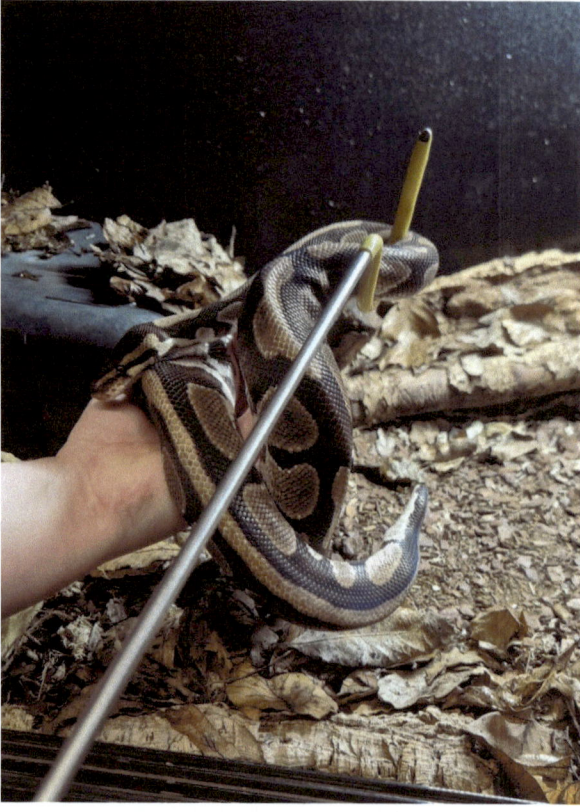

Figure 21.19 Handling a Royal Python with a snake hook.

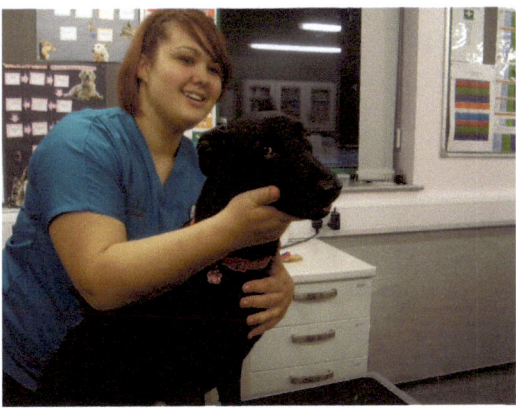

Figure 21.20 Controlling the head, standing to the side.

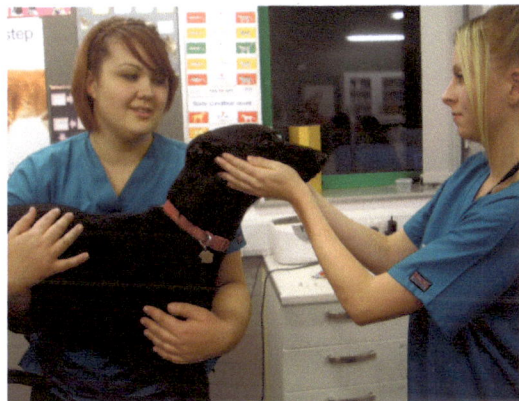

Figure 21.21 Controlling the head, standing in front.

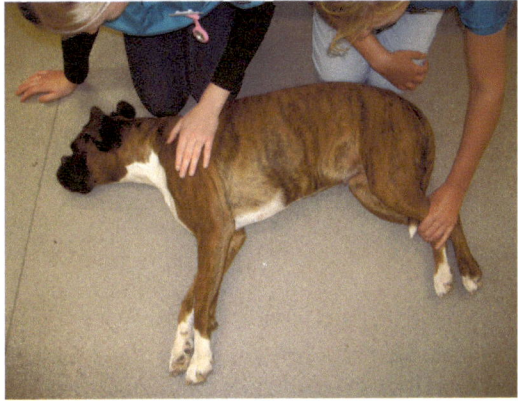

Figure 21.22 Restraint for access to the limbs, chest, or abdomen.

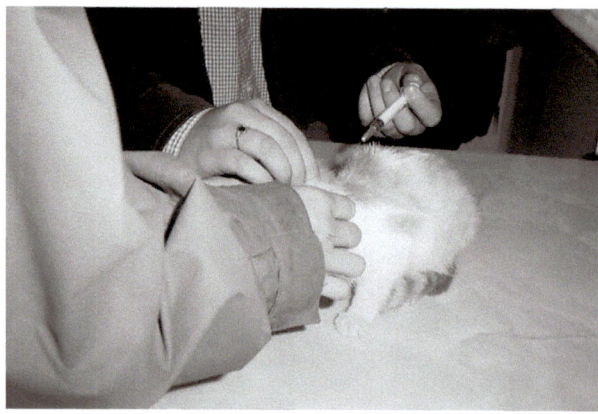

Figure 21.23 Subcutaneous injection for cat in sitting position.

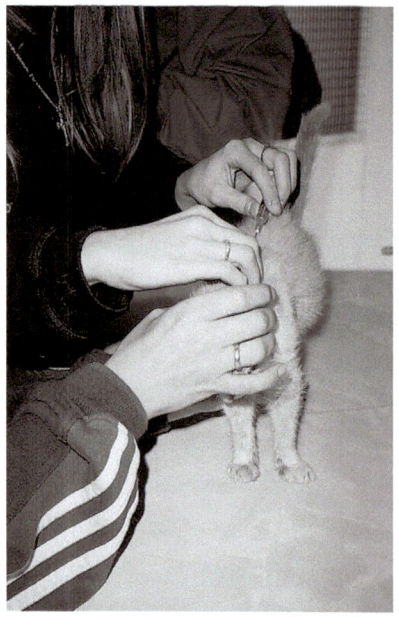

Figure 21.24 Subcutaneous injection for cat in standing position.

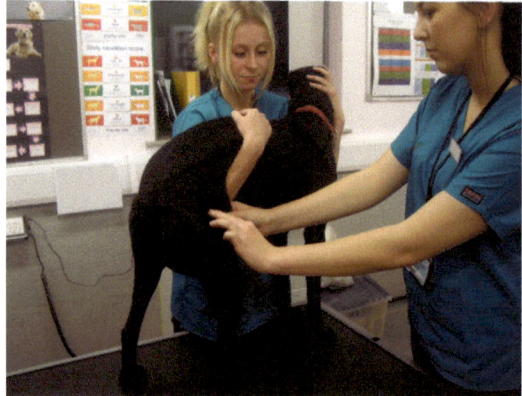

Figure 21.25 Dog standing – restraint for injection into the front/cranial part of the upper hindlimb.

Restraint Equipment for Animals

There is a range of restraint equipment available on the commercial market for different animal species that can aid the handling process, including muzzles, graspers, nets, Y-poles, catch poles, and crush cages. These should not be used without proper training.

A towel is a simple piece of equipment that is widely available and not too costly. Often, wrapping the animal in a towel will help the animal to feel secure and less stressed (Figure 21.30a,b). Placing a towel over a cage can help to calm an animal that may be feeling stressed due to being contained.

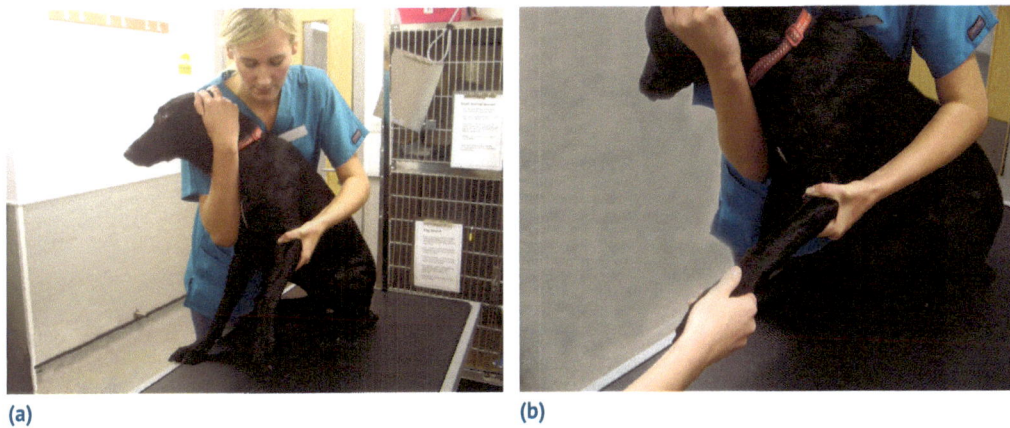

(a) **(b)**

Figure 21.26 (a) Position for intra-venous (i.v.) restraint. (b) Place thumb over the upper part of the leg and rotate the vein from medial to cranial surface.

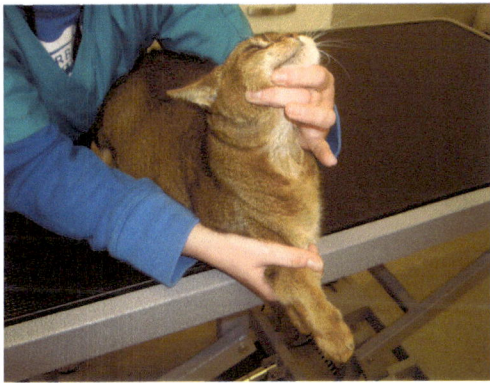

Figure 21.27 Restraint by one person of a cat for (i.v.) injection.

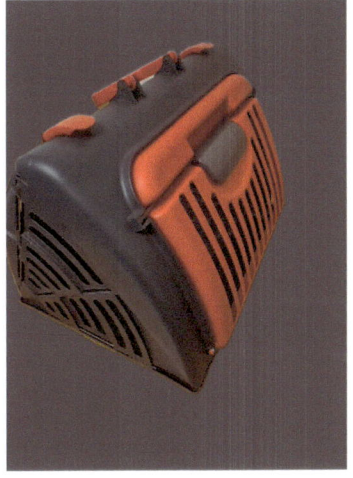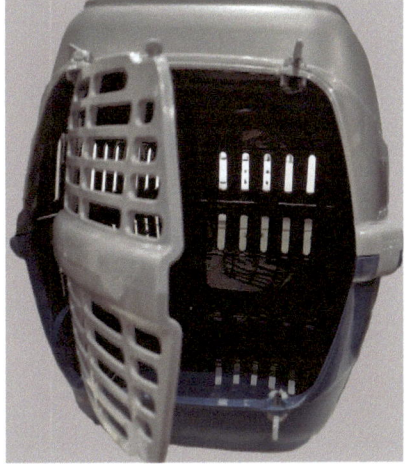

Figure 21.28 Examples of commercial animal carriers.

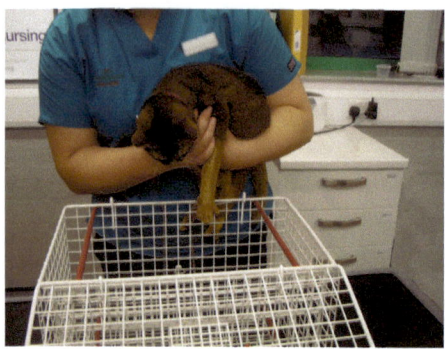

Figure 21.29 Lifting a cat from a carrying cage.

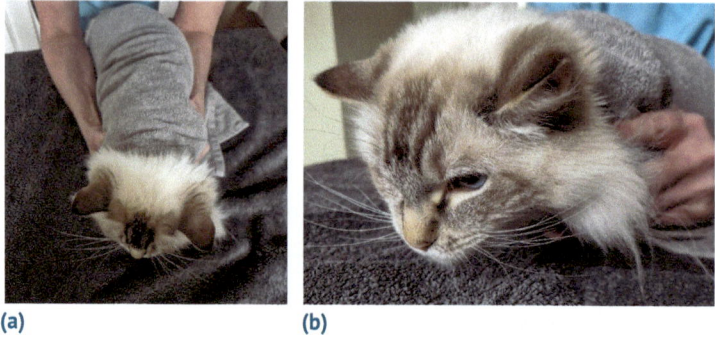

(a)   (b)

Figure 21.30 (a and b) Towel wrap for a cat.

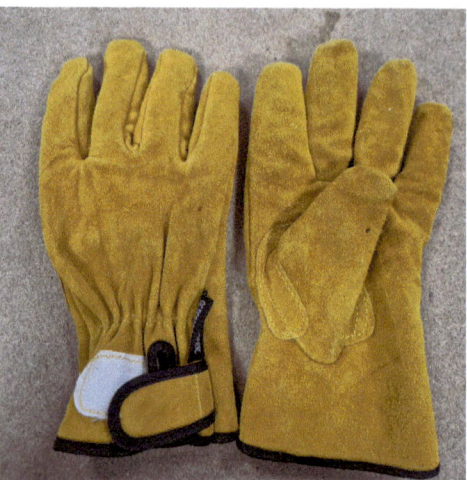

Figure 21.31 Gloves for handling.

Some animals do not want to be handled and will resist. Protective equipment in the form of gloves (Figure 21.31), or leather gauntlets may be used to protect the handler, particularly if they are at risk of being bitten by the animal. Some handlers find that gloves can hamper their ability to get a secure hold on the animal, particularly with smaller species, reptiles, and birds. With smaller rodents, tubes or small tubs can be used to safely capture them from their accommodation prior to handling.

Summary of Animal Handling and Restraint

There are several reasons why animals need to be handled and potentially restrained. The reason for handling will usually dictate the method to be used. For example, if the animal's abdomen needs to be examined, they need to be either flat on their side or held with their abdomen facing upwards.

Before handling any animal, check their behaviour and temperament so that they can be approached sensitively. Ensure the handling environment is secure to prevent escape.

The handling experience should be safe, effective, and as positive as possible for the animal involved.

22

Grooming and Coat Care

Learning goals

In this chapter, the learning goals are:

- To identify the reasons for an animal to be groomed
- To identify the aims of grooming an animal
- To describe the factors affecting coat growth
- To identify and describe the coat types in dogs and cats
- To name and describe the use of a range of grooming equipment
- To describe a grooming procedure including bathing and drying

One of the many responsibilities of an animal owner is that of coat care. This chapter will mainly focus on coat care in dogs and cats as well as touching on small mammal coat care. As breeds of dog and cat were bred for size, character, and colour, their coat length, texture, and density evolved alongside. Careful management of these many and varied coat types is part of the owner/animal interaction. Often, an owner chooses the breed that they want based on an image in a breed book, but it is essential to investigate the amount of time and frequency of coat care required. There is a vast difference in the time it takes to groom a Hungarian Vizsla and an Old English Sheepdog, or a Siamese and a Persian cat.

Reasons for Grooming

There are several reasons for grooming animals:

- For hygiene purposes
- For welfare
- For ease of owner management
- For show
- For work
- For acceptance in society

Animal Biology and Care, Fourth Edition. Emily Jewell.
© 2026 John Wiley & Sons Ltd. Published 2026 by John Wiley & Sons Ltd.
Companion Website: https://www.wiley.com/go/animal/biology4e/jewell

Main Aims of Grooming

There are several aims when grooming an animal:

- To remove dead hair
- To clean the coat and skin
- To remove knots, mats, and tangles

Grooming Dogs

Grooming covers the following factors:

- To encourage bonding and trust between an animal and its handler
- To improve the handling of the animal
- To monitor the general health of an animal
- Allows opportunity for identifying health problems, such as external parasites (fleas/mites) and skin problems (lumps, bumps, etc.)
- To monitor the condition of the nails

The dog's coat

The earliest breeds of dog evolved in the northern hemisphere and so needed a dense coat for protection from the cold. As dogs moved further south to the warmer climates of the world, their coat became thinner and shorter to allow the dog to live comfortably in extreme heat. Selective breeding further enhanced coat features for specific breeds and purposes. Table 22.1 shows different coat types recognised at the time of writing.

Every breed of dog varies in the proportions of the type of coat hair it has. Hairs grow in hair follicles with several hairs to each follicle. Usually, there is an outer coat composed of primary guard hairs and an undercoat made up of secondary hairs. Often, the undercoat is finer and downier than the outer coat. Hair will be shed periodically. The growth rate of hair varies from breed to breed.

Other factors which influence the growth of hair are as follows:

- *Seasons*
  - Spring – triggers production of the summer coat, causing the old winter coat to be shed. The coat is oily, due to an increase in the sebaceous gland activity in the skin.
  - Autumn – triggers the production of the much denser winter coat, causing the summer coat to be shed. The coat is less oily due to reduced sebaceous gland activity.
- *Environmental temperature*
  Dogs kept in centrally heated housing will shed their coat continuously. Dogs kept in outside kennels will shed in spring and autumn.
- *Health*
  - The coat can be affected by skin infections, ectoparasites (e.g. fleas/mites), and metabolic conditions such as Cushing's syndrome. The growth cycle of the coat can be interrupted.
- *Hormone levels*
  - Levels of hormones change during the oestrous cycle of an animal, and this can slow the rate of growth in a coat. The coat texture can alter in some disease conditions making it feel rougher to the touch. Some diseases that affect hormone levels such as Cushing's disease can also affect the quality of the animal's coat.

Table 22.1 Examples of coat type in the dog.

Type	Hair length	Breeds	Grooming frequency
Smooth (Figure 22.1)	Short and fine	Chihuahua	Minimal grooming
		Boxer	Twice weekly
		Doberman	Weekly
		Whippet	Weekly
		Pointer	Weekly
Short (Figure 22.2)	Short and dense	Labrador	Twice weekly
		Corgi	Weekly
Double (Figure 22.3)	Medium to long	Border Collie	Daily and weekly
		German Shepherd	Daily and weekly
		Old English Sheepdog	Daily and weekly
Wiry (Figure 22.4)	Short	Dachshund	Weekly
		West Highland White	Weekly
	Long	Airedale	Daily and weekly
		Schnauzer	Daily and weekly
Silky (Figure 22.5)	Short	Spaniel	Daily and weekly
		Pekinese	Daily and weekly
	Long	Afghan	Daily and weekly
		Yorkshire	Daily and weekly
Woolly/curly (Figure 22.6)		Bedlington	Daily and weekly
		Poodle	Daily and weekly
		Kerry Blue	Daily and weekly

Daily indicates the coat should be briefly groomed once a day.
Weekly means the coat should be thoroughly groomed once a week.

- *Nutrition*
  - A poor diet or poor digestion/absorption issues can be reflected in the animal's coat condition. Ensuring the animal receives a balanced diet with all essential nutrients required will ensure normal coat growth and condition.

Grooming for different coat types

There are several different coat types in dogs (Table 22.1). The coat type depends on the proportion of different hair types within the coat. Knowing the coat type of a dog is important as it allows the right products to be selected during the grooming process.

Smooth coat

A true smooth coat is smooth and sleek in appearance with minimal undercoat. Examples include the Whippet and the Hungarian Vizsla.

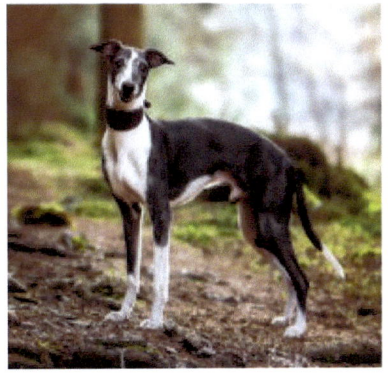

Figure 22.1 Smooth coat – Whippet.

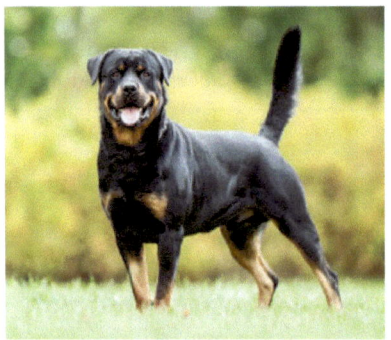

Figure 22.2 Short coat – Rottweiler.

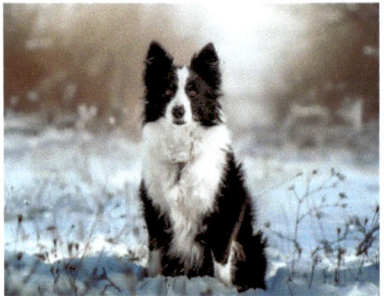

Figure 22.3 Double coat – Border Collie.

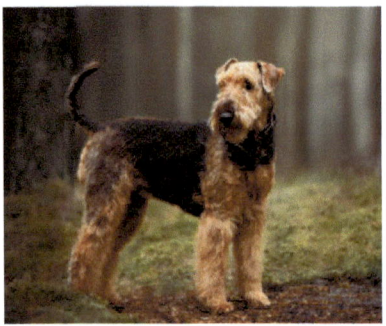

Figure 22.4 Wire coat – Airedale.

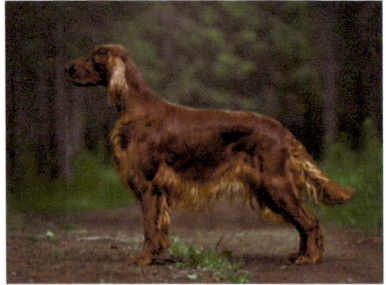

Figure 22.5 Silky coat – Irish Setter.

Equipment required:

- Use a hound glove

Short coat

The short coat has more undercoat than a smooth coat, e.g. in a Labrador Retriever. As a rule of thumb, if running fingers through the coat in the opposite direction reveals hair that is longer than the width of the fingers, it is considered a short coat. It is rare for matting to occur in this type of coat, but the coat can become clogged with dead hair when moulting. Increased grooming at this time will keep the skin in good condition. To prevent loss of natural oils in the coat, only bath twice a year unless very dirty.

If the coat is muddy, brush the mud out once the coat is dry.

Equipment required:

- Use a comb and a bristle brush
- A slicker brush can be used if needed to remove undercoat

Double coat

In a double coat, the topcoat and undercoat are of equal length. The coat tends to stand off the skin to create a fluffy appearance. The coat is usually waterproof. This coat type can matt and tangle if not groomed frequently. Regular grooming sessions of up to three-quarters of an hour to one hour are necessary to prevent the coat tangling.

Some breeds in this category, for example, the Old English Sheepdog, are clipped to about 2.5 cm in length, which makes grooming easier and the dog's coat more manageable. This clip also allows dogs to cope better in hot weather.

Bath a maximum of three to four times yearly, ideally in spring and autumn to condition the coat and clean the skin. Brush out mud once dry and regularly comb out the undercoat during the moulting season.

Equipment required:

- Bristle brush
- Slicker brush
- Comb

Wiry coat

A true wiry coat (e.g. Border Terrier) feels harsh to the touch. The coat is dense in nature. To avoid matting of the coat, these breeds need regular combing. To keep the coat wiry, the topcoat should be hand stripped and plucked two to three times per year. Alternatively, it may be machine clipped at 3-month intervals, followed by a bath to condition and clean the skin. It should be noted that clipping will make this type of coat become softer to the touch. Should mats occur in a wiry coat, work them out carefully with the correct de-matting equipment. As a wiry coat grows, if it is not hand-stripped in time, it gets softer and is said to have blown.

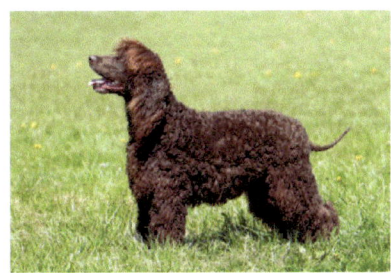

Figure 22.6 Woolly/curly coat – Irish Water Spaniel.

Equipment required:

- Slicker brush
- Comb
- De-matting comb

Silky coat

A silky coat is usually medium long in length and soft and fine to the touch. Without frequent attention, these coats become very tangled. The coat is so fine in these breeds that it is hard to untangle even with de-matting combs. Spaniels, Setters, and Afghan Hounds must have the dead coat hair stripped out every 3–4 months. At the same time, the coat is usually trimmed, paying particular attention to ears and feet. The fine hair in the ear canals should be plucked at regular intervals and the foot hair trimmed to reduce mud and the attachment of barbed grass seeds. Some owners prefer these breeds to be clipped to make the coat easier to manage. Bath as required to help both grooming and skin condition, using an appropriate shampoo.

Equipment required:

- Pin brush
- Slicker brush
- Comb
- De-matting comb
- Clippers and blades

Woolly/curly coat

Woolly/curly coats are often referred to as a non-shedding coat. The coat tends to be dense and pro-fusely curly. The coat doesn't moult but grows continuously. As the hair grows, it becomes trapped, and so, regular grooming is a must for this coat type. These breeds need clipping and bathing every 6-8 weeks. If not groomed out, the dead hair will form a feltlike mass. The ear canals need regular plucking to prevent mats which soon plug with earwax and may lead to infection if not attended to.

Equipment required:

- Comb
- De-matting comb
- Slicker brush
- Scissors
- Clippers and blades

There are some breeds of dogs who have coats that don't fit into these six main categories of coat type. Examples of these include the Mexican Hairless (Figure 22.7) and the Hungarian Puli (Figure 22.8).

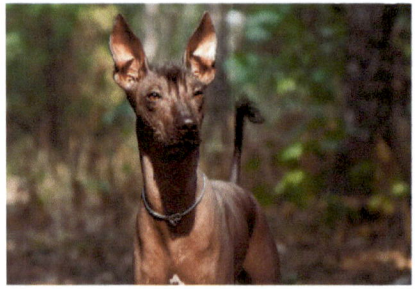

Figure 22.7   Mexican Hairless.

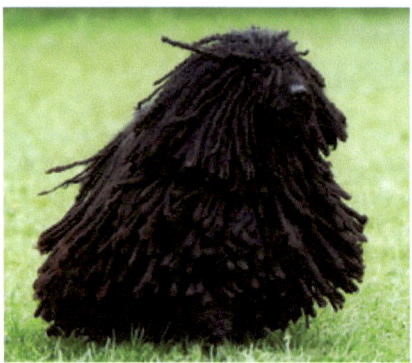

Figure 22.8   Hungarian Puli.

Coat care and grooming requirements in such breeds need to be researched before acquiring any of these breeds.

Grooming equipment

Every dog needs its own grooming equipment, normally bought when getting up a new puppy. There is a great deal of grooming equipment available on the commercial market. Equipment to choose from includes the following:

- *Brushes:*
    - Bristle brush
    - Slicker brush
    - Hound glove
    - Rubber brush
- *Combs:*
    - Fine tooth comb
    - Wide-toothed comb
    - Rake comb
    - Flea comb
    - De-matting comb
- *Cutting equipment:*
    - Stripping knife or comb
    - Thinning scissors
    - Scissors
    - Electrical clippers
    - Nail clippers

Brushes
- *Bristle brushes* are available in a range of sizes and shapes. The handle is made of either wood or rigid plastic, with synthetic or natural bristles. The bristles are set close together, making this an ideal surface-only brush. It is unable to penetrate dense coats but is ideal for smooth and short coats and for the removal of mud or other surface material stuck to the hair. The main effect of this surface brushing is to stimulate the skin and distribute the natural oils from the skin to the hair shaft ends, giving a shine to the coat.
- *Pin brushes* are available in a range of sizes. The handle is made of either wood or rigid plastic. The pins are set in a flexible rubber-backed cushion and usually have plastic-coated tips to prevent scratching the animal's skin. The pin brush will separate hairs and lay the coat in position, which is useful for long silky coats and double coats. These brushes also stimulate the skin, distributing the natural oils from the skin to the tips of the hair. If the coat has tangled hair or knots, then use a comb first to gently remove these before brushing. This will prevent the coat being pulled or broken when the pin brush is used.
- *Slicker brushes* are available in a range of sizes. They have wooden or rigid plastic handles (Figure 22.9). The pins are hooked and set in a rubber-backed cushion, giving some flexibility to the grooming movement. The function of these hooked pins is to remove dead undercoat. Pressure should not be applied when using the slicker brush because the pins can easily scratch or damage the skin surface. Slicker brushes can be used on a range of coat types from silky to double and in some body areas of curly and wire-coated breeds. Slicker brushes should

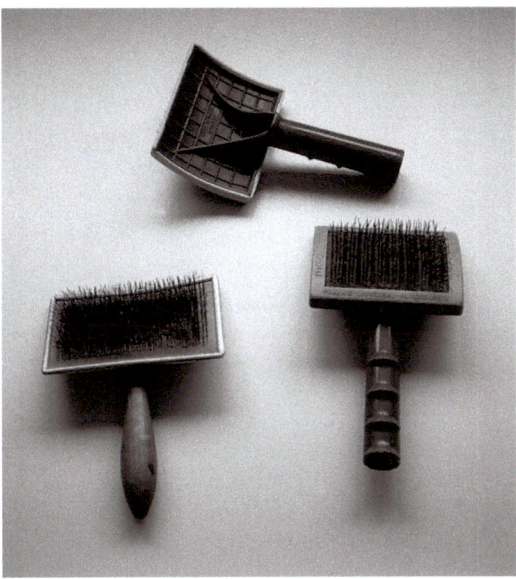

Figure 22.9 Slicker brushes.

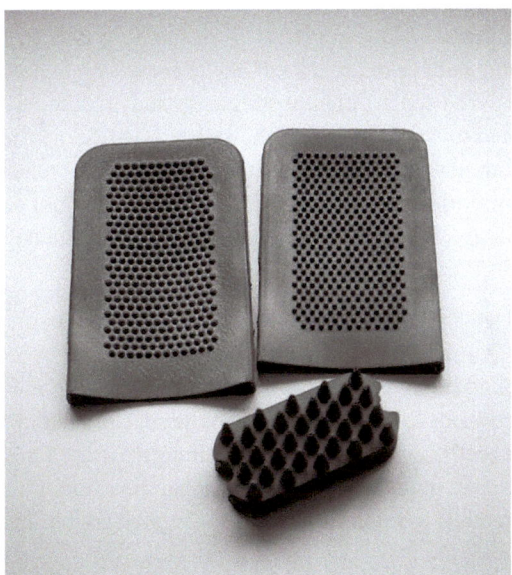

Figure 22.10 Hound glove (top) and rubber brush (below).

never be used on areas of the body where the coat is normally thin such as the stomach, groin, or armpits.

• *A hound glove* fits over the groomer's hand like a mitten or glove (Figure 22.10). They are made of flexible plastic or rubber with short bristles made from wire or plastic, and some have a velvet-type surface on one side and bristles on the other. They are used to remove dead or moulting hair (bristle side) and to polish the coat (velvet side) in smooth coated breeds. Care should be taken when using the bristle side if the bristles are made of wire, in case too much pressure is used and the skin is damaged.

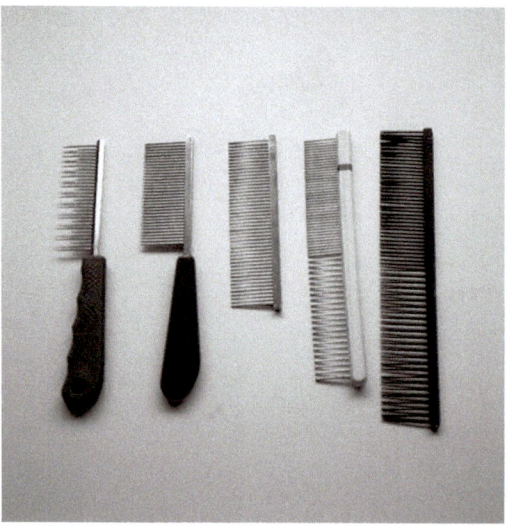

Figure 22.11 Comb types.

Combs

Combs are used to remove dead hair and prevent mats forming behind the ears, in the neck/collar area, and over the hindquarters. Combs are made from metal or plastic, with or without handles (Figure 22.11) and with solid teeth or rotating teeth. Some combs are half wide toothed and half fine toothed, so that each half can be used in different body areas and on different coat types. The teeth tips are rounded or plastic coated to avoid damaging the skin surface. Some combs also have individual rotating pins that roll individually and prevent coat damage when in contact with a mat or tangle.

Combs should be used carefully, especially when encountering a knot or tangle. Slowly tease the hairs and never rush this stage or the coat will be pulled, hurting the dog and causing a negative experience for the dog.

- *Rake combs* have ridged metal teeth with round tips, set perpendicular to the handle, and resemble a small garden rake (Figure. 22.12). They should not be used by pressing into the coat. Their function is to break up mats and, in dense coats, lift and remove dead undercoat hair. They are pulled towards the groomer through the coat and in the direction of the coat hair.
- *Flea combs* have fine teeth set close together, with a grip area. These are pulled slowly and carefully through the coat, going with the normal coat direction. If a parasite is encountered, the gap between the teeth is too small for it to pass through so it is lifted onto the comb for the groomer to remove.
- *De-matting combs* have wooden handles and teeth which on one side are rounded and blunt and on the other side are a series of cutting blades (Figure 22.13). These combs are used, with extreme care, to cut through large mats of hair by placing the blunt side against the dog's skin surface and with a gentle sawing action cutting away from the skin surface and through the mat. This will allow the matted areas to either be combed out or further subdivided for combing and removal of the dead hair.

Cutting equipment

- *A stripping knife* is used to remove dead hair and at the same time trim the live hair (Figure 22.14). The comb has a serrated metal cutting edge, set against a guard plate on one side for the removal

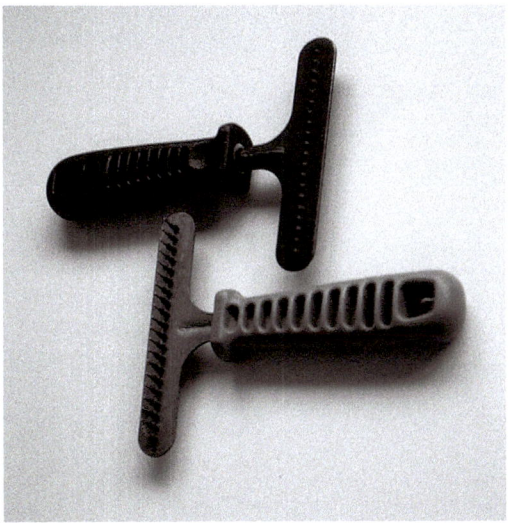

Figure 22.12 Rake comb.

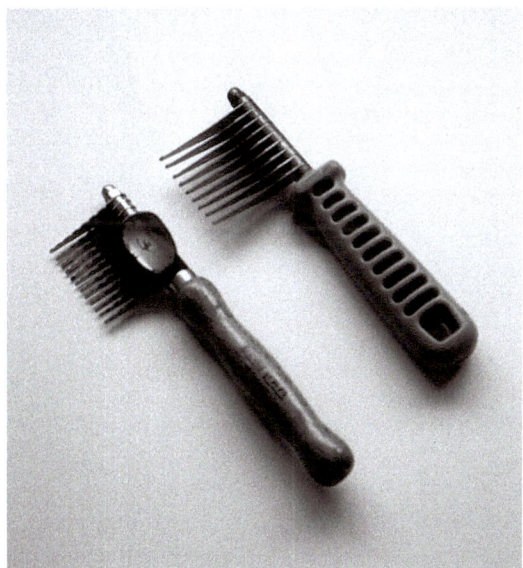

Figure 22.13 De-matting comb.

of dead hair. The stripping knife has a metal handle and blade. Sections of coat hair are held between the operator's thumb and the blade, and the blade is pulled away from the skin with a twisting movement. At the same time, dead hair can be pulled or plucked. This is known as hand stripping and is used on wire-coated breeds such as Border Terriers, Wire-haired Dachshunds, and Schnauzers. If done correctly, hand stripping should not be painful for the animal.

- *Thinning scissors* (Figure 22.15) have one regular and one serrated blade or both blades serrated. They are used to thin the coat without affecting its appearance and so are used on the undercoat, preserving the appearance of the outer topcoat.

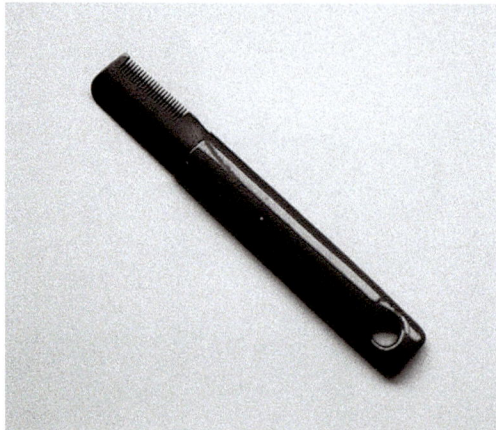

Figure 22.14 Stripping knife.

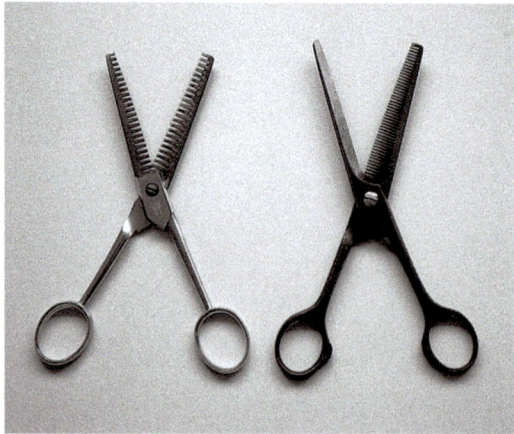

Figure 22.15 Thinning scissors or shears.

- *Scissors* (Figure 22.16) are available in many sizes and shapes for use on various body areas, from long, sharp, tapering blades to short, blunt-ended blades, depending on the area that requires a trim. Blunt-ended scissors are used to trim between toes and in delicate areas around the eyes, ears, lips, and genitals.
- *Electrical clippers* (Figure 22.17) are used by groomers in conjunction with scissors, particularly in the curly-coated breeds such as the Poodle or Labradoodle. These coats keep growing all year round and need constant attention. The clipper cuts away the excess hair more rapidly than scissors and is used with a variety of detachable blades. The blades vary from fine-toothed for close trims to ones set with wide-spaced blades or teeth, which leave short hairs against the skin surface. The blades are snapped onto a post on the clipper only when the clipper is running. The clipper is held like a pencil, which gives a firm grip, allowing the groomer to move over the coat lightly and keep the blade flat against the section being clipped. Always keep the blade of the clippers flat to the coat to avoid cutting the skin.

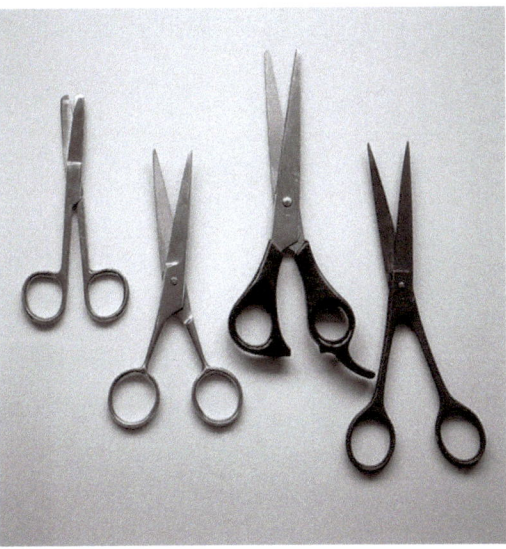

Figure 22.16   Scissor types.

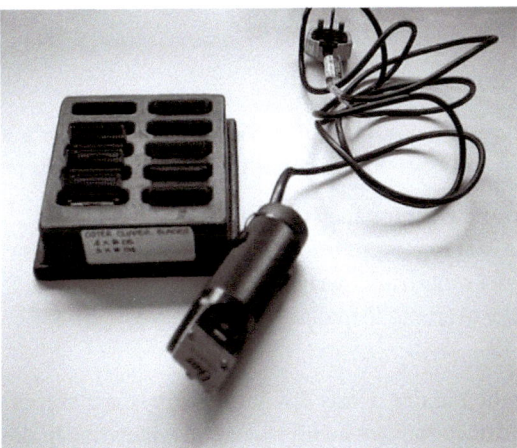

Figure 22.17   Electrical clipper with range of blades.

Clippers will get hot during use, so it is important to closely monitor the blade temperature to prevent a clipper burn or rash developing on the skin surface. There are several ways of avoiding this:

- Spray hot blades with aerosol lubricant spray to reduce temperature.
- Change the hot blade for a new cool blade.
- Use a second clipper, allowing the first to cool.
- Keep the blades in use sharpened.
- Only clip hair that is completely dry.
- *Nail clippers* are only used to cut nails which are overlong. A range of clippers is available (Figure 22.18), from the guillotine clipper (also useful in small mammals) to the double blade scissor type. The choice of nail clipper will depend on the length and position of the nail presented. In recent times, nail grinders have become popular to use with dogs as it is claimed that they cause less stress than guillotine or pliers type nail clippers.

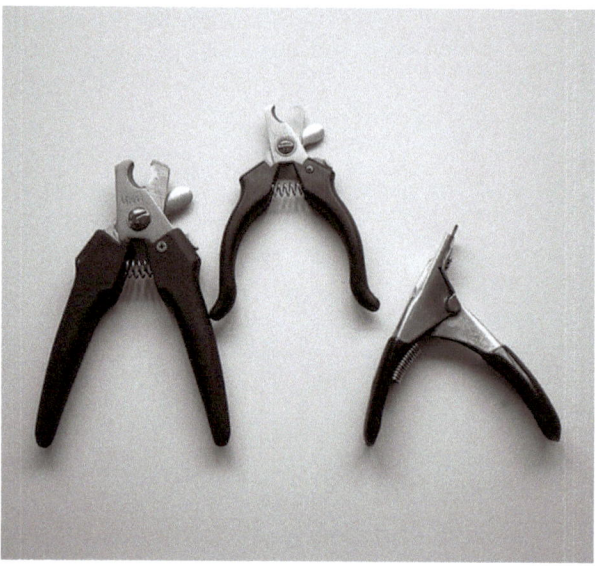

Figure 22.18 Types of nail clippers.

Grooming procedure in dogs

Depending on the coat type of a dog, grooming will be a daily and/or a weekly event. It provides the owner with the opportunity not only to condition the coat and skin but to:

- Clean any discharge and examine the eyes
- Check and clean the ears to prevent infection developing
- Clean and examine the mouth and particularly the teeth
- Examine and trim any overlong toenails
- Check the anal region

The eyes should be bright and free of any discharge. If any discharge is seen in the corner of the eye, moisten a clean piece of cotton wool with water and wipe away in the direction of the nose. If the discharge is not a clear colour, check for signs of inflammation. Use a separate piece of cotton wool for each eye. Eye wipes are commercially available if preferred to cotton wool.

The ears should be free of wax, a dull pink colour, and without odour. In the curly-coated breeds, the ears need to be plucked free of hair, which, if left in place, attracts wax, parasites, and infection. Check for signs of discomfort or reluctance by the dog when the flap is being examined, which may indicate a problem.

For the mouth, the gums and tongue should be pink (pigmented in the Chow Chow) or partly pink with pigmented areas. The gums should be well defined around each tooth, with no food or other materials attached. To prevent any build-up of tartar on the teeth, pet toothpaste in various flavours and toothbrushes can be used as part of the daily grooming examination.

The feet or paws should be clean around the nail bed, nails just in contact with the ground, and excess hair cut short between the pads and nails to prevent mats and grass seed barbs penetrating the skin and causing an abscess.

The anal region under the tail and around the anus needs to be checked daily in dogs, whether short or long coated. The area should be free of any faecal material and show no signs of redness or inflammation. Should the dog start licking excessively around the anal region or scooting on its rear end, the anal glands should be checked for a blockage. These glands are situated on either side of the anus and may not empty as expected when the dog defaecates, leading to infection.

Nail clipping

Healthy, active dogs do not need frequent nail clips. The nails will wear down naturally with everyday walks on paved surfaces. The exception may be the dewclaw, which can grow round into the nail bed if left unchecked, although they tend to be slow growing in most breeds.

The nails may need attention if:

- The dog is exercised only on soft ground or grass
- The dog is elderly
- The dog walks with uneven gait – this may be due to injury or skeletal abnormalities
- A nail becomes broken or damaged

Nail clipping is a process that many people are scared to do, but once you have learnt, then it is quite straightforward. Care must be taken not to cut the *"quick"* in the nail. The quick is the blood vessel running down the centre of the nail. If this blood vessel is caught, then bleeding can be stopped quite quickly. It is better to cut a small amount at a time if you are unsure. Once an animal has had a bad experience during nail clipping, then it can react badly on future occasions.

Equipment needed:

- A pair of nail clippers.
  - There are a range of styles on the market from small scissor type nail clippers to plier type and guillotine type. There are also electric nail grinders that can be used. Use the type that you feel most comfortable with.
- A coagulant powder should be available.
  - A coagulant powder or gel helps to stop bleeding if clipping causes the nail to bleed. There are several brands commercially available, e.g. Kwik Stop, Styptic Powder, and Trimmex.
- A nail file.
  - Nail files can be used at the same time as clipping to smooth off any rough edges. They can also be used on claws in between trimming sessions to smooth any breaks or flaked nail edges. Nail files can be used to trim the sharp ends of claws, particularly dew claws.

Nail clipping process

- Choose the right type of nail clipper for the job – one that you feel comfortable with – plier type or guillotine types are commonly used.
- The size of clipper used will relate to the size of claw being cut. If you use clippers that are too big for the claw, then you can damage the claw. If the clippers are too small, then you will not get a full cut through the nail which can be painful for the animal.
- Restrain the animal appropriately and reassure throughout by staying calm, being confident and talking in a calm manner to the animal.
- Locate the 'quick' in the animal's claw. This can be easily seen if the claws of the animal are white, but it is trickier in animals with dark claws. If the animal has dark claws, it is necessary to examine the shape of the claw and identify a cutting position approximately 0.5–1 cm in front of the quick. A rule of thumb is to identify a triangular shape at the end of the claw (Figure 22.19).

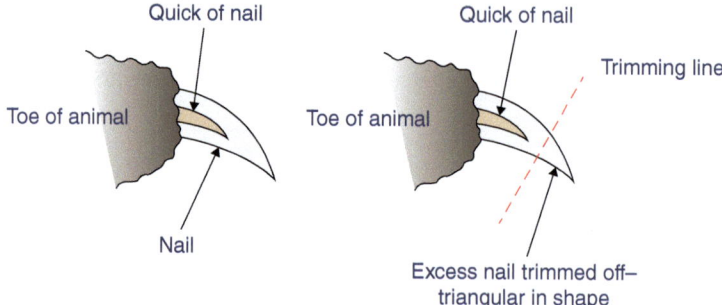

Figure 22.19   Nail trimming.

- Holding the claw firmly at the base to prevent any twisting, quickly cut the claw using firm pressure to minimise any trauma for the animal. Avoid cutting the 'quick'. Always ensure you can see where the blades of the claw clippers are to avoid cutting too much off at once.
- If the quick is cut, apply a coagulant powder or gel to the bleeding claw. If no powder is available, apply firm pressure to the end of the claw until bleeding stops.
- Check the nail afterwards for sharp edges and if any are present, then use a nail file to gently smooth the sharp edges.

Brushing the coat

Once the general checks are complete, brushing and combing in preparation for the bath can begin. It is essential to brush and comb before the bath to remove all matted and tangled hair. Shampoo and drying make matting much worse in some coat types. Check through the coat with a wide-toothed comb to ensure no tangles are left.

Start the brushing procedure with:

- The hind legs
- Then the forelegs
- Back to the tail section and tail
- The body coat, one side at a time
- Chest area
- Lastly the head, face, and ears

When brushing, pay particular attention to the groin area and the armpit area on the forelegs where mats may develop. The head and ears in breeds such as Poodles, Spaniels, Lhasa Apso, and Afghan Hounds needs particular attention. The ear hair is long and fine and tends to form small mats.

The eye area on breeds such as Pekinese and Shih Tzu need particular attention and care as these are short-nosed breeds (*brachycephalic*) with protruding eyes. As a last resort, it may be necessary to remove mats and tangles with scissors or electrical clippers, especially if it is clearly painful to the dog or the dog is becoming aggressive due to the grooming.

Bathing

Reasons for bathing:

- To control skin parasites
- To clean a soiled coat

- To remove odours
- To improve coat appearance for showing
- As part of a medical treatment
- To mask the scent of oestrus

Equipment needed for bathing includes:

- Cotton wool to plug ears (optional)
- Shampoo/conditioner
- Mixer hose or jug
- Bath with non-slip mat
- Towel or dryer
- Ear plugs – after brushing and combing, ear plugs may be placed in the ear canal to prevent the entry of shampoo and water. This is optional and should not be used if upsetting to the dog.
- *Shampoo* – there is a wide range of shampoo on the commercial market available for different coat types, different coloured coats, etc. If in doubt, use a general-purpose shampoo unless the coat requires otherwise. Shampoos available include the following:
  - *Mild* – have only low levels of detergent to avoid eye or skin irritation.
  - *Medicated* – prescribed by a veterinary surgeon in cases where the dog has skin problems. These shampoos contain antiseptics such as iodine to reduce skin bacteria levels or drugs to assist a specific skin condition.
  - *Insecticidal* – for control of surface/skin parasites such as lice, fleas and ticks. These are often used in combination with parasite control programmes that use spot-on, tablet or injection methods.
  - *Colour enhancing* – used to improve the appearance of coats, particularly white ones.
- Always transfer the shampoo being used into a plastic container (such as an old washing-up liquid bottle) as this allows easy application of the shampoo and if the shampoo bottle should be knocked and fall, there is no risk of broken glass, and the noise of the container falling will not frighten the dog. Follow the instructions on the shampoo bottle to determine whether it should be used in concentrated form or diluted.
- *Conditioners* may be used to improve the coat texture and make it more manageable for final brushing when dry. Conditioners can help to prevent tangles in long-haired coats.
- *Mixer hose or jug* – the use of a hose with a shower head allows the water pressure and temperature to be regulated (Figure 22.20). If a hose is not available for rinsing, then use a jug.
- *Bath* – a household bath can be used, with a hair catcher over the plughole to prevent blockage or a child's paddling pool. Always provide a non-slip surface to prevent the dog from damaging the bath surface if it slips or panics. Rubber bathmats or car mats can be used.
- *Towels or dryer* – several towels are needed for any breed. Always have more available than required to avoid having to leave a half-dry dog. In winter, place the dog in a warm area to dry once excess water has been removed from the coat using towels. Hand-held hair dryers (Figure 22.21) may be used but be careful

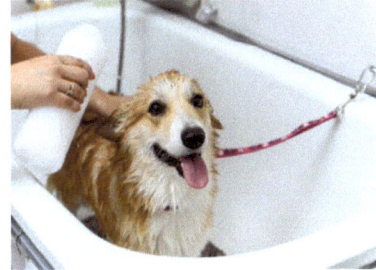

Figure 22.20 Dog bath with shower hose.

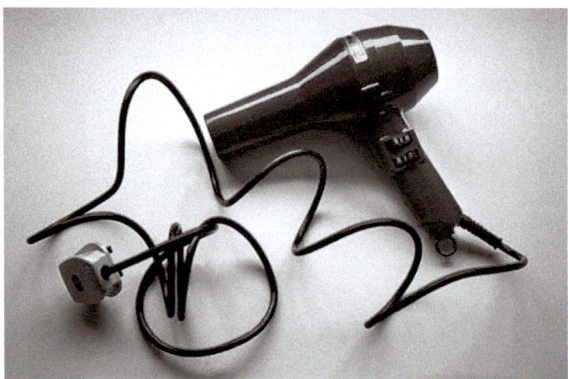

Figure 22.21 Hand-held dryer.

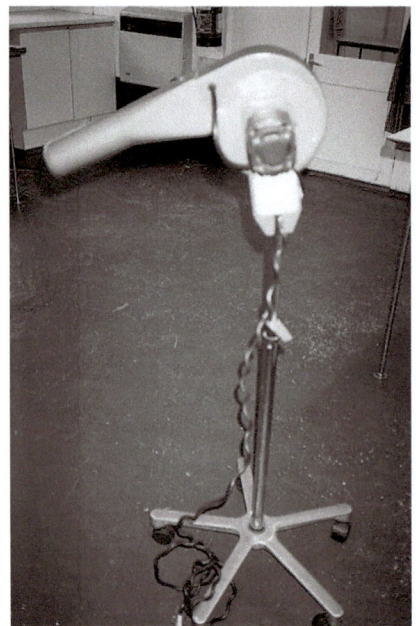

Figure 22.22 Type of standing floor dryer stand.

to gradually introduce the dog to the dryer as the noise and warm airflow may frighten it. Never hold dryers too close or use a high-temperature high-flow setting.

- *Floor dryers* – mounted on stands and are powerful, quickly drying heavy-coated breeds (Figure 22.22).
- *Cage dryers* – attach to the front of holding kennels and cages. These are used after towel drying.
- *Wall-mounted dryers* – like hand-held dryers but more powerful and space saving. A hose applies the 'blow dry' effect when directed on to the dog's coat.
- *Cabinet dryers* – box cages with a false, vented floor, containing the blow dryer (Figure 22.23). Warm air flows, fan assisted, into the box area where the dog sits.

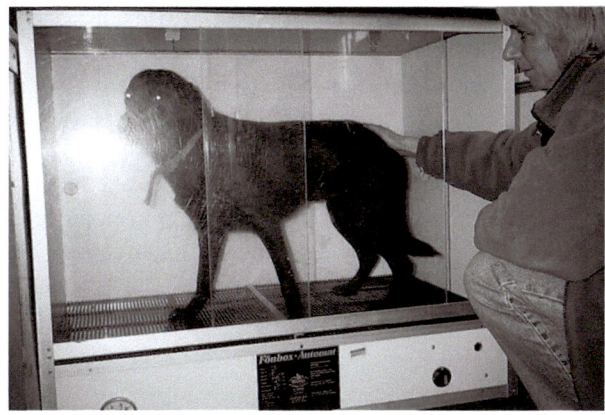

Figure 22.23   Cabinet dryer with false vented floor.

Bathing technique in dogs

- Make sure before bathing starts that all the equipment required is to hand. Never encourage a dog to jump into or out of a bath in case of injury – always lift the dog safely into the bath, ensuring the correct lifting technique is used. Do not leave an animal unattended in the bath in case the animal panics.
- Use a collar restraint to attach the dog to the bath, leaving both the groomer's hands free. A nylon collar and lead should be used, never a chain. If the dog panics or slips, the nylon lead can be cut quickly, preventing injury.
- The groomer should wear protective clothing and non-slip soles to shoes or boots, for safety. When using medicated and parasite shampoo, gloves should be worn by the groomer to protect their skin.
- Carry out the bathing process as follows:
    1. Dilute the shampoo as required.
    2. Place a non-slip mat into the bath area.
    3. Lift the dog into the bath and secure the restraint. Two people may be required to lift medium and large breeds.
    4. Regulate water flow and temperature.
    5. Soak hindquarters first, using the hands to force water through heavy coats.
    6. Continue soaking, moving last to the head and face, protecting the eyes and ears from the water.
    7. Once the dog is soaked, introduce the shampoo, using hand and sponge. As before, start over the hindquarters and move towards the head, including the abdomen, under the tail and between the foot pads but always protecting the eyes.
    8. Hold the head up to encourage water and shampoo to drain back along the spine while attending to the face and chin.
    9. Rinse off the shampoo.
    10. Repeat the application of shampoo (if medicated or parasite shampoo, leave in contact with the skin for correct amount of time).
    11. Rinse thoroughly from head to toe.
    12. Squeeze water out of coat using hands or chamois-type cloth.

13. Towel dry on a non-slip surface and place in a warm area to finish drying or dry using a dryer.

14. Pat dry to absorb excess water. Never rub long coats vigorously as this will create tangles.

- During the drying stage, the coat can be brushed out. The objective of using the dryer to dry some breeds is to get the coat as fluffy as possible. To achieve this, the coat is dried in sections, brushing constantly to straighten curls.
- Finally, trim nails if necessary and clip hair between foot pads.
- Professional groomers would continue with the plucking, stripping, clipping, and scissoring required by certain breeds, depending on coat type and requirements. This would be done on a grooming table (Figure 22.24). The dog would then be transferred to the holding kennel to await collection by the owner (Figure 22.25).

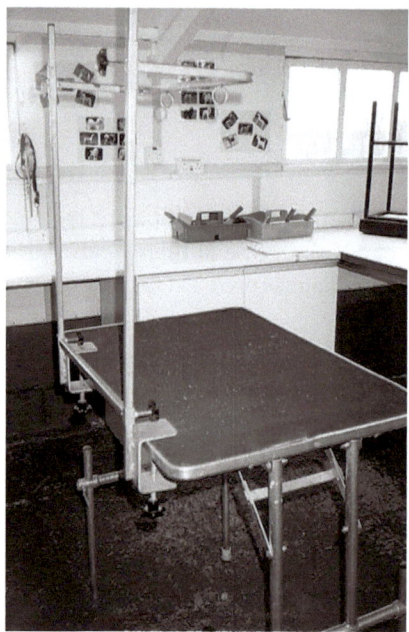

Figure 22.24   Grooming table.

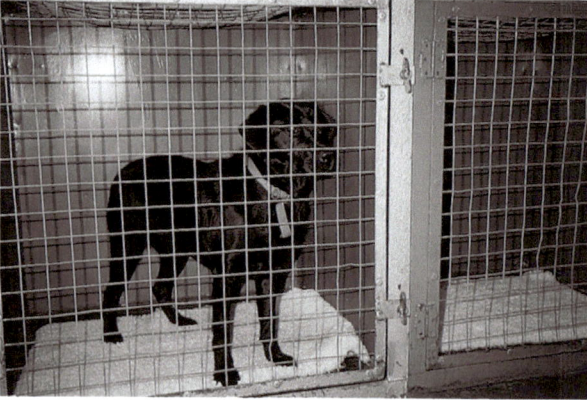

Figure 22.25   In the holding kennel awaiting collection by owner.

Cats

In cats, the grooming process provides the owner with the opportunity not only to condition the coat and skin but to:

- Clean any discharge and examine the eyes
- Clean the ears and check for signs of infection, excess wax or ear mites
- Examine the mouth and check the teeth for build-up of tartar and for gum disease
- Examine and trim claws and clean claw bed of caked-on dirt
- Clean dirty coat
- Check for skin parasites

Grooming should begin from the time of weaning to accustom a kitten to short but daily coat care. As with the dog, this also becomes a bonding/playtime session between the owner and the animal. This attention is particularly important if the kitten is to be a show animal.

Cats spend a considerable part of every day in self-grooming. They have a specially adapted tongue with backward-facing barbs for the removal of dead hairs from the coat.

Grooming in cats will:

- Remove dead hair
- Remove material from coat surface
- Stimulate skin and distribute secreted oils for coat condition
- Provide a feeling of well-being

Constant grooming in long-haired cats can cause health problems. During self-grooming, the cat will swallow large quantities of saliva and wet hair, which forms *hair balls* or sausage-shaped plugs in the stomach. This ingested hair can cause an obstruction in the digestive tract. In the event of loss of appetite, weight loss or constipation, contact a veterinary surgeon for advice.

The cat's coat

Selective breeding and genetic mutation have enhanced cats' coats or caused coat loss. The cat has a topcoat of *guard hair* and an undercoat, which consists of coarse, bristly *awn* hairs and soft downy hairs.

Examples of coat types in cats are as follows:

- *Shorthair*, e.g. British short hair, has short guard hairs with even shorter but slightly curly awn hairs as a sparse undercoat.
- *Longhair*, e.g. Persian, has extremely long guard hairs with a thick undercoat of downy hair, which gives this breed its full, dense coat.
- *Semi-long hair*, e.g. Ragdoll – like a long-haired coat but mid-length. Possesses a thick undercoat of downy hair, which thickens further during the colder months.
- *Curly coat*, e.g. Cornish Rex, has very short curly awn and downy hairs of the same length and no guard hairs at all.
- *Wire hair*, e.g. American Wirehair, has short curly, even coiled guard hairs, down, and awn.
- *Hairless*, e.g. Sphinx, which has a coat so sparse as to appear hairless but in fact has a covering of downy hairs on the legs, tail, and face only.

The cat has three kinds of skin glands to care for its coat. Two types are sweat-producing glands, some located only on the pads of the feet and others over the entire body, used to leave their scent and mark territory. Territory marking is seen when the cat rubs against objects. The third type of gland is the sebaceous gland near the hair follicles, which secretes sebum to help waterproof the coat.

Moulting occurs in the spring and autumn, when the coat comes out in what seem like handfuls at a time. Long-haired coats will moult all year round due to the constant room temperatures in which these breeds of cat tend to live. It is essential that the long-coated breeds have owners who realise the necessity of daily grooming routines.

Grooming procedure in cats

Short coat
These cats are efficient self-groomers, with the normal-shaped head giving a slightly longer tongue than in the long-coated breeds. Two half-hour grooming sessions per week are ideal. In between, continue to condition the coat by stroking along the lie of the hair or polishing the coat using a piece of silk, velvet or chamois leather cloth.
Equipment required:

- Fine-toothed comb
- Soft bristle brush
- Rubber brush (see Figure 22.10)
- Chamois cloth

Long-haired and semi-long-haired coat
These cats tend to have shorter faces resulting in shorter tongues, therefore making these breeds less efficient self-groomers. Moulting all year round, the coat tends to mat. Grooming is needed daily, split into two half-hour sessions during the day to check for mats. Start with a normal comb to remove dead hair and then use a fine comb to fluff up the coat. A toothbrush is used to brush the facial hair, keeping well clear of the eyes.
Equipment required:

- Wide-toothed and fine-toothed combs
- Slicker brush
- Bristle brush
- Toothbrush – medium bristle

Curly coat
Curly coats should not be overgroomed as this could result in baldness. A soft brush with short bristles is sufficient for removal of dead coat. Groom twice weekly.
Equipment required:

- Soft bristle brush

Wire coat
These cats have a crimped, woolly coat which is coarse to the touch. Removal of the dead hair in a wiry coat is essential but ensure that the curls spring untangled back into position. This is achieved by minimum brushing with a soft bristle brush and hand stroking at least twice weekly.
Equipment required:

- Soft bristle brush

Hairless coat

With hair only on the extremities, skin conditioning is more essential in these breeds. Do not brush these breeds. The skin needs daily sponging to remove dander (small scales from the hair and dried skin secretions). A sponge moistened with warm water wiped over the body daily or more frequently if required will remove the dander which, if left, could cause a skin allergy.

Equipment required:

- Sponge

Bathing a cat

1. Groom out all mats and hair contaminated with faeces. If these mats cannot be groomed out, it may be necessary to cut them off with scissors.
2. Dilute the shampoo as required and make sure all equipment is to hand before starting the process.
3. Place a non-slip mat into the bath area.
4. Unless bathing is a routine experience, cats can find it very traumatic so only bath them if necessary.
5. Two people are required, one to hold and reassure and one to bath:
    i. Fill the bath with about 10 cm of warm water into which the cat is lowered gently.
    ii. Use a mixer hose and/or a sponge to soak the cat's fur from hindquarters to head (protecting the eyes and ears).
    iii. Apply the shampoo, rubbing it into the coat.
    iv. Rinse the shampoo out thoroughly from head to toe.
    v. Proceed with a thorough rinse and then wrap the cat in a towel.
    vi. At all times, make sure water or shampoo never gets close to the eyes, ears or mouth.
    vii. Pat dry to absorb excess water or use a chamois-type cloth. Never rub long coats vigorously as this will create tangles.
6. Wipe over the face with cotton wool moistened in warm water.
7. Towel dry and keep in a warm area until fully dry or dry using a handheld dryer if the cat will tolerate it. The dryer should be on a warm setting and held at a safe distance away from the cat.
8. Once the coat is dry, comb out gently and brush.
9. Finish with the grooming of the coat hair.
    - Short hair – start at the head and comb/brush towards the tail, including chest and abdomen. Then, rub down with a chamois or nylon pad to polish the coat.
    - Long hair – comb the legs free of tangles; then the abdomen, flanks, back, chest, and neck; and then the tail section, fluffing out the coat hair by brushing the wrong way. Finally, using a toothbrush, groom the facial hair.

Once all grooming is complete, remove the dead hair from the combs and brushes, wash, disinfect, and rinse before storing to prevent cross infection between grooming sessions or infecting another animal groomed with the same equipment. Equipment should be sterilised on a regular basis, e.g. monthly.

Warning

- If a cat's coat is dirtied by chemicals, such as tar, creosote, paint, or oil, remove as soon as possible to prevent absorption through the skin or self-grooming and ingestion of the chemical, which may be a poison.

- Never use chemicals to remove these substances.
- On a dry coat, use soft margarine, washing-up liquid or liquid paraffin to work the substance free of the hairs and then proceed with a bath and dry thoroughly.
- If the cat has self-groomed, contact a veterinary surgeon immediately for advice.

Grooming Small Mammals

Small mammals will usually groom themselves and need no assistance with coat care except for long coated breeds such as the Angora rabbit and Sheltie guinea pigs. These long-coated breeds must be checked daily in spring and summer for signs of fly strike (a condition where flies lay their eggs in the sensitive skin around the genital areas).

Small mammals rarely need to be bathed except for long haired guinea pigs breeds to remove urine stains from the coat and occasionally ferrets to remove the excess oil from their coats

Species such as chinchilla, gerbils, hamsters, and degus require an additional sand bath to clean their fur and help manage the oil content of their coats as their fur is very dense.

Claws can be clipped with either scissor type or plier type clippers that are a suitable size for the animal's claws.

Summary of Grooming and Coat Care

There are several reasons why an animal may be groomed with the main aims of grooming being health, hygiene, good welfare, and bonding.

Coat care is important in all species and the growth of the coat can be affected by several factors.

Different breeds of cats and dogs have distinct coat types, and it is important to care for the coat correctly and be able to recognise a healthy coat and when there may be problems.

There is a wide range of grooming equipment on the commercial market. The equipment needed for basic grooming to be carried out is combs, brushes, and nail clippers and toothbrushes.

Bathing and drying procedures must be undertaken with care to ensure the safety of the animal.

Grooming is an essential aspect of good animal welfare.

23

Feeding Animals

Learning goals

In this chapter, the learning goals are:

- To identify types of feed and supplements
- To identify types of feeding equipment
- To identify feeding routines
- To identify guidelines for food storage

There is a wide range of commercial feedstuffs that can be provided for animals. Owners/carers/keepers will have preferred products and brands to feed their animals, but the key consideration should be whether the food being provided meets the dietary requirements of the animal. If the animal is being fed a suitable balanced diet for its life stage and activity levels, then there is no need to provide additional supplementation. The diet provided should provide sufficient energy for the animal via fats and carbohydrates.

General Considerations for Feeding Animals

- Read instructions carefully before feeding any food
- Type of food
- How the animal should be fed
- Equipment needed to feed the animal
- How the food should be stored
- Amount of food an animal should be given
- How often an animal should be fed
- Activity level of the animal
- Life stage of the animal

Before feeding

- Ensure that food and water containers are cleaned
- Check that the food is suitable for the animals, its age, life stage, and activity levels so that it is receiving the right types and proportions of nutrients for maintaining good health
- Feed only fresh foods in the right quantities to prevent overfeeding

Animal Biology and Care, Fourth Edition. Emily Jewell.
© 2026 John Wiley & Sons Ltd. Published 2026 by John Wiley & Sons Ltd.
Companion Website: https://www.wiley.com/go/animal/biology4e/jewell

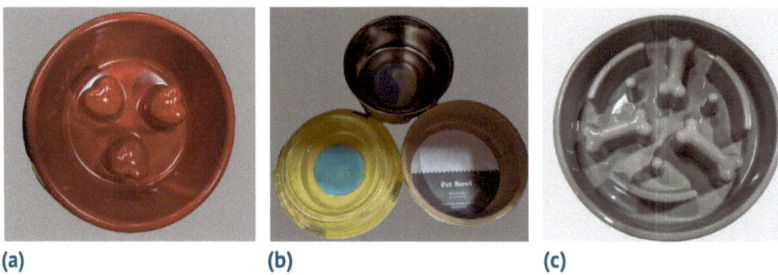

(a)   (b)   (c)

Figure 23.1 Commercially available food bowls.

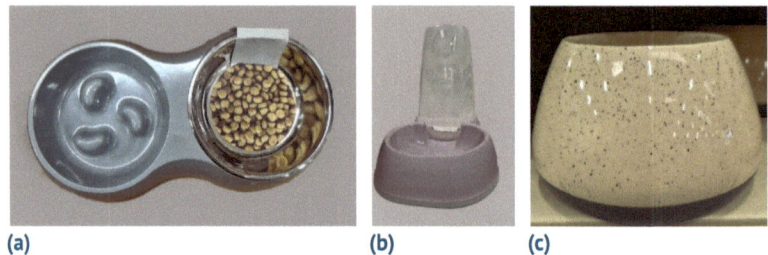

(a)   (b)   (c)

Figure 23.2 Commercially available water bowls.

- Check that the feed provided is in date, has not been broken open or damaged, and is not contaminated by anything
- The food should be stored in closed containers at room temperature and kept dry
- Water is fresh and always available

Figures 23.1 and 23.2 show a variety of commercially available food and water bowls. Slow feeder bowls are a recent introduction to the commercial market and they help to reduce the speed at which animals eat their food and can drink their water. Water bowls with higher sides have been designed for different breeds such as spaniels to avoid their ears getting wet when drinking from the bowl.

Types of Food

There are a wide range of commercial foods available for animals, which can be split into the following categories:

- *Live*
  - It is only legal to feed live invertebrate food such as mealworms, crickets and locusts, and bloodworms.
  - Reptiles, amphibians, fish, and birds are usually fed invertebrate diets. Rodents may also be given mealworms as a source of protein in their diet.
  - Feeding live insects encourages the display of natural hunting behaviours in reptiles and amphibians.

- **Commercially prepared**
  - *Tinned food* — meat and vegetable protein–based foods usually mixed with biscuits or meal to make up a complete diet. Protein levels in cat food are usually much higher than in dog food.
  - *Frozen food* — foods for fish such as bloodworm are frozen. Reptiles may be given rodents and day-old chicks but they must be fully defrosted prior to feeding. There are also frozen meat foods available for dogs and cats that must be defrosted before feeding.
  - *Semi-moist foods* — complete foods that contain three times the number of calories of tinned foods.
  - *Complete dry foods* — concentrated foods that contain four times the calorie content of tinned foods. These have virtually all water content removed and therefore fresh water must always be available when feeding dry foods. Some dry foods need water adding to them before feeding.
  - *Biscuit meal* is usually cereal based and designed to be fed with tinned food.

- **Fresh/natural**, e.g. forage, vegetables, fruit, herbs, nuts, and seeds.
  - These foods are included to increase vitamins, minerals, and vegetable oils in the diet. Birds require different seed types in their diet. Rabbits and guinea pigs need high-fibre diets with approximately 90% being fibre based e.g. Timothy hay. All omnivores can have a range of fruits and vegetables adding to their diets for variety.

- **Home-produced diets**
  - Home-produced diets must still be balanced, but they can be time consuming to prepare. It is important to either mince or chop up food into small pieces for smaller animals such as cats and ferrets.
  - Bones should not be fed as part of a home-produced diet
  - All foods included should be of good quality
  - Uneaten food should be removed daily
  - Fresh water should always be available and changed at least once a day
  - Serve at room temperature
  - Raw egg white should not be fed as it makes biotin (vitamin B7) unavailable to the animal.
  - All foods supply energy. This is measured in units of heat (kJ/g or kcal/g). Protein and carbohydrate are equal in energy content, but fat will provide twice this amount of energy for every gram of weight.
  - Examples of nutrient sources in a home-produced diet could include:
    - Proteins – check levels are suitable for the animal's life stage. The protein content of a diet must make up at least 20% of the total energy present:
      - Liver (high in phosphorus but low in calcium and rich in vitamins A and B)
      - Heart (high in fat, therefore used only in small quantities)
      - Chicken and turkey are lower in calories than other meats and easily digested
      - Fish is a good protein source, but all bones must be removed (grill or steam but do not boil)
      - Egg (scrambled) is useful for recovery from illness and restoring appetite
      - Minced beef or lamb will include animal fat
      - Pulses such as lentils could also be included
    - Fibre, vitamins, and minerals
      - Vegetables (cooked carrot, cabbage, green beans, pumpkin)
    - Fats
      - Animal fats – Meat of animal origin can contain animal fat, e.g. lamb
      - Vegetable oils

    ○ Carbohydrates to supply energy (usually need flavouring)
      – Cereals
      – Potato
      – Rice
      – Pasta
      – Noodles
- Avoid adding salt or sugar to any home-produced foods

Animal supplements

Supplements are foods that are provided in addition to the normal ration given. Some supplements may correct a deficiency in an animal with a medical disease or be given to prevent disease from occurring:

- Reptiles and amphibians usually need additional vitamin D and calcium added to their diet in the form of a powdered supplement to prevent metabolic bone disease. This can be added to live invertebrate feed so that they are gut loaded before being fed to the reptiles or amphibians. Alternatively, the insects can be dusted with the supplements prior to feeding.
- Guinea pigs must be given vitamin C in their diet to prevent scurvy as they are unable to manufacture it.
- Birds require an additional source of calcium (particularly in breeding season for egg formation) and this is usually fed in the form of cuttlefish (Figure 23.3).
- Birds also require additional grit in their diet to help with the crushing of seeds in the gizzard.

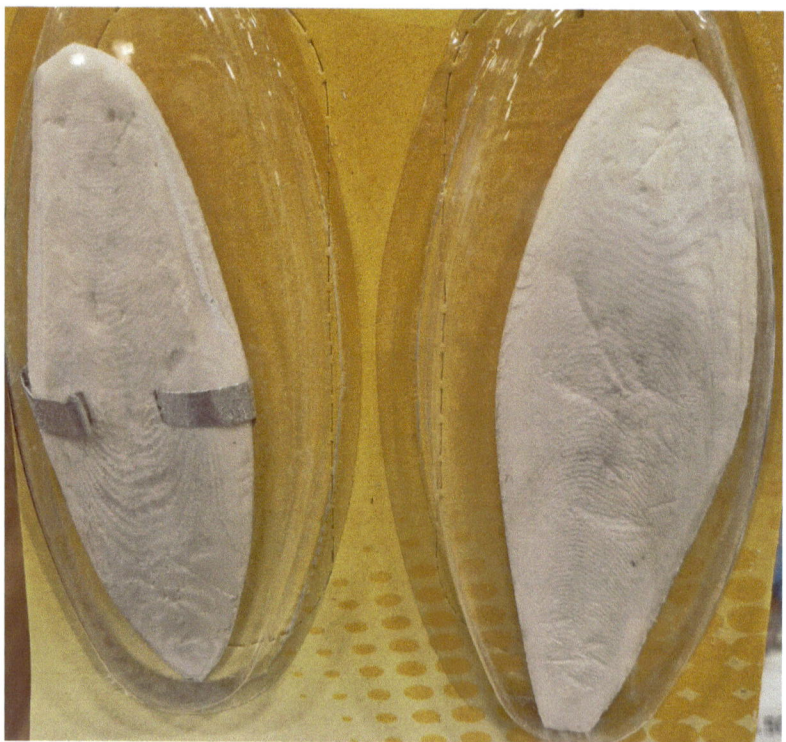

Figure 23.3   Cuttlefish for birds.

Animal treats

- There are a vast range of animal treats available on the commercial market.
- Treats are often used for rewards in training or as additional snacks and are often high in calories.
- Treats are often overfed by pet owners, leading to overweight animals.
- Branding and marketing of treats is aimed at getting owners to feel that their animals are missing out if they are not given treats. Treats exist in many different shapes, textures, colours, smells, and flavours (Figure 23.4a,b), with some representing human food items and flavours that would normally exist in the human diet, not the animal one.
- Treats should not be used to improve a poor diet or be supplied in excess. A good-quality complete and balanced food will provide the nutrients required for health and fitness.

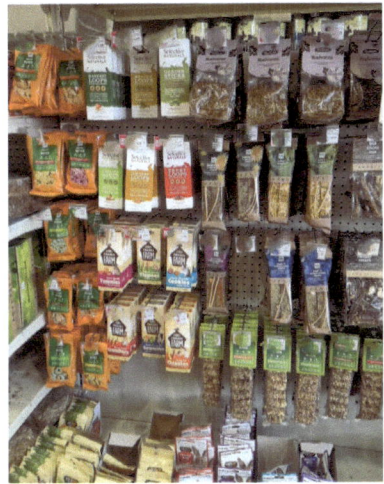
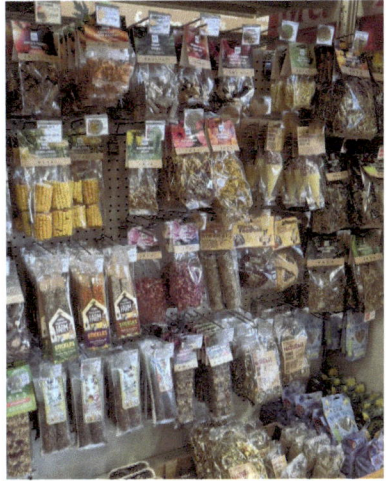

(a)

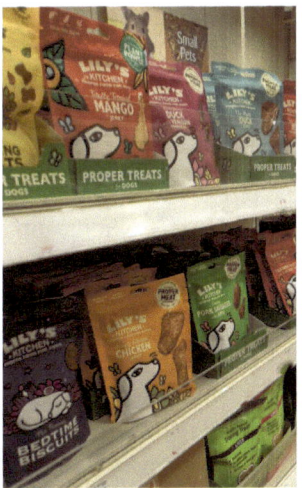
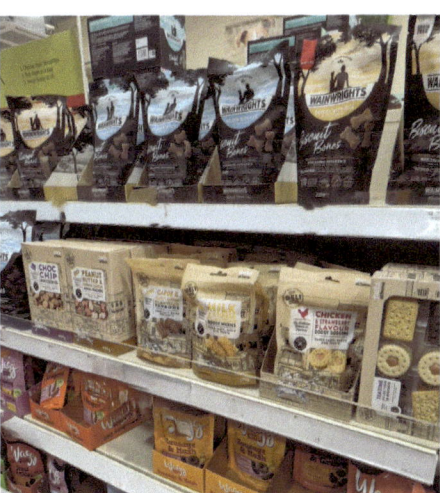

(b)

Figure 23.4   Commercially available treats for (a) rodents and (b) dogs.

How much food to provide?

The amount of food to be provided is based on energy needs and the rate of conversion of food to energy (metabolism) by the individual animal. The frequency of feeding is also based on nutritional demands for the animal. Requirements can be affected by:

- *Age/life stage* – geriatric animals need lower energy diets than young animals to prevent weight gain due to lower levels of activity. Young animals need high-protein, high-calorie diets due to their rapid growth rates. It is important that calcium and phosphorus are balanced to support bone development in young animals. Young birds need high-protein and high-fat diets for growth. Young animals need more frequent meals than adults, for example, puppies and kittens usually start with four meals a day once weaned and then progress to one or two meals a day as adults. Juvenile reptiles will usually be fed daily, adults may be fed less often, depending on species.
- *Activity levels* – a working gun dog or farm dog will need more energy in its diet than a non-working breed such as a Papillon.
- *Physiological condition* – the stages of gestation and lactation require more energy and protein than those animals not in that physiological state. Lactating animals require additional calcium in their diets and plenty of fresh water available.
- *Season* – calorie intake may need to be increased in colder months to maintain body temperature, particularly in animals kept outdoors. In reptiles, calorie intake may need to decrease as their metabolism will slow at lower temperatures. Additional fruits and vegetables can aid with providing extra water in the warmer months.
- *Temperature* – extreme high and low temperatures can affect an animal's appetite and their metabolism. Fresh water should always be available.

All commercially available food will have instructions on quantities to feed. The manufacturer will use the kcal/day requirements to suggest the amount in weight (grams) of the diet to feed regarding the percentage value of nutrients in that food.

Methods of feeding

There are different methods of feeding animals, and it should be specific for the species.

- *Bowl feeding* — the food is provided in a bowl. Whilst this keeps the food contained in a bowl, it does not encourage display of natural feeding behaviours for animals but does keep the environment tidy.
- *Scatter feeding* — scattering food around an enclosure promotes foraging behaviours in animals. It provides enrichment for the animal to find the food in its environment. Be aware that some animals hoard food and so the accommodation must be regularly checked to ensure that there is no rotting food anywhere.
- *Bottle/syringe feeding* – young mammals such as puppies and kittens may need to be hand reared and fed commercially produced formula milk via bottle or syringe.
- *Hand feeding* – animals that are recovering from illness or surgery may need hand feeding to stimulate their appetite. Small amounts should be offered frequently. Foods with a strong smell are useful when trying to encourage an animal to eat, e.g. cats and tuna fish.
- *Enrichment* — Licki mats make an animal work for their food and should be given as a reward (Figure 23.5). Timed feeders can be used to stimulate foraging behaviours.

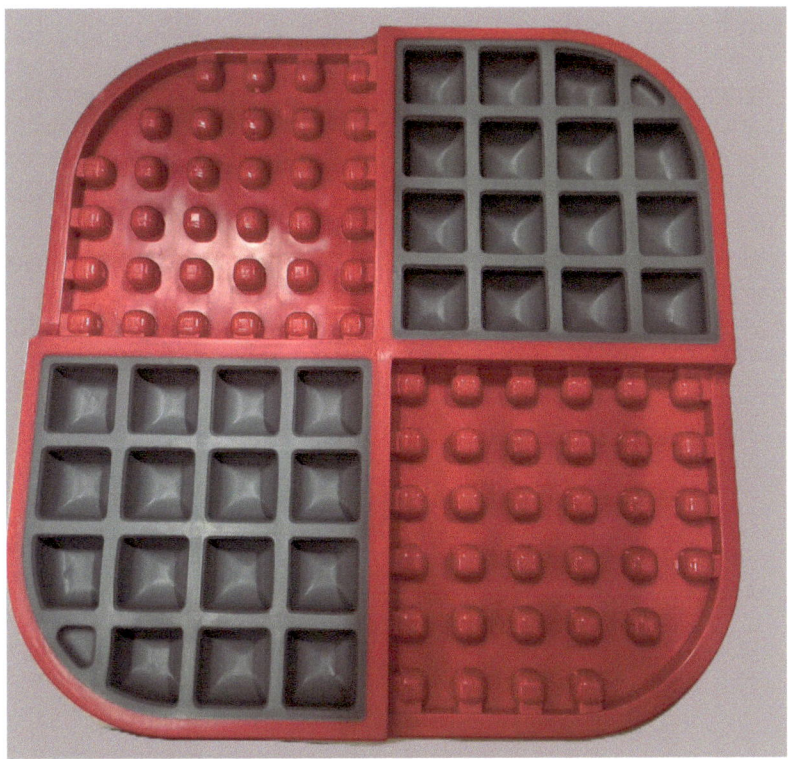

Figure 23.5 Commercially available product to provide treats for dogs.

Fresh water can be provided in bowls or in bottles, according to what is suitable for the animal species. Reptiles have their vivaria sprayed to maintain humidity and some will drink these droplets from the foliage and furniture within their accommodation.

Food storage

Animal foods should be stored in cool, dry places.

- Secure, airtight containers are ideal for food storage to deter insect pests and vermin, such as wild rats and mice. If vermin have access to foodstuffs, then they can contaminate it with their urine.
- If foodstuffs are not stored properly, then they can spoil, and either be wasted or cause problems if fed to animals. For example, if foods are stored in a damp environment, the *Aspergillus fungus* can develop, and if fed to animals, they could develop aspergillosis.
- Food quality can be affected by:
  - Humidity
  - Temperature
- Frozen foods should be thoroughly defrosted prior to being fed.
- When receiving deliveries of food, it is important to check the use by dates of stock and rotate stock (oldest fed first providing it is within its use by date).

Summary of Feeding Animals

There is a wide range of foodstuffs on the commercial market for animals. Some animals may need supplements provided as part of their dietary provision. Any treats provided should be incorporated into the daily energy ration for the animal.

Just as with foodstuffs, there is a wide range of feeding equipment commercially available and often the choice is down to the owner/carer/keeper.

Frequency of feeding and amount to feed depend on several factors, but the key reason is to ensure that the animal receives an appropriate amount of energy via its diet.

Food storage is often an area that is overlooked, but it is essential that it is kept with hygiene in mind to prevent spoilage, wastage, and contamination of food.

24

Other Animals Kept as Pets

Learning goals

In this chapter, the learning goals are:

- To identify and describe basic husbandry considerations for a range of animals kept as pets including:
  - Small mammals
  - Birds
  - Fish
  - Reptiles, amphibians, and invertebrates

Across the United Kingdom, cats and dogs make up the major proportion of pets kept in UK households; however, small mammals, birds, tortoises, and fish are also kept in large numbers. At the time of writing, keeping reptiles, amphibians, and invertebrates as a hobby has continued to increase over the last decade. If working in the animal industry, it is likely that, at some point, all these animals will be encountered within a collection, and so having knowledge of their care and husbandry is important. Beyond pet ownership, the care of some of these species can be very intricate, and it may be necessary to take expert advice in some cases, e.g. reptiles and fish.

Basic Husbandry for Other Animals

Housing

There are a range of housing options (cages, runs, tanks, pens, vivaria, aquaria) for small mammals, birds, fish and reptiles available in the current market (2025). Choice *should* be made according to suitability for the species and practicalities of hygiene, but there is often an aesthetic appeal for the owner/carer/keeper that is part of the final decision made.

Whatever housing option is chosen, it must be safe and secure for the animal. The following aspects of the housing should be considered:

- Constructed soundly of materials suitable for the species being housed:
  - No sharp edges
  - No rough surfaces
  - No loose joints

Animal Biology and Care, Fourth Edition. Emily Jewell.
© 2026 John Wiley & Sons Ltd. Published 2026 by John Wiley & Sons Ltd.
Companion Website: https://www.wiley.com/go/animal/biology4e/jewell

- Easy to clean
- Easy to provide food and water
- Comfortable for the animal intending to be housed
- Enrichment can be placed within the housing to mentally stimulate the animal
- Escape proof for the animal intending to be housed
- Prevents other animals from getting in
- Large enough for free movement of the animal and allows a moderate amount of exercise, e.g. a rabbit in a hutch should be able to stand up on its back legs and have space between its ears and the roof of the housing. A bird should be able to sit on a perch in the cage and have head clearance and tail feather clearance and be able to stretch its wings up and out without them touching the sides of the cage
- Dry and well ventilated
- Methods for heating or cooling as required during seasonal changes in environmental conditions, without being subjected to extremes of temperatures, e.g. direct sunlight entering the housing – this is particularly important in the case of reptiles that are not capable of maintaining their own body temperature and so are reliant on external heat sources
- Lighting requirements can be met
- The animal can excrete away from the bedding/food areas
- Suitable drainage

Promoting health

As previously mentioned in the previous chapters, promoting health is of vital importance when looking after animals and this can be summarised in the following way:

- Regularly examine the animal to determine health status or detect injury. If any animal is found to be diseased, it is important to move it to isolation or quarantine areas
- Only purchase animals from reputable and reliable sources to avoid disease being brought into the existing animal establishment
- Clean housing thoroughly and disinfect regularly
- Move any sick animal to isolation
- Apply high levels of hygiene to all equipment used in the housing, regularly using disinfectants
- Have a good airflow through the housing to prevent breathing problems and airborne diseases
- House different species separately where possible unless it is a mixed exhibit, where it is known that animals can exist together
- Change bedding several times a week, depending on species

Small Mammals

Small mammals that may be kept as pets include rabbits, guinea pigs, hamsters, gerbils, rats, mice, and ferrets.

Handling of these species must be done with care to avoid injury to the animal and the handler. If these types of animals are not used to regular handling, then they may bite or scratch, and so a basic knowledge of handling for each species is important to ensure the welfare of the animal. Initial restraint of these species should be firm but gentle to prevent injury (Figure 24.1).

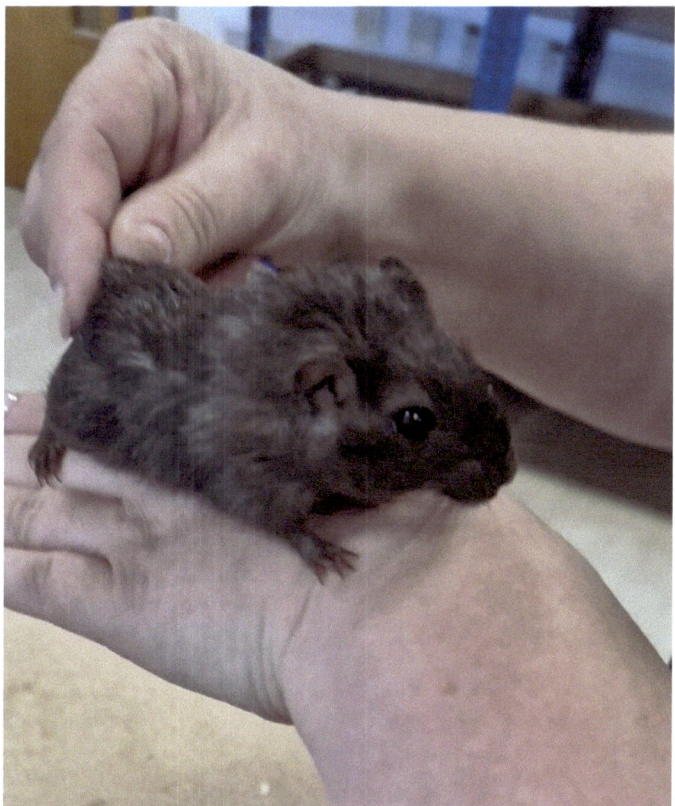

Figure 24.1   Gentle restraint, allowing the gerbil to explore without escaping.

Ferrets

Ferrets are a species that is growing in popularity in the United Kingdom with approximately 100,000 being kept as pets in 2024. Ferrets may be kept as pets, as working animals (for hunting rabbits), or as show animals. Ferrets (*Mustela putorius furo*), belong to the order Carnivora, family Mustelidae, and have descended from the European Polecat. There are three main types of ferrets – standard ferret, micro ferret, and Angora ferrets that can exist in several colours, such as sable, silver, cinnamon, albino, and dark-eyed whites. Ferrets can also be categorised by their coat markings, for example masked, mitted, bibbed, or solid.

Ferrets are sociable animals, and most enjoy living as part of a group (*known as a business*). If keeping a group of ferrets, it is best to ensure they are neutered.

Ferrets sleep for a long time in the day – up to 20 hours daily and are most active around dusk.

Ferrets do have a musky odour due to the oils released from sebaceous glands in their skin. These oils can build up in their bedding and this increases the smell. Entire ferrets also have a stronger smell. Regular cage cleaning and access to the outdoors helps to reduce the smell.

Ferrets use a range of methods to communicate. They use scent to establish if another ferret is part of their group or not along with establishing whether females are in season. Some ferrets can try to be dominant over others and it is important to look out for aggressive behaviours and dragging cage mates around.

Ferrets can be vocal and make a 'dooking' sound. They may also hiss, or they may scream if they feel they are in danger.

Ferrets are seasonal breeders with the mating season usually being between March and October. Jills are *induced ovulators* and must be mated to release eggs from the ovaries. If a female ferret comes into oestrus and is not mated, then she will remain in season and can develop a condition called *aplastic anaemia* which can lead to her death.

It is advised that all ferrets are neutered if they are not to be bred from. Males can be *castrated* or *vasectomised*. An unintended consequence of surgical neutering is the development of a hormonal condition called *hyperadrenocorticism or adrenal disease*. Both sexes may be given a contraceptive implant (Brand name Deslorelin) to suppress sexual activity through reduction of hormone levels. Implants last for between 18 and 24 months.

Biological data

Male	Hob
Female	Jill
Offspring	Kits
Adult weight	0.6–2.0 kg (males are heavier than females)
Maturity	4–8 months
Gestation period	39–42 days
Litter size	8 (average size)
Weaning age	6–8 weeks
Body temperature	37.8–40°C
Life span	6–10 years (average)

Anatomical facts: Ferrets
Teeth
- Dental formula: incisors 3/3, canines 1/1, premolars 3/3, and molars 1/2.

Senses
- Ferrets have poor eyesight. They rely on their senses of smell, taste, and hearing.

Skeleton
- Ferrets have a very flexible skeleton. They have an elongated body and large vertebrae which enables them to move in confined spaces and turn around in narrow tunnels.

Sweat glands
- Ferrets are unable to sweat and as a result are extremely susceptible to heat stroke.

Housing ferrets
Ferret housing should:
- Be escape proof
- Be well ventilated but draught free
- Be between 15 and 21°C in temperature. Outside ferrets will adjust to cold temperatures provided they have plenty of suitable bedding, but they will need additional opportunities to cool down in temperatures above 21°C due to their sensitivity to heat stroke.

- Have a sleeping area, an exercise area, and a toileting area.
- Be spot cleaned every day to avoid a build-up of faecal matter.
- Pet ferrets must have an enriched environment as they need mental and physical stimulation. They like to explore, dig, climb, and investigate everything in their enclosure. Ferrets also like their own space and so hide areas, hammocks and tunnels are essential additions to the enclosure. A range of toys should be available for investigation, such as balls and crinkle toys.
- Some ferrets enjoy a shallow water bath, but this should be supervised.

Feeding ferrets
- Ferrets are *obligate carnivores* as they do not have the enzymes needed to digest plant-based products properly.
- Raw diets are available, as are commercial kibble diets. Raw food or day-old chicks can be provided twice a week in addition to kibble. Raw food should have 15% fat, 30% protein and a low fibre content. It is important that vitamin and mineral content is balanced.
- Ferrets have high metabolic rates and fast transit time through the digestive tract and so food should always be available.
- Ferrets will hoard food. Always check the bedding area and remove uneaten food to prevent it becoming mouldy.
- Encourage ferrets to forage for their food by scatter feeding kibble.
- Avoid too many treats for ferrets although salmon oil is a popular one as it can be used to distract ferrets when handling, clipping nails, examining teeth, etc.
- Monitor the weight of each ferret in a group monthly, to ensure each ferret is getting enough food.
- Water can be supplied in bottles with a sipping spout or in bowls. Ensure ceramic bowls are heavy enough to not be tipped up by the ferrets. Fresh water should be supplied daily.
- Do not house ferrets near prey species.

Handling ferrets
- Daily handling helps strengthen bonds between ferrets and their handlers.
- Ferrets need a firm grip, particularly the larger males.
- The easiest way to handle a ferret is to place one hand under or around the ferret's chest and then support the hind legs with the other hand, The ferret should be held close to the handler's body so that it feels safe. Ferrets should not be held near to the handler's face.
- Ferrets may be trained to walk on a lead although the walk will go where the ferret wants to go rather than where the owner wants to go! If ferrets are walked in areas where many dogs visit, it is recommended that they are vaccinated for distemper.

Sexing ferrets
- Testicles in entire males are obvious.
- The urethral opening in males is further apart from the anus.
- In females there is a Y-shaped slit in the vulva located near to the anus. When a jill is in oestrus, the vulva is very pink and very swollen.

Gerbils

The species most kept as a pet is the *Mongolian gerbil – Meriones unguiculatus*. Gerbils belong to the order Rodentia, suborder Myomorpha, and there are about 80 species of gerbil in the wild. The gerbil is adapted to living in desert and semi-desert areas (Mongolia and northeastern China).

As a result of their wild habitat, gerbils can conserve liquid, producing very concentrated urine and dry faeces, which are odour-free. Gerbils are camouflaged in the wild due to their beige coat colour and reflect heat from their pale underneath to keep cool.

Gerbils are active both day and night (*diurnal*). In body proportions, the gerbil closely resembles the kangaroo, jumping rather than running when attacked. In the wild, gerbils can leap several feet in any direction, especially if startled, which, as a pet, can make them hard to handle although with sufficient handling, they become friendly.

Gerbils are lively, intelligent, and inquisitive animals. They sit up on their hind legs to watch for predators and communicate danger by thumping their hind legs or indicating their dominance. They spend a large part of their day burrowing, shredding bedding, tunnelling, and exploring. They love to burrow and so need a soft, deep substrate to build tunnels and create nests.

Gerbils are very social animals and are best kept together in groups, with same-sex litter mates or in breeding pairs. Gerbils will mate for life and should be introduced around 10 weeks of age. Adult gerbils will fight to the death, so try not to introduce adults to a stable family group.

Biological data

Male	Sire
Female	Dam
Offspring	Cubs
Adult weight	75–130 kg (depending on breed)
Maturity	10–12 weeks
Gestation period	24–28 days
Litter size	3–6 (average size)
Weaning age	21–28 days
Body temperature	38°C
Life span	2–5 years (average)

Anatomical facts: Gerbils
Teeth
- Incisors are open rooted and continue to grow through the gerbil's life. Check regularly.
- Dental formula: incisors 1/1, canines 0/0, premolars 0/0, and molars 3/3.

Scent glands
- Gerbils have scent glands on their abdomen, which are used for identification of members of the same family and marking of territory.

Adrenal glands
- Hormones from these endocrine glands assist the gerbil's ability to conserve water in adverse conditions.

Hind legs
- Longer than front legs; therefore, they can jump to escape from predators.

Tail
- Used for balance and turning.
- Gerbils have a dark tip on the end of their tail which acts as a decoy for predators. The tail can be shed if the gerbil is in danger or if it is grasped away from its base, but it does not re-grow.

Eyes
- Gerbils have relatively large eyes and very good vision.

Hearing
- Gerbils have an acute sense of hearing, due to an enlarged middle ear, to hear birds flying above and avoid being eaten.

Housing gerbils

Gerbils are social animals and will live in groups but can be aggressive to any newcomer. As pets, they are easy to handle, clean and friendly.

Gerbils are adapted to live in extremes of temperature, from 43°C to below freezing. The gerbil is a burrowing animal, creating elaborate tunnel systems and entrances. They do this to find a constant temperature within the ground. The burrowing material, peat, hay or wood shavings, needs to be dampened slightly to allow tunnels to be constructed that keep their shape. Sand must not be used on its own as a substrate as it may cause eye problems or respiratory problems. Shredded paper or hay can be provided so that the gerbil can build a nest/bed area.

The ideal housing is a glass tank of at least 90 cm in length, approximately 30cm deep, with a close-fitting mesh lid. Allow enough room between the lid and the tunnel material for above-ground or surface activity and prevent condensation.

Gerbil housing should:

- Be escape proof
- Contain only non-toxic materials, as gerbils will gnaw anything in their environment
- Be in a warm environment; 18–29°C is ideal. Gerbils are best kept at 15–20°C/59–68°F. Gerbils do not hibernate but may enter a state called *torpor* if the temperature is too cold
- Be washed, disinfected and rinsed every 2 months
- It is vital that substances for gnawing are provided for the gerbil to keep their teeth in good condition. Gnaw blocks may be bought from pet shops, or alternatively, natural non-toxic branches, such as apple twigs may be used instead. Putting branches in the cage also allows the gerbil to get exercise by climbing but ensure that they are not too near to the roof or gerbils may escape
- Have good light levels in the daytime to encourage activity
- Gerbils may occasionally be provided with a dust bath filled with chinchilla sand, as this help keep their coats in good condition
- Gerbils produce only a few drops of urine and faecal pellets are dry and odourless, so bedding only needs to be changed about every 2–4 weeks, unless particularly dirty

Feeding gerbils
- Gerbils are omnivores.
- Food can include grain (e.g. wheat, maize, oats, barley), seeds (e.g. millet, sunflower) and greens (e.g. dandelion, groundsel, chickweed).

- Sunflower seeds should be restricted as these are too rich in fat and calcium, which can lead to dietary imbalance and ill health.
- An animal protein source may be included in a commercial gerbil food or boiled egg can be added to the diet. The protein content of the food should be approximately 20%.
- The diet can be supplemented with fresh fruits and vegetables, such as apple, banana, and carrot, but too much can cause diarrhoea.
- A gerbil will eat approximately 1 tablespoonful of food/day.
- Gerbils will hoard food. Always remove the uneaten food to prevent it from becoming mouldy. It is better to scatter feed the food as an enrichment, but if bowls are provided, then they should be metal or ceramic so that gerbils cannot chew them.
- Water must be supplied in bottles with dispensing spouts. The bottles can be attached to the side of the tank or the lid, but ensure it is suspended above the level of the substrate, or the dispensing spout will become blocked. The water should be supplied fresh daily.

Handling gerbils
- To handle a gerbil, it is better to scoop it up in cupped hands or an appropriate container. Do not attempt to lift a gerbil by the tail as it may be shed, which will cause pain to the gerbil (Figure 24.1).

Sexing gerbils
- The distance between the urethral opening and the anus is longer in the male gerbil than in the female.

Guinea pigs

Guinea pigs (*Cavia porcellus*) are also known as cavies. They belong to the order Rodentia, sub-order Hystricomorpha, which also includes chinchillas, degus and porcupines. There are three main coat types of guinea pig, within which there are many colour and marking variations. These can be grouped as:

- *Smooth* or short hair (also referred to as self-varieties), e.g. Self Golden or Dutch
- Containing whirls, ridges and rosettes, e.g. Abyssinian, Coronet
- *Long coated* (up to 50 cm in length) with long hairs, e.g. Peruvian, Texel, and Sheltie. Long coats require a lot of grooming and are mostly kept for showing, therefore not recommended for beginners

Guinea pigs are popular pets but can be nervous. They are generally docile, rarely bite, and are easy to handle and tame. They should not be kept on their own because they are very sociable animals. All-female or all-male groups can live together; however, the males must not be housed anywhere near the females as once they are sexually mature, they will fight for dominance. Females and males can be neutered if non-breeding mixed groups are to be kept as pets.

Guinea pigs are not as agile as many other rodents, but they are able to run quickly, especially when startled, despite their short legs and stocky body. To communicate, guinea pigs can make a range of noises, from squeaks and squeals to grunts. Guinea pigs are also known for their 'chattering'. Although guinea pigs do not dig, they are at home in dense undergrowth and enjoy making 'runs' through long grass. The main difference between guinea pigs and other rodents is the length of gestation and the subsequent advanced stage of their young at birth.

Biological data: Guinea pigs

Male	Boar
Female	Sow
Offspring	Piglets
Adult weight	75–100 g
Maturity	Males: 8–10 weeks
	Females: 4–5 weeks
Gestation period	60-72 days
Litter size	2–6 (average size)
Weaning age	3–4 weeks
Body temperature	38–39°C
Life span	4–7 years

Anatomical facts: Guinea pigs
Teeth
- Dental formula: incisors 1/1, canines 0/0 (diastema), premolars 1/1, and molars 3/3.
- The teeth of a guinea pig are open rooted, and chisel shaped, continuing to grow throughout their lifetime. Guinea pigs do not have a second small pair of incisors (*peg teeth*) found behind the main pair as in rabbits; however, they do have a gap behind the incisors called the *diastema*. This allows the sides of the cheeks to be drawn in behind the incisors, enabling the animal to continue gnawing while regulating what it swallows.

Tail
- Born without a tail.

Scent glands
- Sebaceous glands are located on the rump and used to mark territory. In older animals, these glands can become blocked and infected, and this is something to watch out for.

Pelvis
- The pubic symphysis (floor of the pelvic joint) will separate under the influence of hormones during parturition, to allow the newborn passage through the birth canal. Newborn guinea pigs are referred to as *precocious*, meaning that within a few hours of birth, they are self-sufficient, eating and drinking from feeding dishes. They are born with a complete coat, with eyes and ears open and with a set of teeth in place.

Housing guinea pigs
Guinea pigs are sociable and can be housed as a colony. A single animal can be housed with another species such as a rabbit breed of similar size (Figure 24.10a) although there are different viewpoints about this. Guinea pigs can be housed inside or outside providing it is a sheltered environment.
Housing should:

- Protect from extremes of temperature in summer and winter
- Protect the animal from getting wet and exposure to draughts

- Be well constructed from good-quality materials which have not been treated with any toxic chemicals
- Be the correct size with separate compartments for eating and sleeping; housing intended for rabbits can accommodate two to three guinea pigs
- Provide good airflow and ventilation
- Protect from predators by being raised and fitted with a sturdy catch/lock system
- Contain materials for gnawing to reduce the teeth length. A supply of bark-covered branches from non-toxic trees (i.e. fruit trees) should be regularly changed
- Have a summer run for natural grazing or wire off a part of the garden to allow for space and freedom to exercise. Ideally, this run will be portable to allow movement onto different areas of grass. Be careful not to place the run in direct sunlight and provide a shaded area
- Be easy to clean. Use similar bedding as that used for rabbits, but it must be clean, dry and dust-free. Ideal types of bedding include wood shavings to absorb urine and straw and hay for warmth. Guinea pigs tend not to toilet in one area, so more frequent cleaning is required than for a rabbit. If feeding and water bowls are used, these need daily washing as they tend to be fouled
- Disinfect at least monthly to remove the scale and odour from housing

Example of indoor and outdoor guinea pig housing is shown in Figure 24.2a,b.

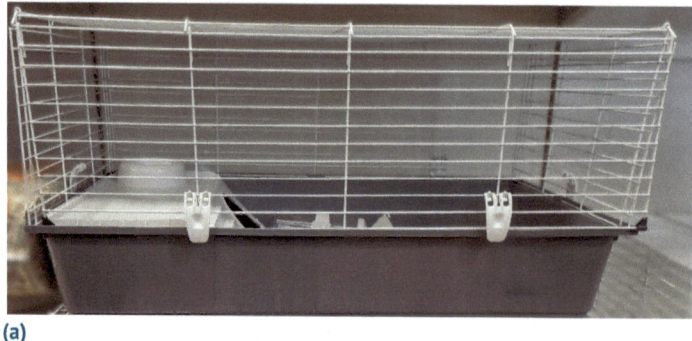

(a)

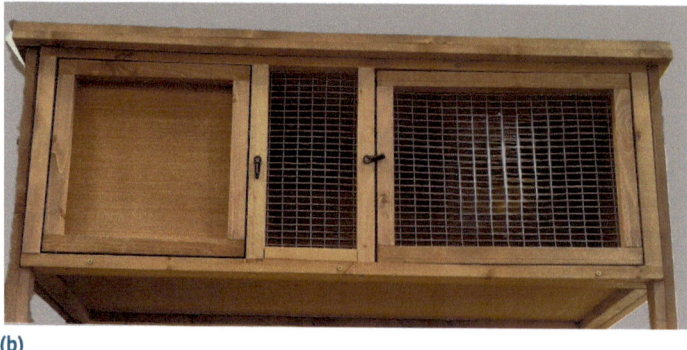

(b)

Figure 24.2 (a) Indoor and (b) outdoor housing commercially available for guinea pigs.

Feeding guinea pigs

Guinea pigs are herbivores and spend most of their waking hours grazing if permitted. By nature, guinea pigs dislike any change to their routines, so introduce any changes gradually and monitor afterwards. Guinea pigs often chew feed and water containers and so choose metal or ceramic containers rather than plastic ones. A water bottle is better for providing water to a guinea pig than a bowl.

Commercially available pelleted guinea pig feed can be used. If any other prepared diet is used, then it is essential to supplement vitamin C, as ascorbic acid, in the diet, for skin and coat condition. *Guinea pigs are unable to manufacture vitamin C and must receive it in their diet.* Although some vitamin C can be obtained from natural grazing, they must have a daily supply of 10 mg/kg body weight. During pregnancy, the quantity of vitamin C can be increased by three times the normal daily amount to maintain a healthy animal.

Rabbit diets are generally not suitable for guinea pigs as they may contain levels of vitamin D that are too high for the guinea pig. Read the packaging and ask the supplier for advice. This is one reason why a discussion exists around housing rabbits and guinea pigs together.

Good-quality hay should be provided. Pelleted food can be supplemented with fresh vegetables (swedes and carrots) and fruits. Useful green foods include broccoli, dandelion, and groundsel. Always provide fresh drinking water daily.

Handling guinea pigs

Handling of guinea pigs should be carried out quietly and confidently to avoid unnecessary struggling which could result in injury to the guinea pig or to the handler. Talk quietly to the guinea pig in a reassuring voice to minimise any distress. If a guinea pig feels secure during handling, there should be no problems.

When lifting a guinea pig, it is important to be gentle:

- Place one hand over the guinea pig's shoulders and back and using the other hand to support the back end of the guinea pig, lift the guinea pig up.
- Once lifted, a guinea pig should be turned towards you so that it feels secure with its feet on your chest.
- Alternatively, a guinea pig can be cradled along the arm.
- A guinea pig will struggle if it does not feel secure, and this can cause injury to both the handler and the guinea pig.

Sexing guinea pigs

Once the technique is learnt, it is very easy to distinguish between the males and the females. The guinea pig should be lying supported on its back with its back legs facing away from you. Place gentle pressure on the lower abdomen in the genital area. In a male animal, the penis will be displayed. In females, a 'Y' shape tends to be observed (Figure 24.3). Once guinea pigs have been sexed, they should be kept in separate groups to avoid unnecessary breeding.

Hamsters

Hamsters are one of the most popular small pets. Belonging to the order Rodentia, suborder Myomorpha, there are over 20 species of hamster. However, those most kept as pets are:

- *Syrian hamster – (Mesocricetus auratus) – must be kept on their own once mature.* They are aggressive to other hamsters, both male and female, once they reach puberty. They may

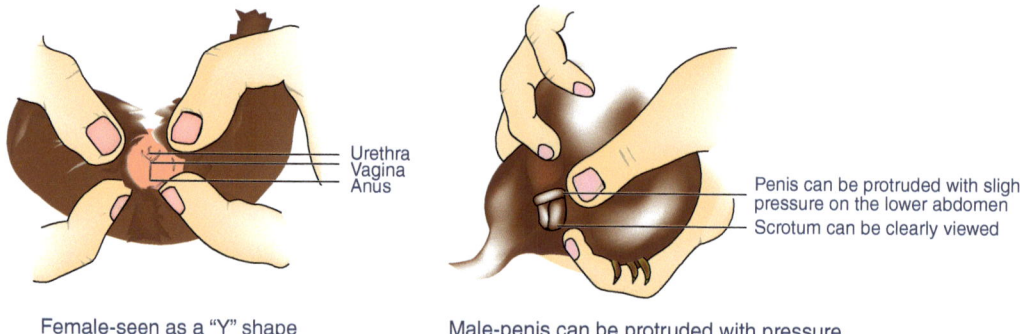

Urethra
Vagina
Anus

Penis can be protruded with slight pressure on the lower abdomen
Scrotum can be clearly viewed

Female-seen as a "Y" shape

Male-penis can be protruded with pressure

Figure 24.3 Sexing guinea pigs. *Source*: Ferris, 2003 / John Wiley & Sons.

hibernate if their environmental temperature falls below 5°C. There is a wide range of colours of Syrian hamster available, and they are referred to as individual breeds, e.g. black-eyed cream, Swedish Black and Cinnamon. Coat types also contribute to different hamster breeds, e.g. Satins and long hairs.

- *Russian hamsters* – (*Phodopus sungorus*) – the most sociable of all the hamsters. In the wild, they live in family groups rather than alone. They should be kept in pairs or as small groups, but if not handled regularly, they can become aggressive. They have a similar shape to the Syrian hamster but are much smaller. Colours include cinnamon, grey, sapphire, spotted and winter white.
- *Chinese hamsters* – (*Cricetulus griseus*) – less sociable than the Russian hamster but can be kept in pairs or small groups if introduced to each other when young. They are slightly smaller in size than the Russian hamster but have a longer body with a small visible tail.
- *Roborovski hamsters* – (*Phodopus roborovskii*) – are the smallest of all the hamsters and must be kept in pairs or groups. They resemble a Russian hamster in appearance with a white moustache. The Roborovski is not recommended as a pet for children because it is so small and active and therefore hard to handle.

Hamsters are active at dawn and dusk (*crepuscular*) but sleep most of the day. Dwarf hamsters show more activity during the day. Hamsters are escapologists and any cage needs to be secure. Dwarf hamsters, such as the very small Roborovski hamster, are best kept in tanks. Hamsters can bite if disturbed from their sleep, and when feeling threatened or aggressive, they sometimes squeal, screech, or hiss. Their sense of smell is their primary sense, and they become accustomed to the scent of the group if not living singly. If one animal has been handled extensively or placed in the company of another hamster, the group may attack it.

Biological data: Hamsters

	Syrian	Chinese	Russian
Male	Sire	Sire	Sire
Female	Dam	Dam	Dam
Offspring	Pups	Pups	Pups

	Syrian	Chinese	Russian
Adult weight	85–150 g	27–35 g	27–35 g
Maturity	6–10 weeks	14 weeks	14 weeks
Gestation period	15–18 days	20–22 days	19–20 days
Litter size	3–7	3–7	3–7
Weaning age	21–28 days	20–22 days	20–22 days
Body temperature	37–38°C	37–38°C	37–38°C
Life span	1.5–2 years	1.5–2 years	1.5–2 years

Anatomical facts: Hamsters

Teeth
- Incisors are open rooted and continually grow. They must be regularly checked to ensure they are not overgrown.
- Dental formula: incisors 1/1, canines 0/0, premolars 0/0, and molars 3/3.

Mouth
- Hamsters have large cheek pouches, reaching almost to the scapula area of the shoulder, used to transport food or store it temporarily.

Eyes
- Hamsters are short-sighted and rely on scent within their enclosure.

Scent glands
- Situated in the flank region and used to mark territory, these are seen as darker patches of skin and are also known as *flank glands*. They can be obvious in older animals leading owners to think there is a skin problem.

Housing hamsters

Syrian hamsters are naturally solitary animals and will fight other individuals if not closely supervised. Dwarf hamsters will happily live in pairs or small groups if raised together from a young age. When awake, hamsters have a lot of energy. Hamsters in the wild will dig tunnels close to the surface and in the wild, hamsters can cover up to 11 km, daily.

There is a wide variety of accommodation available for hamsters. Hamster housing should be as big as possible so that the hamster can gain adequate exercise. Hamsters need plenty of living space and a smaller area for sleeping. A rough size guide is 2400 cm^2 × 30 cm high.

To prevent boredom, housing should include playthings such as cardboard tubes, empty jam jars, and exercise wheels of a solid construction. If the temperature of their environment drops below 5°C, hibernation for survival may occur, particularly with the Syrian hamster.

Hamsters will chew soft metals, plastic and wood, and so it is best to avoid these materials in the housing if possible.

Hamster housing should:

- Be constructed from materials that are non-absorbent, easy to clean and relatively non-chewable

- Have side access to the cage so that the hamster doesn't think that the owner/carer/keeper is a predator and so attack them
- Have only safe bedding materials, such as peat or wood shavings as a base, covered with untreated paper or cardboard for shredding and nesting
- Be kept inside
- Not be in direct sunlight. The temperature should be approximately 22°C. Remember, hamsters may try to hibernate if the temperature drops too low
- Be well ventilated but not draughty
- Include a sleeping house
- Be cleaned at least two to three times a week
- Provide exercise equipment, such as a wheel, tunnels, ladders, and plenty of safe materials for shredding
- Bedding – wood shavings can be used in the bottom of the cage and shredded paper for the resting area. Hay should not be used as it can damage the hamster's pouches. Nylon bed material should not be used as it can get twisted around the hamster's legs and also get stuck in their pouches, and this can cause them to become infected

Feeding hamsters
- Hamsters are relatively easy animals to feed although a lot of hamsters are overweight due to a lack of exercise and being given too much food.
- The hamster is an omnivore and can be fed a commercially produced 'hamster mix' food, which contains maize, corn, alfalfa, dried peas, sunflower seeds, and peanuts. The diet should contain animal protein. Vegetables and fruits (e.g. carrot, apple) will help to improve health status, with small quantities given daily. Hamsters need a supply of food to gnaw on to prevent incisor overgrowth. As well as the nuts in the diet, dog biscuits and wholemeal macaroni can be provided.
- Watch out for selective feeding where the hamster will only choose specific parts of a mixed food to eat.
- Hamsters will attempt to eat and hoard anything; therefore, they must not be given sweet treats. The adult hamster will eat its own droppings, particularly for vitamins B and K formed in the gut by bacteria.
- Food can be provided on an *ad-lib* basis for hamsters, but the bowl should not be filled up until the bowl is empty so that the hamster does not become fussy. Check for areas of stored food in the housing and clean them up before re-filling the bowl.
- Provide fresh drinking water daily using a water bottle and sipper tube. Ensure the bottle is suspended where the hamster can reach it and out of the way of the substrate, so the dispensing tube does not become blocked.

Handling hamsters
Once a hamster is awake, let it explore its surroundings and come to you. Stroke a hamster first so it gets used to your smell. Do not rush a hamster or it may bite. Either let the hamster climb into the handler's hand, scoop it up in cupped hands or in a small container, or place one hand firmly over its shoulders and back and lift into the other hand (Figure 24.4). Once lifted, let the hamster wander between the handler's hands. To restrain a hamster, place the thumb and forefinger to either side of the head and hold still or scruff gently at the back of the neck. Never handle a hamster or scruff a hamster that has full cheek pouches – allow them to empty them first.

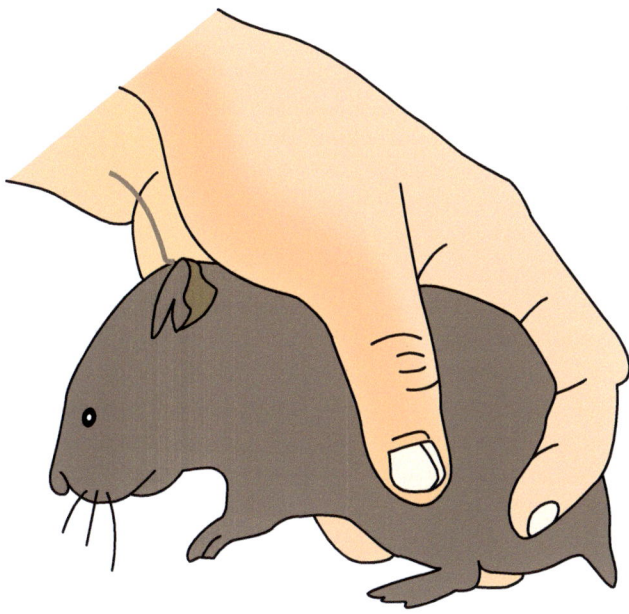

Figure 24.4 Handling a hamster. *Source*: Ferris, 2003 / John Wiley & Sons.

It is important to be confident when handling hamsters as they can sense nervousness and will bite. Regular handling is good for hamsters as it gets them used to humans.

Sexing hamsters
- Male and female hamsters are sexually mature at an early age and so should be separated from 6 weeks of age.
- Adult hamsters are relatively easy to sex as when viewed from the above; the male has a more pointed look to the back end of his body due to the presence of testicles. In females, the end of their body is more rounded although the tail can look more prominent.
- Young hamsters are not so easy to sex, but it can be done by observing the distance between the anus and the genital areas – in males, the distance is greater than in females (Figure 24.5).

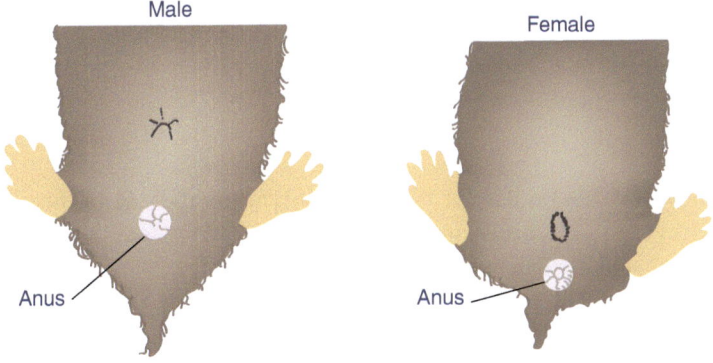

Figure 24.5 Sexing hamsters. *Source*: Ferris, 2003 / John Wiley & Sons.

Mice

Mice kept as pets are known as fancy mice and they belong to the order Rodentia, suborder Myomorpha – *Mus musculus*. They are initially categorised according to their coat type (varieties), and then, they are grouped into sections within each variety according to their colour and body markings. Varieties include long hairs, Rex and Satins.

Mice are very social animals and should live either as a breeding pair or in a grouping of two or more females. Male mice will fight if kept together. Mice have a very high reproductive rate, and so a pair should only be kept together if you can guarantee homes for the offspring. Mice are very agile and quick to move. They can make good pets and are lively, friendly, intelligent and inquisitive animals. Mice are easy to tame and rarely bite unless threatened. Aggression is signalled by drumming the tail on the ground and stamping the hind legs. Mice are efficient climbers, clinging to surfaces and clothing of handlers, making handling easy. Mice do tend to be more active at night, communicating with each other by body language and voice, squeaking (high-frequency, high-pitch sounds) when frightened. Odour can be a problem, particularly with male animals, and so it is important to clean them out at least once a week.

Biological data: Mice

Male	Buck
Female	Doe
Offspring	Kittens/pups
Adult weight	20–40 g
Maturity	3–4 weeks
Gestation period	19–21 days
Litter size	5–11 (average size)
Weaning age	18 days
Body temperature	37.5°C
Life span	1–2.5 years

Anatomical facts: Mice
Teeth
- Dental formula: incisors 1/1, canines 0/0, premolars 0/0 and molars 3/3.
- A mouse's teeth are open rooted and continue to grow (incisor teeth only). The lower jaw is adapted in movement to allow gnawing or chewing.

Eyes
- Vision is not good, but because of their eye position (on the side of the head), the field of vision compensates. As a result, mice navigate their environment through smell and touch. Mice see better at night than in the day.

Feet
- Mice have scent glands on the soles of their feet that they mark their territory and food location.

Housing mice

The best accommodation for mice is a glass tank of at least 1200 cm^2 area and approximately 60 cm deep with a close-fitting wire mesh lid to prevent condensation from building up. Mice enjoy climbing and so need relatively tall cages. Plastic cages are a potential alternative and are easy to clean but are chewable.

It is important that any housing for mice is environmentally enriched with tubes, ropes, exercise wheels and compartments. Plenty of enrichment will enable the mouse to exercise and keep busy to maintain health and fitness (Figure 24.6).

Housing for mice should:

- Be escape proof, using commercial glass or plastic cages or tanks
- Be kept indoors, with an activity area and nest box containing a variety of bedding materials (shredded paper, hay or straw)
- Have no direct sunlight or draughts, thus avoiding extremes of temperature. Mice are best kept at 15–27°C/59–81°F. If the temperature rises above 30°C, then the mice can suffer from heat stroke
- Be dry and easy to clean
- Be cleaned at least once a week, preferably twice a week to reduce odour and accumulation of urine and faeces
- Contain plenty of enrichment
- Contain materials for gnawing to promote good tooth condition. Gnaw blocks may be bought from pet shops, or natural non-toxic branches such as apple twigs may be used instead

Feeding mice

- Mice are omnivores.
- Pelleted commercial balanced mouse diets are available. Mice require some animal-based protein in their diet, which the commercial foods will provide. They benefit from other additions to the diet, such as small quantities of dog biscuit, wholemeal bread, pieces of fruit (apples, grapes and strawberries) and vegetables (especially green vegetables) in small amounts, several times a week. If peanuts and sunflower seeds are given, monitor their intake as they

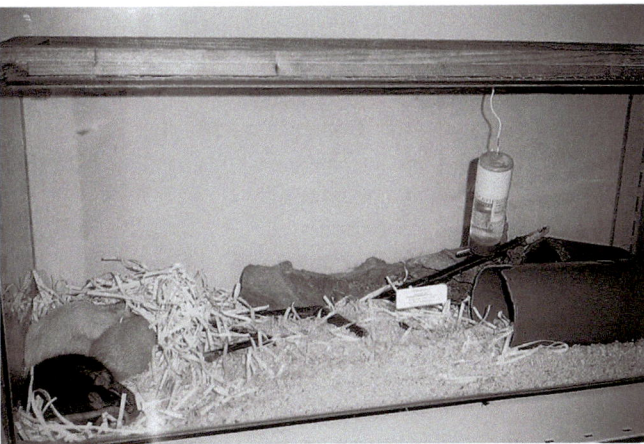

Figure 24.6   Housing with plenty of compartments.

can be fattening for the mouse due to their high lipid content. Too much fruit will result in diarrhoea.

- A mouse will eat approximately 3–6 g of food/day. Mice will store their food and so it is necessary to check for uneaten food that may go mouldy. Remove any uneaten food materials each morning.
- Food bowls may be provided and should be made of metal or ceramic so that the mice do not chew them. Alternatively, it is better to scatter feed for enrichment purposes.
- Water must always be provided, via a water bottle and sipper tube. Ensure the bottle is suspended above the level of the substrate or the dispensing spout will become blocked. Fresh water should be provided daily.

Handling mice

- Scoop the mouse up in cupped hands or in a small pot.
- Place the mouse onto an outstretched palm for stability and hold by the base of the tail for security.
- To restrain the mouse, place the forefinger and thumb of one hand on either side of the mouse's head to keep the head still and cup the body of the mouse in the hand.

Sexing mice

- An adult male mouse will be easy to sex due to the obvious visual presence of testicles. However, the most reliable method to use is to examine the distance between the anus and the urethral opening. In a male, there is a longer distance between the two.
- Younger mice are more difficult to sex, but females are likely to have more obvious nipple presence.

Rabbits

Rabbits (*Oryctolagus cuniculus*) belong to the order Lagomorpha, and since their domestication, there have been many different characteristics selected for. Rabbits are popular pets and there are over 80 breeds to choose from, with variation in shape, colour, size and character. Rabbits can usually fall into three main categories:

- *Normal* – these breeds have a coat type of short, dense fur like that of the wild rabbit, and were bred originally for meat, e.g. New Zealand White, Chinchilla, Dutch (Figure 24.7) and Californian
- *Fancy* – mainly bred for show, with distinguishing features, e.g. Lop for their large ears, Netherland Dwarf and Flemish Giant for their size and Himalayan for their coat markings
- *Rex and Satin* – noted for their velvet- or satin-like coats in which the guard hairs are missing or below the under-hair level, giving the coat a smooth, dense appearance

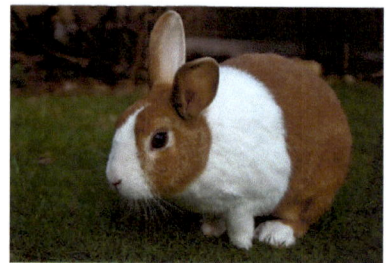

Rabbits are social animals if reared with their littermates and should not be kept on their own if possible. In the wild, they live in groups with a well-defined hierarchy. The males will fight to defend territory if kept in the same housing, as they would in the wild. Females will live together happily but are likely to show dominant

Figure 24.7 Dutch rabbit.

aggression once maturity is reached. Most owners pair up male and female, with one or both neutered if not intending to breed from them. Sometimes, rabbits can be paired with other species, such as guinea pigs, but this is not always ideal because the rabbits can bully the guinea pigs (being a smaller animal); also, the two species have different nutritional requirements, making feeding difficult. A rabbit kept alone needs a lot of human interaction to prevent development of fearful or aggressive behaviour. To enable this, some single rabbits are trained to use litter trays and are kept as house pets.

Biological data: Rabbits

Male	Buck
Female	Doe
Offspring	Kits (kittens)
Adult weight	1–10 kg (depending on breed)
Maturity	12 weeks onwards
Gestation period	28–32 days
Litter size	2–7 (average size)
Weaning age	6 weeks
Body temperature	38.5°C
Life span	6–8 years (average)

Anatomical facts: Rabbits

Eyes
- Rabbits have a wide field of vision, 190° for each eye. Dilation of the pupil means their night vision is about seven to eight times more effective than that of humans.

Ears
- Have a good blood supply and assist with body heat regulation and sound gathering.

Teeth
- Dental formula: incisors 2/1, canines 0/0 (diastema or gap), premolars 3/2, and molars 3/3.
- Rabbit's teeth are open rooted, continuing to grow throughout their life. If the correct foods and environment are provided, the teeth are continually worn down, which is essential for health. Rabbits are classified as herbivores; this effectively means that their diet consists mostly of plant matter. Therefore, the diet must be high in fibre (approximately 90%).
- The teeth are adapted to bite, chew and grind the high-fibre diet. It is because of constant wear and tear that the teeth continue to grow during the animal's life.
- The upper incisors are chisel shaped and grow roughly at a rate of 2 mm/week. The two pairs of upper incisors (Figure 24.8) are situated one behind the other. The upper hind incisors are called peg teeth. They are intended to be worn away by the lower incisors; in a normal, healthy rabbit, this effect gives the teeth their sharp chisel edge (Figure 24.9).

Body cavities
- The thoracic cavity is small, allowing for a large abdomen, which houses a lengthy intestinal tract with a large caecum.

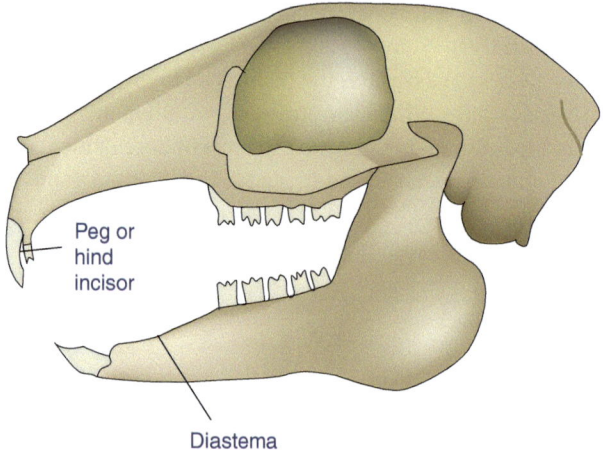

Figure 24.8   Rabbit skull – detail of mouth.

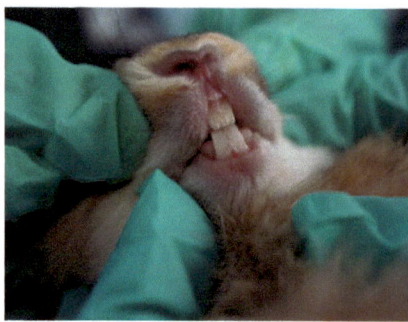

Figure 24.9   Examining a rabbit's teeth.

- The digestive system of rabbits has evolved to ensure that maximum benefit is derived from their diet. Digested foods pass through the stomach, into the small intestines and onto the caecum. This is a sac-like structure near the junction of the small and large intestines. It contains active bacteria that break down plant fibre (cellulose) for digestion and absorption. Many nutrients would be lost to the body at this point; however, the rabbit overcomes this loss by passing these nutrients in the form of soft caecal pellets (produced at late night/early morning) from the anus and eating them directly from the anus (*coprophagia*). The swallowed caecal pellets are mucous covered and stick together to pass through the digestive tract, allowing further breakdown and absorption of any useful nutrients. The rabbit then passes their characteristic dry, hard faecal pellet. This process of passing nutrients twice through the digestive system allows for maximum extraction of nutrient material. One way of observing that a rabbit is unwell is to see if soft sticky faeces is present in the housing.

Skeleton
- Rabbits have light, delicate bones covered with a powerful muscle system, especially to the hind legs. This can mean that the limbs and spine are prone to fracture, if handled carelessly. Rabbits can also cause substantial injury with their hind legs due to the power transferred through the limb.

Scent glands

- Located in the anal region for marking of territory.

Housing rabbits

There are many information sources providing plans and layouts for both inside and outside housing for rabbits. They provide construction details for housing and runs and safe materials to use. It is important to ensure that any housing is of the right size for the eventual size of the adult rabbit and allow sufficient head clearance space for the rabbit to sit up on its hind legs. Rabbits and guinea pigs of similar size can be kept together, but this is a concept that is continually debated, and the animals must be monitored carefully to ensure that there is no bullying from either animal species (Figure 24.10a). Figure 24.10b,c show enriched housing for individual species.

Rabbits do need regular exercise, ideally in an enclosed section of grass in the garden or a mobile run or in an assault course with wide plastic pipes in the hutch area. Fruit tree logs (safe for rabbits) can be included in both run and hutch to add interest.

Housing for rabbits should:

- Protect from extremes of heat, cold and draughts. The preferred temperature is 12–20°C
- Be well constructed from good-quality materials. If materials have been treated, check that the chemicals used are non-toxic
- Be the correct size, with separate compartments for living and sleeping
- Protect from predators by being raised and fitted with a sturdy catch/lock system
- Contain materials for gnawing to reduce the teeth length. A supply of bark-covered logs from non-toxic trees (i.e. fruit trees) should be regularly changed

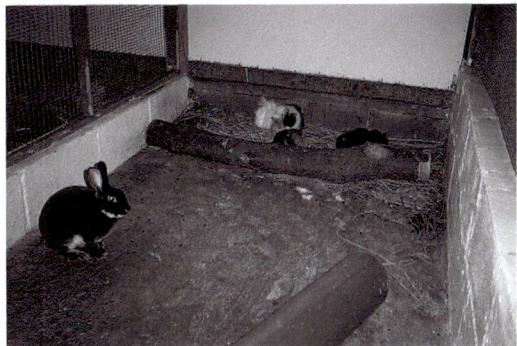

(a)

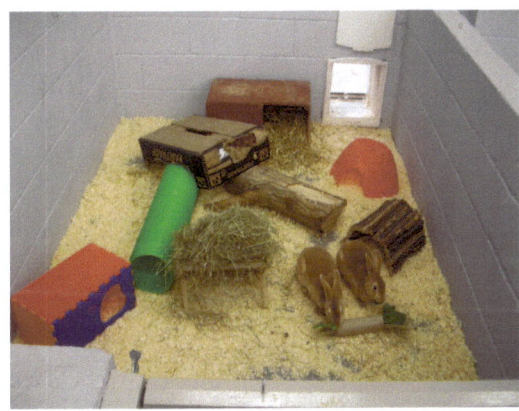

(b)

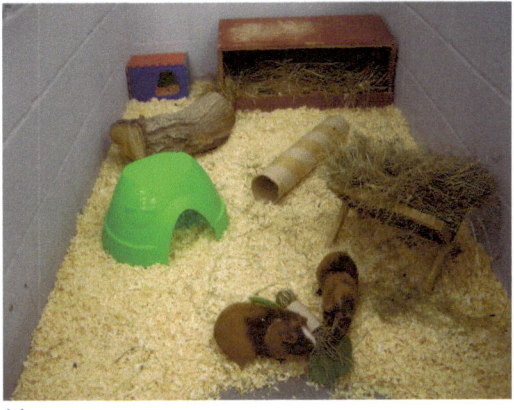

(c)

Figure 24.10 (a) Example of group housing of rabbit and guinea pig. (b) Enriched rabbit-only housing. (c) Enriched guinea pig-only housing.

- Include an escape-proof portable outdoor 'summer' run for natural grazing and exercise
- Provide good ventilation
- Be easy to clean. Remove all soiled bedding daily (spot clean) and carry out a full clean on a weekly basis. Rabbits tend to use one spot in the hutch as a toilet and can be trained to use a litter tray. Ideal types of bedding include wood shavings to absorb urine and straw and hay for warmth. Disinfect at least monthly to remove the scale and odour from housing

Feeding rabbits

- Many rabbits are fed on commercially produced pelleted foods which may contain anti-coccidial agents which could be harmful to some species. Check the packaging if rabbits and guinea pigs feed together as these additives would be harmful to the guinea pig.
- Rabbits are herbivores, so most of the diet should consist of roughage: good-quality hay or grass, supplemented by herbs, leafy greens and vegetables. Select vegetables and greens carefully. Do not feed if any of the following are suspected or present:
  - Greens are not freshly picked
  - Mould is visible
  - The feed is frozen or unwashed
  - The feed has been sprayed with chemicals or weedkillers
  - Plants that may be poisonous
- When selecting and feeding greens and vegetables, ensure that they are as fresh as possible and pesticide- and herbicide-free.
- Muesli-type (cereal-based) foods were once popular as diets for rabbits, but it is now known that these should not be fed as they can cause dental and digestive problems in the rabbit as well as provide potential for selective feeding which can then lead to an unbalanced diet being eaten. Complete foods are like the rabbit mixes but with the addition of alfalfa to balance the cereals and provide the required dietary fibre content. These foods are useful for rabbits living in environments where there is no access to weeds, vegetation or hay.
- Rabbit treats are manufactured commercially to exercise teeth; however, it is still important to provide natural sources, such as hay and twigs, to encourage gnawing to wear down the constantly growing teeth.
- Some wild plants are poisonous to rabbits and should never be used for feed; these include:
  - Any flowers or leaves from bulbs, i.e. tulip, bluebell or crocus
  - Lily of the valley, laburnum or lupins
  - Buttercups
  - Deadly nightshade
  - Scarlet pimpernel
  - Bracken
  - Hemlock (easily confused with hedge parsley)
  - Foxglove
  - Privet or yew
  - Bindweed
- Fresh water must always be available, from a water bottle with spout or a drinking bowl. If water bottles are used, the spout must be of a non-chewable material. Water bowls can be difficult to keep free of hay, food and droppings. Whichever method is used, a change of water must be made at least once daily.

Handling rabbits

If handled regularly, correctly and gently, a rabbit will become tame quite quickly.

- Rabbits are easily frightened and must be handled carefully and securely.
- If a rabbit feels insecure or is handled badly, it will struggle violently potentially, causing serious injury to both the handler and itself.
- Rabbits should never be picked up by their ears as this will cause them pain and distress and potentially severe injury.
- Nervous rabbits should be lifted gently with one hand over the shoulders, while the other hand lifts the rump. Once lifted, nervous rabbits can be supported along the forearm of the handler with their head tucked against the body under the elbow until the rabbit can be placed on a non-slip surface (Figure 24.11).
- Tame rabbits can be lifted by putting one hand under the chest and holding the forelegs separately between the thumb and the two fingers while supporting the rump with the other hand. Once lifted, support the rabbit by holding against your chest before placing it onto a non-slip table. Keep control of the rabbit on the table by placing your hands around its body.
- Rabbits must not be allowed to struggle violently as they may break their backs by kicking and twisting.
- It is advisable to replace a rabbit in its housing backwards to avoid a last kick back as it is released.

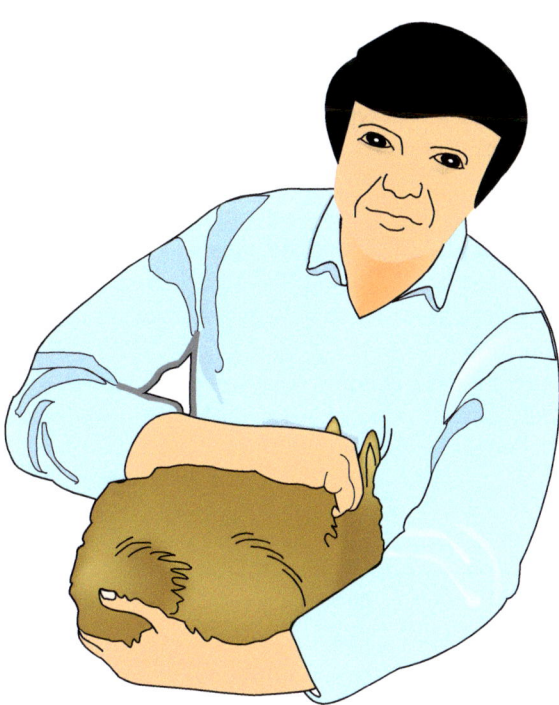

Figure 24.11   Handing and restraining a rabbit. *Source*: Ferris, 2003 / John Wiley & Sons.

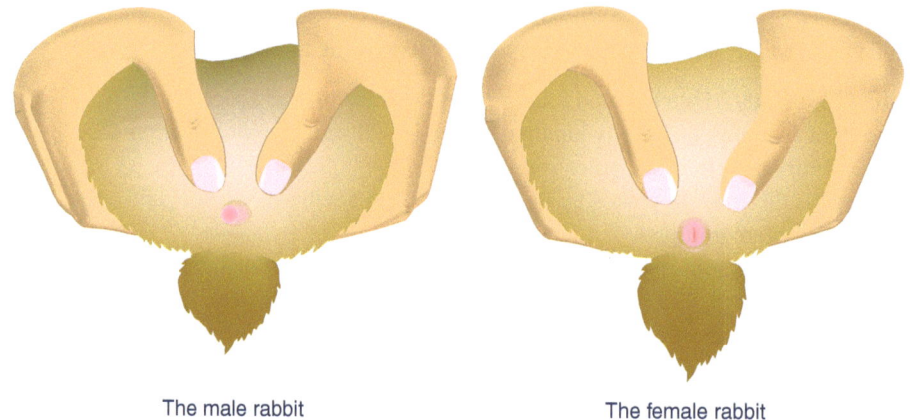

The male rabbit   The female rabbit

Figure 24.12   Sexing rabbits. *Source*: Ferris, 2003 / John Wiley & Sons.

Sexing rabbits

Adult rabbits can be sexed quite easily as testicles are easily observed, but determination of sex in young rabbits can be difficult. Figure 24.12 shows the difference between the appearance of the genitals in a male and female rabbit.

Rats

Rats kept as pets are also known as fancy rats. Belonging to the order Rodentia and suborder Myomorpha, the fancy rat species is descended from the wild brown rat, *Rattus norvegicus*. They are categorised first according to their coat type (varieties, e.g. hooded or self) and then grouped into sections by colour and body markings. Varieties available include albinos, hooded, Rex, and Siamese.

Rats are very social animals and will happily live together, although they can be kept on their own if they have plenty of human attention. Rats can be housed as breeding pairs or groups of the same sex, although adult males may fight after puberty. Rats are highly intelligent and require plenty of enrichment. They can be trained to respond to their name and learn a variety of tricks. Unlike other rodents, they need at least an hour a day of play time outside their cage or housing. A single rat would require more.

Rats can make good pets for older children. They are good climbers and very inquisitive. They make little noise, but odour can be a problem, particularly if groups of males are kept together, and so they must be cleaned out once a week as a minimum.

Biological data: Rats

Male	Buck
Female	Doe
Offspring	Pups
Adult weight	400–800 g
Maturity	6 weeks onwards
Gestation period	20–22 days

Litter size	6–12 (average size)
Weaning age	21 days
Body temperature	38°C
Life span	3 years

Anatomical facts: Rats
Teeth
- Dental formula: incisors 1/1, canines 0/0, premolars 0/0 and molars 3/3.
- Rats have open-rooted incisor teeth, which continue to grow throughout their life.

Long bones
- Ossify in the second year of life. This means that under 1 year of age, their bones are quite soft.

Digestive tract
- Rats have a divided stomach, large caecum, and no gall bladder.

Housing rats
The best accommodation for rats is a cage that allows for plenty of exercise. Rats enjoy climbing and so need relatively tall cages. Rats will live in small groups or alone, but do need plenty of space for activity, toys, and environmental enrichment. They can become attached to their owners, are quick to learn, and are easy to train. Rats will burrow given the opportunity and can be nocturnal.

Housing should:

- Provide enough space for a nest box and activity areas
- Be inside but not in direct sunlight or draughts. Rats are best kept at 15–27°C/59–81°F. If the temperature rises too high, then rats can suffer from heat stroke
- Rats should be provided with toys, as they like to spend a lot of time investigating equipment and exploring their enclosure. Toilet rolls and large plastic pipes make good toys for rats as well as wooden toys, knotted ropes, ladders, etc. Non-toxic branches are excellent for allowing the rats to climb in their cage. The environment should be interesting, with different levels (Figures 24.13 and 24.14)
- Be easy to clean and be cleaned two to three times per week to reduce odour, urine, and faeces. Use a dust-free, absorbent litter in the cage, with shredded paper for bedding in the nest area
- Have a solid floor to avoid injury to the rat's feet
- Be gnaw proof and made of materials not treated with toxic chemicals

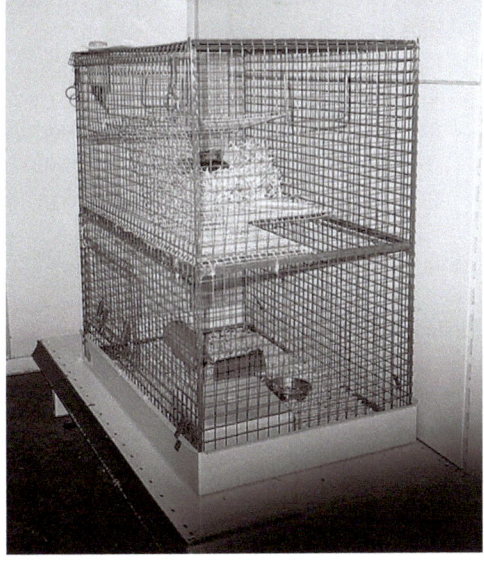

Figure 24.13 Type of housing with two levels for a rat.

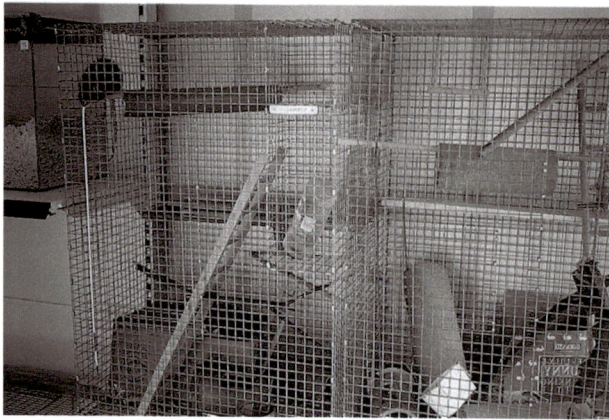

Figure 24.14   Close-up view of a two-level house.

- It is vital that substances for gnawing are provided for the rat to keep their teeth in good condition. Gnaw blocks may be bought from pet shops, or natural non-toxic branches such as apple twigs may be used instead

Feeding rats
- Rats are omnivores.
- Diets can be bought in pellet form, and these contain balanced nutrition for the rat. The protein content of the food should be 25–40%. Lean meat scraps or dog food, wholegrain cereals, fruits, and some vegetables can be added to the rat's diet. If sunflower seeds or peanuts are given, then the amount should be monitored as they are fattening due to their high lipid content and so should not be given in excess.
- Rats do not eat strange or new foods readily.
- Provide fresh water daily, using a bottle and sipper tube to prevent contamination. Ensure it is suspended above the level of the substrate, or the dispensing spout will become blocked.
- Rats will eat approximately 25 g of food/day.
- Food bowls may be provided and should be made of metal or ceramic so that the rats do not chew them. It is better to scatter feed to enrich their environment.

Handling rats
Rats can be lifted across their shoulders or scooped up under their abdomen, or when young, they can be lifted by the base of the tail and placed onto outstretched palm for stability.

To restrain the rat, place the forefinger and thumb of one hand on either side of the rat's head to keep the head still and support the body of the rat in the other hand unless it is small enough to cup in the same hand that is holding the head still.

Sexing rats
An adult male rat will be easy to sex due to the obvious visual presence of testicles. However, the most reliable method to use is to examine the distance between the anus and the urethral opening. In a male, there is a longer distance between the two. Younger rats are more difficult to sex, but females are likely to have more obvious nipple presence as in mice.

Birds

Birds are kept either as pets, for breeding or for exhibition. They can be housed singly in cages of suitable size or in groups in large outdoor aviaries. There are many different species of bird (class: Aves), which are assigned to 27 orders.

The orders most in animal collections/establishments are:

- *Anseriformes* – ducks, geese and swans
- *Falconiformes* – diurnal hawks and falcons
- *Galliformes* – domestic fowl and pheasants
- *Passeriformes* – finches and canaries (passerines) (Figure 24.15)
- *Psittaciformes* – parrots and budgerigars (psittacines)
- *Strigiformes* – owls
- *Columbiformes* – pigeons and doves

Most caged pet birds come from one of two main orders:

- Passerines – perching birds (e.g. canary, finch)
- Psittacines – climbing birds (e.g. budgerigar)

The two main features of anatomy which distinguish these two groups are:

- beak conformation – passerines peck at seeds, whereas psittacines open fruit and nuts
- foot conformation – passerines have three outer toes facing forwards and one inner toe facing backwards (Figure 24.16), whereas psittacines have two middle toes facing forwards and two outer toes facing backwards (Figure 24.17).

Anatomical facts: Birds
Skeleton
- Bones are thin, some containing air sacs (linked to the respiratory system) making up a light-weight structure for flight.

Digestive tract
- Food is stored in the crop; the gizzard then grinds the food to pass to the intestines. The cloacal opening is a common end to the outside for the digestive, urinary and reproductive tracts.

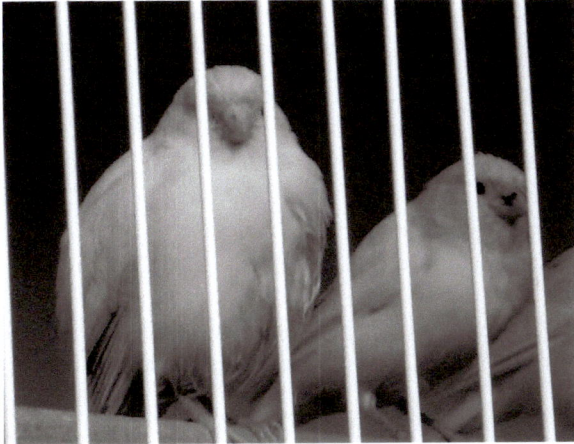

Figure 24.15   Canaries.

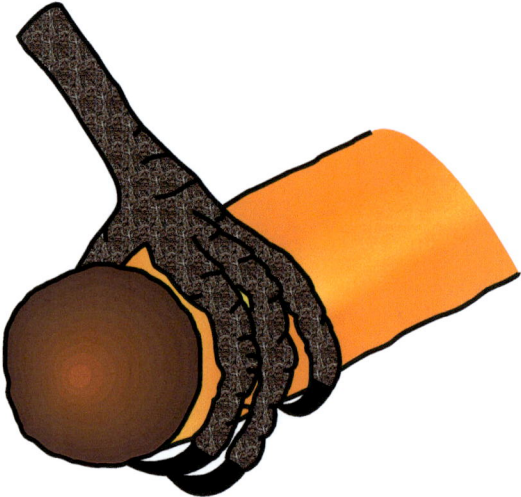

Figure 24.16   Passerine foot.

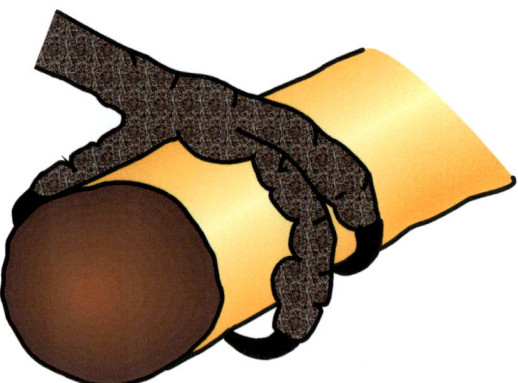

Figure 24.17   Psittacine foot.

Respiratory system

- Birds have no diaphragm; the lungs are set out in pairs through the thorax and abdomen area (Figure 24.18). The bird's respiratory system is complex for improved flow of air to the tissues.

For many pet owners, their choice is the budgerigar, which belong to the parakeet family. Budgerigars have a chattering call and can be taught words and simple tunes. They are easy to keep, in terms of both housing and feeding needs. If budgerigars are let out of their housing into a room, they will normally return to the accommodation quite readily. Some birds are valued for their song, such as the canary (particularly the male bird). Canaries belong to the finch family of birds, which are quick moving, hard to catch and usually kept in an aviary-type housing and as a group.

If pet birds do share the house uncaged, it is important to remember that birds like to explore and should not be left unattended. Precautions to take before letting the bird out of its cage include:

- Close all windows and doors
- Do not allow flight or access to the kitchen area, because of hot surfaces and fumes that may be fatal to a bird

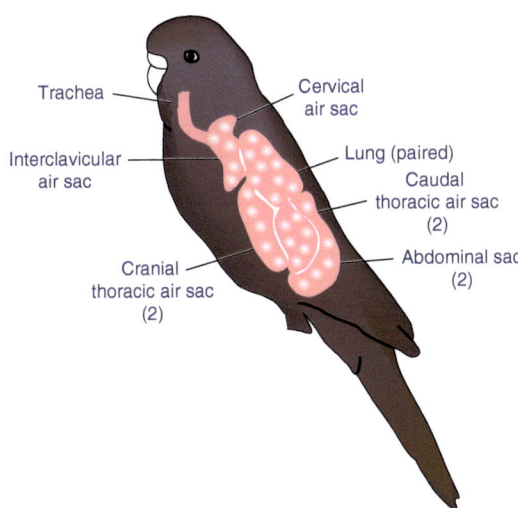

Figure 24.18 Avian respiratory system.

- Check that electrical cables are not exposed and that electrical fans are switched off
- Remove houseplants that are toxic to birds, such as cacti
- Remove other pets, such as dogs or cats

Housing for pet birds must be easily cleaned, both daily to remove droppings and, more thoroughly, monthly. Birds are kept as pets for many reasons, one of which is to display their beauty, achieved by keeping them in:

- Cages
- Aviaries

Housing for birds
Cage system
There are many types of cages available, with a variety of costs, sizes, and designs. However, many are unsuitable for the many varied species kept as pets. A cage should be as large as possible, especially if the bird is going to be confined for much of the day in it.

A bird cage must:

- Be large enough to allow the bird to stretch its wings up and out without touching the sides of the cage
- Not cause the bird to fly in an artificial way, i.e. circular cages
- Be strong and well-constructed with no sharp edges (especially around the cage base)
- Have safe cage fittings, i.e. materials that cannot be chewed used for food containers
- Have good door fastenings so that the bird(s) can't get out and nothing else can get in
- Be easy to keep clean
- Have meshwork or bars on one side to give a feeling of security to the bird
- Be placed well above the ground level, i.e. at eye height
- Provide environmental enrichment (toys/activities)
- Have a variety of perches (not covered with sandpaper as these can damage the feet)
- Be sited away from draughts, direct sunlight, and any harmful fumes (cooking fumes, i.e. over-heated oil, cigarette smoke, and room sprays)
- Be cleaned daily (removal of unwanted fresh foods, seeds, and droppings)

Aviary system

There are many advantages to pet birds when housed in a larger space such as an aviary. Flight becomes possible, providing a more natural environment, complete with plants and secluded areas. There are disadvantages as well. Aviaries are more difficult to clean as it is more time consuming to remove dropped foods, but this must be done to reduce the risk of disease being introduced to the pet birds by wild birds, mice, and rats that are attracted by the uneaten foodstuff. The most obvious concern for birds housed outside is their exposure to hot and cold weather conditions.

An aviary must:

- Be well designed, with a safety door, as large as possible in size and high enough for good flight but be easy to clean
- Be made of materials that will cause no harm (to include gauge of the netting and wood types used)
- Have a floor/base that is easy to clean, i.e. concrete
- Have perches of different diameters and heights
- Have shallow baths or a misting system for bathing
- Be covered in part (or one entire side) to avoid wind and rain
- Have an inside shelter of boxes to encourage roosting at night
- Be secure to avoid bird escapes and entry by other species
- Ideally have a double door entry system
- Ensure a 12-hour period of daylight, using lighting systems in the winter, to encourage food intake in the correct amounts
- Never have food containers placed under perches; preferably, they should be off the floor

Budgerigars

The budgerigar (*Melopsittacus undulatus*) is available in a wide range of colours, but in the wild, it is green. It originates from Australia, where its natural habitat is semi-arid (hot) grassland with trees, near water holes. All budgies originated from the light-green variety found in the wild. Other colours started to appear late in the nineteenth century as birds showed an increase in popularity. Varieties include the Lutino, Grey Winged Sky Blue, Crested Opaline Cobalt, Grey, Recessive Pied Violet, and Spangle Light Green.

Budgerigars are the most practical of the cage birds. They are lively, colourful, quite hardy, and diurnal and can be brought up to mimic human speech. Although they need daily attention, they are reasonably cheap to house and feed.

Biological data: Budgerigars

Male	Cock
Female	Hen
Offspring	Chick
Adult weight	30–35 g
Sexing	A male bird has blue cere
	A female has brown cere
Maturity	5 months onwards
Clutch	3–6 white eggs

Incubation time	18 days to hatch (up to 3 weeks)
Fledgling	Further 35 days
Body temperature	40–42°C
Life span	6–8 years

Anatomical facts: Budgerigars
Beak
This is a hinge joint between the skull and upper beak. With no teeth, this allows increased movements suitable for slicing through nut shells, with the help of a flexible tongue to obtain food (Figure 24.19).

Feeding budgerigars
- Budgies are hard-billed birds and so eat seeds.
- Seed mixes containing various types of millet and linseed, fruit and occasional insects can be fed. It may be necessary to give or provide an iodine supplement if one is not already included in the seed mix given.
- Fresh fruits, vegetables and green foods (dandelion, chickweed, groundsel and lettuce) add interest and nutrients to the diet.
- Vitamin D must be supplemented if there is no access to sunlight.
- The seed and fruit should be given in bowls but do not place bowls directly under perches to prevent contamination with bird droppings.
- A supply of calcium as cuttlefish should be held in the cage clips for the bird to consume.
- Fresh water should be readily available from drinkers.
- Grit mixture (oyster shell and particles of stone/rock) should be available to aid digestion.
- When feeding, blow husks off the top of the bowl to see how much actual feed is left.
- Food bowls should be metal or plastic not ceramic, as they get broken easily.
- Water containers should be cleaned thoroughly to prevent algal growth.

Handling budgerigars
Ensure all doors and windows are shut before attempting to catch the budgie. The method of catching will vary according to whether the bird is housed in an indoor cage or an outdoor aviary. A bird net may be needed in the latter case.

Once the bird has been caught, place one hand over the bird's back and use the thumb and forefinger on the same hand to restrain the head. Hold the bird firmly but gently to prevent struggling. If the bird is held too tightly, then it can suffocate.

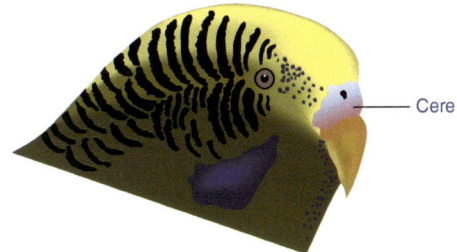

Cere

Figure 24.19   Budgerigar beak.

It is important to keep the head still to prevent injury to the handler. A budgie can give a very hard bite – remember that the beak is designed to eat seeds!

Sexing budgerigars
Determining the sex of the bird is relatively easy in adult birds. Males have a blue cere and females have a brown/pink cere. Young birds have brown ceres. Alternatively, DNA sexing can occur.

Canaries

Canaries are found in a wide range of colours and markings but in the wild are in greenish-yellow colour only. The canary (*Serinus canaria*) is part of the finch family of birds and belongs to the order Passeriformes (passerines).

Canaries originate from the Canary Islands and parts of Europe. The natural habitat for the canary is scrubland, fields, and pastures, and it is diurnal. Passerines are perching birds, best kept in aviary flocks because it is rare that they are tame enough to handle.

Biological data: Canaries

Male	Cock
Female	Hen
Offspring	Chick
Adult weight	20 g
Sexing	When mature, both sexes look alike. The male bird song is the best identifier. To be sure of obtaining a male, birds are usually bought several months after fledging, by which time the cock birds will be distinguished by their song
Clutch	3–6 eggs are laid every other day
Incubation time	14 days
Fledging	Further 14 days
Body temperature	40–42°C
Life span	6–9 years

Anatomical facts: Canaries
Beak
- This is short and conical in shape and used to crack seeds when feeding (Figure 24.20).

Feeding canaries
- Canaries are hard-billed seed eaters. Their food contains both cereals and oil seeds such as canary seed, millet, rape seed, and hemp. It is important to remove the husks from the feed container every day to enable feeding. Appropriately sized grit (soluble and insoluble) must be available to grind the seeds in the gizzard.
- Commercial complete diets are available, but some fresh green foods (lettuce, dandelion, chickweed, and alfalfa), fruits and vegetables should also be offered.
- Remove any uneaten fresh foods or soaked seeds daily. Soaking enables germination of seeds, which improves the nutritional value, but it is important that these are well drained and removed after a few hours if not eaten to avoid fungal growth, which could be harmful.

- Ensure a fresh supply of water, changed daily in the housing (cage or aviary), and thorough cleaning of the water containers to prevent growth of algae.

Fish

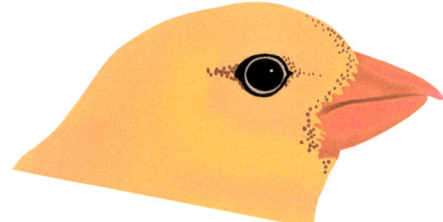

Figure 24.20   Canary beak.

Fish make excellent pets, and in terms of numbers, they are the most kept pet. Fish are attractive, colourful, and interesting to study or just watch. Fish do not demand much time (depending on the complexity of the tank or the species kept) and do not make any noise. Feeding costs are relatively low and equipment can be reasonably simple or as elaborate and expensive as you wish to make it.

Types of fish commonly kept as pets fall into four main groups:

- Coldwater (10–26°C)
- Tropical freshwater (21–29°C)
- Tropical marine (21–29°C)
- Coldwater marine (10–26°C)

Of the three groups, cold water and tropical freshwater fish are normally kept by pet owners and hobbyists. Tropical and cold water marine fish are complex to keep, and a good understanding of their requirements is essential.

Marine fish live in sea water, and they are hypotonic (i.e. less salty than the sea water that is their environment); this causes water to be drawn out of these fish by osmosis (see Chapter 2). To counteract this dehydration, they must continuously take in water by drinking. The fish will die rapidly if the water they drink is not:

- Filtered of excretions (containing ammonia and nitrite)
- The same salt concentration and pH of sea water all the time

Anatomical data: Fish

External anatomical features
Fins

- Give stability in the water, control the direction of movement and can be divided into (Figure 24.21):
  - *Single* – tend to be *dorsal* (top fin for balance), adipose (in some fish only), *caudal* (tail fin for propelling forward) and *anal* (for balance)
  - *Paired* – *pectoral* and *ventral* (pelvic fins) both used for steering
- Fins, combined with body movement, are used for moving through the aquatic habitat. In some fish, the fins are modified for a purpose other than movement, such as ensuring egg fertilisation (the fused anal fin is called a *gonopodium*) and protection from predators. The fin positions on the fish body often indicate lifestyle (as predator or prey may need to be capable of continued speed or only short bursts, respectively).
- The position of the mouth may also indicate where that fish feeds, which, in turn, indicates where in the aquarium it will spend most of its time. For example, fish with *barbels* (feelers)

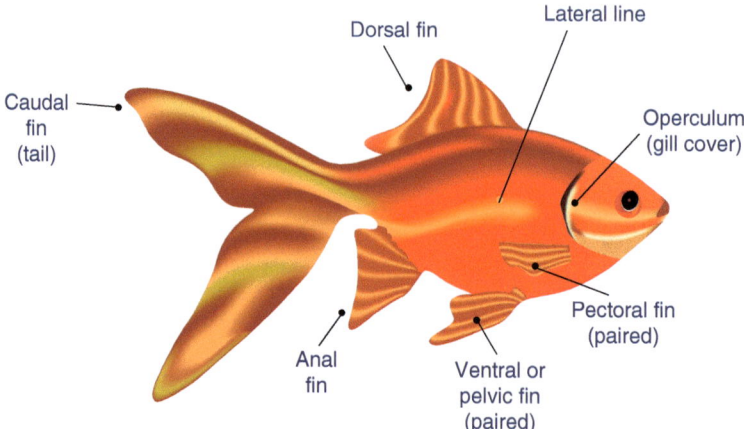

Figure 24.21   Fish: external fins.

around the mouth parts feed on or near the bottom and others feed and swim in the top layer of the water, whereas fish that live in shoals live and feed in the middle layer of water.
- The eyes vary in size and sight ability, depending on lifestyle. Plant eaters have poor eyesight but a good sense of smell to find food. Predatory fish have good eyesight, enabling them to catch their prey.
- Nostrils, connected to the brain by nerves, provide a sense of smell for food location.
- Gills are located beneath the gill cover (*operculum*), allowing the fish to extract oxygen from the surrounding water.
- The *lateral line* is a fluid-filled tube below the skin surface on the sides of the fish, seen as a line of tiny pores opening to the water outside. It is unique to fish and is an organ of hearing. It detects vibrations in the water, alerting the fish to danger, obstacles in its way, and food location.

Head types
- The shape of a fish's head can indicate its location in the aquarium.
- Those with an undershot mouth, fringed with barbels, tend to feed on the bottom of the tank.

Internal anatomical features
- The heart has only two chambers.
- The *swim bladder*, which is filled with gas, helps to maintain buoyancy in the water in most fish.

Tropical freshwater fish

- Tropical freshwater fish have a life span of approximately three years.
- Tropical freshwater fish are found in waters around the world, the temperature of which will vary (21–29°C) depending on altitude, i.e. mountain stream, lake, river pool or sea-level swamp.
- Some fish species in the wild may be found in many continents or only in one lake or river.
- Tropical freshwater fish can be divided into two main groups:
  - *Egg layer*, hatching into fry (i.e. gouramis, tetras, barbs)
  - *Live-bearer*, giving birth to fully formed young which are larger than fry (i.e. platies, guppies)

Coldwater fish

- Coldwater fish have a life span of approximately 6–20 years.
- Coldwater fish are found in a range of habitats in the wild. The water temperature (10–23°C), the oxygen levels, the speed of the water current, and the water chemistry will vary depending on location, i.e. lakes, ponds, streams, and mountain streams.
- The two fish commonly kept from this group are:
  - Goldfish
  - Koi carp

Goldfish

Goldfish varieties are increasingly diverse as a group.
Ideal conditions for a goldfish are:

- Water – neutral pH to slightly alkaline
- Temperature – 10–26°C
- Region – bottom, top, and middle

Goldfish fall into three main categories:

- *Common* – the most popular in terms of the number owned; they are a hardy fish, able to live in aquarium or pond
- *Single tailed* – known for fast swimming ability; the Shubunkin is ideal for a home aquarium, whereas the Comet is better in a pond or large aquarium
- *Double tailed* – are more unusual and a less hardy type. They are only suitable for deep aquaria and indoor pools. They tend to have a shorter life span due, in part, to their egg-shaped bodies and flotation problems, i.e. Veiltail

Koi

Koi originated from Eastern Asia (Caspian and Aral Seas) and China. They are ornamental varieties of the common carp and can be very valuable.
Ideal conditions for Koi:

- Water – neutral pH and moderately hard
- Temperature – 10–24°C
- Tank region – top, middle and bottom

Koi are messy feeders, requiring a good filtration system to keep the water clear. They tend to destroy plants; therefore, the furnishings in an aquarium tend to be bogwood or smooth rock. Koi can be mixed with fancy goldfish if required.

Considerations when setting up an aquarium

1. *Size of aquarium*
   Standard aquaria can be bought in various combinations of length, width and depth, depending on:
   - The species being kept, e.g. the Veiltail goldfish requires a deeper tank because of the size of its double tail
   - Stocking density of fish to be kept

2. ***Positioning of the aquarium***
   - Firm foundation – the floor must be able to support the weight of the water-filled tank, ideally over joists not just floorboards
   - Away from draughts, heaters and direct sunlight, i.e. not near a window or in a conservatory
   - In an area of a room that has no passing traffic
   - In a quiet area, too dark for a house plant
   - Next to more than one electrical socket
   - Level the tank and place polystyrene or a foam mat under the tank on the stand to cushion it from any unevenness in the metalwork of the stand

3. ***Substrates***

   Substrates are materials placed on the bottom of the tank (Figure 24.22). They include:
   - *Coarse gravel* – best for large tanks; it is used to recreate the bed of a river or stream
   - *Medium and fine gravel* – often mixed and can be used with under-gravel filtration
   - *Coloured gravel* – gaudy but fun; buy from reputable sources to ensure the dyes used are not poisonous
   - *Sand* – very useful for bottom-dwelling species of fish (there are no sharp points that can injure the fish) and a good substrate for plant growth

   Ensure that, whatever the substrate used, it is washed to remove dust particles, dirt and other impurities.

4. ***Filtration system***

   Filter systems are used to clean the water, filtering out waste products such as excess food materials, sections of plants, and fish excretions. A variety of filtration systems are available:
   - *External power filters* draw water through the various filter media and pump the clean water back into the tank.
   - *Internal power filters* also draw water through the various filters but are located inside the tank. These are useful for a smaller aquarium set-up.
   - *Under-gravel filters* consist of one or more perforated plates that cover the base of the aquarium. An air stone or line is attached to a length of tubing, and the plates are covered by substrate material. The flow of oxygenated water through the gravel allows filtering.

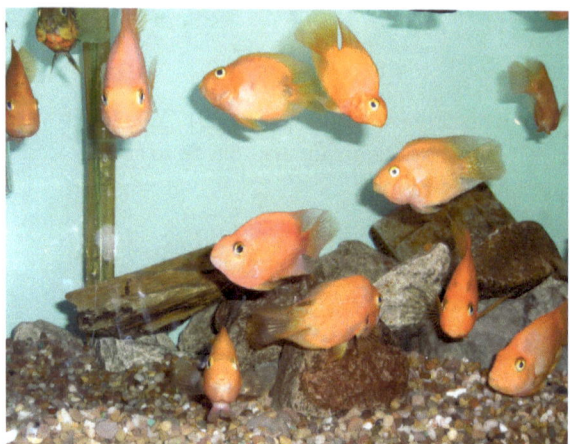

Figure 24.22   Marine tank substrate.

5. *Heating*

Heating is used in both cold water and tropical freshwater tank systems, which require a stable water temperature whatever the environmental temperature may be (even in centrally heated houses, the temperature alters between day and night). Various designs of heater are available (always read the manufacturer's instructions on adjusting the temperature):
- Combined electronic heater/thermostats are located inside the tank (Figure 24.23)
- Submersible heaters controlled by external or internal thermostats
- Under-tank heating mats controlled by external or internal thermostats

6. *Aquarium hood or cover*
- Prevents dust and dirt particles from falling into the tank
- Prevents fish from escaping
- Keeps out predators such as other household pets
- Helps to retain the tank temperature
- Reduces evaporation

7. *Lighting*

Lighting supported in the aquarium hood is essential for the health of the fish and live plants in the tank. Fluorescent tubes have been developed in a few different colours to imitate daylight and can be used in combination to show off the fish colours.

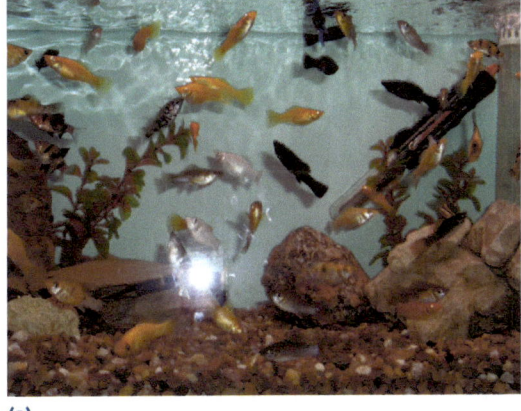

(a)

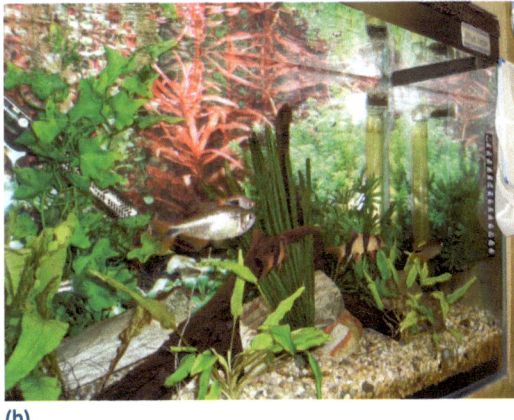

(b)

Figure 24.23   (a) Aquarium heater located in the tank. (b) Fish in an established tank.

Setting up the aquarium

- The aquarium tank is cleaned with dilute detergent to remove any chemicals, rinsed thoroughly and put into position.
- To hide the electrical cables and filter pipes, choose a decorative plastic background to suit the type of ornament in the tank, the plants, and the fish, or have a plain black background. This is a personal choice.
- Next, the filter, substrate (gravel or sand), the heater if required, thermometer, prepared wood, rocks, and other furnishings are placed.
- Using cold or warm water poured from a clean measuring jug onto a saucer to prevent disturbance of the substrate gravel, begin to fill the tank. Water can be pre-conditioned by allowing it to stand for several days or by adding a conditioner. This allows evaporation of any chlorine gas.
- If the substrate gravel has been washed properly, there should be little or no clouding of the water as it is added. Once the gravel has been covered, water can be poured in quite quickly to about 10–12cm from the final water level. Plants (plastic) can be placed when the tank has matured, without overflowing.
- It is important to wait at least 24 hours after the set-up has been run before placing any living plants. This allows time to check that the heater and filter are working properly.
- Before the fish can be added, the tank must be at the correct temperature, maturity, and pH. Depending on which water company provides the water, it is either:
  - hard: a measure of the mineral salts dissolved in the water
  - soft: indicating fewer dissolved mineral salts
  - acid: pH up to 7
  - alkaline: pH from 7 up to 14
- Coldwater fish are adaptable to a wide range of pH but are most stable in water with a reading of pH between 7 and 8.5.
- Most tropical freshwater fish will live in water with a pH value between 6.5 and 7.5, which is about neutral in value, and from slightly soft to slightly hard water. There are kits available to check the pH levels.
- Once the tank is set up, it is best for it to be left for at least 3–4 weeks for the filtration system to mature; however, after 10 days the first few fish can be added, waiting a week to introduce the next few. The final number should be in place by 6 weeks, to give a healthy aquarium environment.
- Bacteria will develop in the filter sponge and assist in the breakdown of waste produced by the fish (ammonia is converted to nitrites by bacteria; nitrites are converted to nitrates in the filtration system). To ensure that both fish and live plants are healthy, maintenance of water quality must take place weekly. A check on the nitrite level using a commercially available test kit will indicate whether a partial water change is required.

The nitrogen cycle in an aquarium

- Waste matter from the aquarium plants, uneaten food, faeces and urine from the fish will all contaminate the tank.
- As they decompose, ammonia is formed, which is poisonous to the fish.
- The bacteria in the water break down the ammonia into nitrites and then nitrates, which are harmless to fish and act as a fertiliser for the live plants in the tank. This completes the nitrogen cycle.

Feeding fish

Types of food:

- Live food (daphnia, brine shrimp, and bloodworm)
- Commercial food (freeze dried, tablet, dried flakes, floating food sticks, and sinking granules)

The most convenient foods are the commercially produced flake or pellet foods. These provide the correct nutrient requirements and, unlike live foods, are free from the hazards of parasite or disease introduction.

Most cold water fish kept in aquariums are omnivorous (feeding on insects and plant material). A good-quality flake food will provide the nutrients, vitamins, and minerals required, but to keep the fish in good health, alternate this diet with other safe live food, such as daphnia or bloodworm.

Tropical freshwater fish also benefit from variety in their diet. Use of dried flake foods combined with frozen or live foods offered once or twice per week will maintain condition and health. If the fish are herbivorous, offer green foods, such as lettuce leaves, regularly.

Aquarium tank maintenance

Daily
- Check the fish
- Check all the tank equipment
- Make sure that the temperature is correct
- Remove any uneaten food

Every 2 weeks
- Test for pH and nitrite levels
- Do a partial water change
- Remove any dead plant material
- Remove any algal growth from the glass front and sides
- Suction off any debris seen on the sand or gravel substrate

Once a month
- Clean the filter

Every 8–12 months
- Replace fluorescent tube lights and air stones
- Service filter motor and air pump
- Take out and scrub all furniture and plastic plants to remove algae

Reptiles

Keeping reptiles, amphibians and invertebrates as pets has increased greatly over the past twenty years. Data collected in 2024 indicates that there are approximately 1.3 million reptiles kept as pets in the United Kingdom. The notion of having a pet that is slightly different along with a greater number of hobbyists and the increase of allergies in children has contributed to this increase in keeping these species as pets. Whether or not these species can be classed as pets is debatable as they have not been domesticated, and neither are they kept specifically as companions. The keeping of these species of animal as pets could be widely debated.

Keeping reptiles, amphibians, and invertebrates brings husbandry demands that can be greater than for any other species except for fish species. Consideration must be given to:

- Dietary needs
- Size of adult animal
- Lighting and heating needs of the species
- Daily management requirements
- Appeal to all household members

Of the animals in this group, reptiles are the most popular – these can be broadly divided into lizards and snakes.

Housing reptiles

Reptiles are housed in accommodation called a vivarium. There are many different styles on the market at the current time (2025), and consideration should be given to the needs of the animal intending to be kept in it before choosing the type of vivarium. Buying the cheapest/most expensive vivarium or the one that looks most appealing to the owner may not be the one that suits the needs of the animal.

Consider the following:

- *Construction material* – Wood, plastic, moulded fibreglass, and glass are common construction materials for vivaria – all have their advantages and disadvantages.
- *Size of the adult animal* – Be wary of saying that biggest is best for reptiles – some reptiles do not like to have lots of space and so be aware of the species' needs.
- *Lifestyle of the animal* – An arboreal or burrowing animal will need a taller or deeper enclosure than a ground dwelling one.
- *Security of the vivarium* – Snakes can be experts at escaping from accommodation and so the vivarium should be easily secured to avoid escapes and avoid other animals or young children from entering the accommodation.
- *Provision of life-sustaining systems* – heating and lighting – how will these be provided for in the vivarium intending to be chosen?
- *Ability to provide the necessary substrate for the species* – There are a range of substrates available on the market, and not all of them are suitable for all species of reptile as they can be ingested and cause impaction problems. Substrates are often used for aesthetic appeal to provide a natural-looking environment rather than to meet the needs of the animal. Newspaper is considered by some to be the most suitable substrate (most newspaper inks are now non-toxic).
- *Ease of cleaning and maintaining hygienic conditions* – There are many furnishings and decorations that can be purchased for vivaria but consider whether they are needed for aesthetic appeal or for the animal itself. Some furnishings can be provided that make the vivarium more interesting for the animal, e.g. rocks can be provided to hide behind/under or to use for assisting with skin shedding.
- *Ease of feeding/water changing* – Consider the diet of the animal and how it can be met and provided for. Also, consider how water should be provided in the vivarium and whether a bowl is needed for bathing or swimming in.
- *Access point into the vivarium* – Just as with mammals, the access points should be at a place where the reptile will not perceive you as a predator.

Heating the vivarium

Heat provision is one of the most important aspects in reptile husbandry as reptiles are unable to maintain their own body temperature. They are *ectothermic* and so rely on the external provision of a heat source to maintain their health and activity levels. A reptile that is too cold will enter a state of *torpor* and may well appear to have died. Too much heat can cause the animal to become stressed if it cannot move away from the heat source, and this can also result in death or injury.

There are different sources of heat (Figure 24.24) that can be provided for a reptile, and all have their advantages and disadvantages.

- Spot lamps are popular choices as they can be used to provide a 'basking hotspot' for the animal, but care must be taken to ensure that the animal cannot touch the bulb in any way or that the bulb is securely fixed so as not to fall onto the animal; otherwise, burn injuries could occur. An alternative to a spot lamp is a ceramic bulb, which emits heat to the surrounding

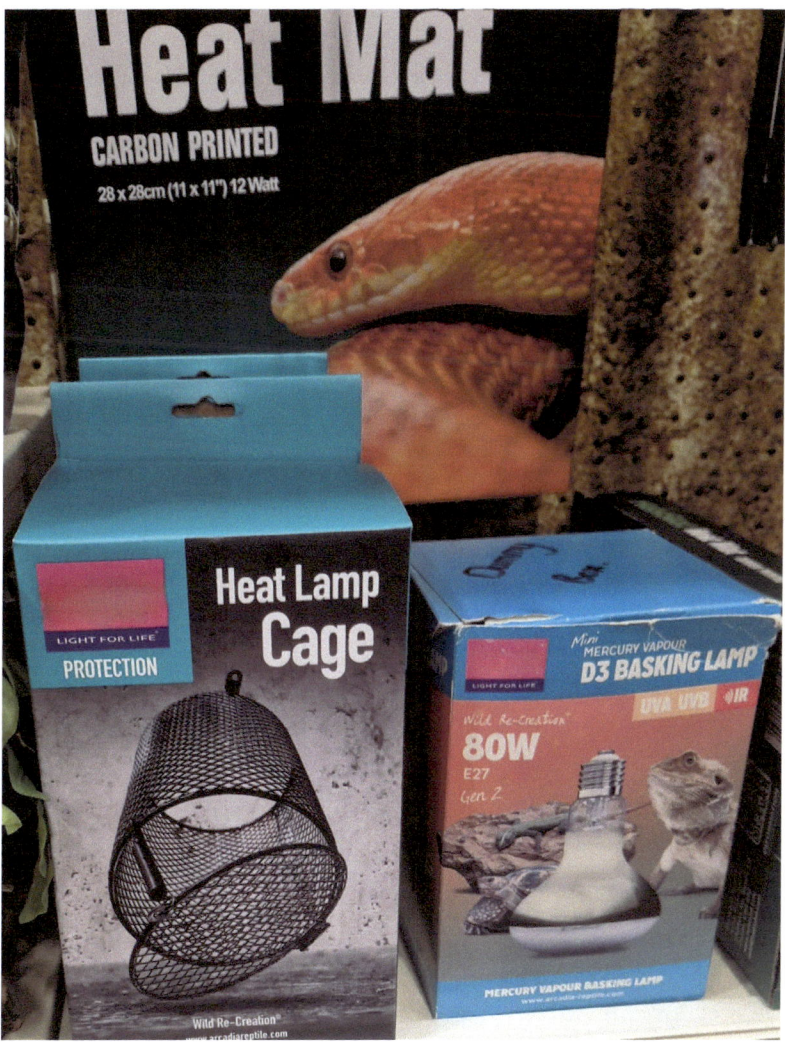

Figure 24.24   Heating options for reptiles.

area, but again, the same precautions must be taken. It is also worth noting that the siting of the bulb in the vivarium should not be in a place where the owner/carer/keeper could injure themselves as they can cause serious burns to humans also. Cages should be fitted around bulbs for protection of both animal and owner.

• Heat mats/pads are useful as a heat source, but instructions must be carefully followed to ensure they have maximum effect without compromising the animal. Heat rocks should not be used as there have been many reported incidences of burn injuries caused to animals.

Within a vivarium, whatever heat source is provided, it is essential to have a *thermal gradient*. This means that the vivarium will be hotter at one end than at the other. This enables the reptile to have a choice of where to be in the enclosure to regulate its body temperature.

A thermostat can be used to regulate the temperature of the heat source provided, and additionally, a timer can be used to replicate the natural temperature cycles in the animal's natural environment.

Humidity in the vivarium

Humidity is an important factor to consider when housing reptiles, and if incorrect, it can affect the health of the animal either by causing cracked skin if too dry for the animal or encouraging fungal infections if too damp. It is essential to research the humidity levels required for the species intending to be kept.

Lighting in the vivarium

Lighting may be provided in a vivarium for several reasons, from allowing the animal to be seen to mimicking the light cycles of the natural environment, but the most important reason is to provide ultraviolet rays, which aid in the metabolism of calcium. Many captive reptiles suffer from metabolic bone disease due to having incorrect lighting combined with provision of an incorrect diet.

When choosing lighting for a vivarium, research how much light the animal intending to be housed requires in terms of strength of light and time required/day (Figure 24.25). Lights in a vivarium will generally need to be on for 10–12 hours each day.

Light source provision can be controlled through using a timer to replicate the light cycles of the animal's natural environment.

Light sources should be replaced on a regular basis – every 6 months as a minimum as the strength of a light source diminishes over time.

Hygiene and cleaning in the vivarium

Hygiene is important to both the animal and its owner/carer/keeper. Many reptiles are known to carry the *Salmonella* bacteria which can be transferred to humans as it is zoonotic. High standards of hygiene are therefore vital.

Faeces should be removed daily. A full clean should be carried out according to the number of animals kept in the vivarium. Substrate should be removed and refreshed on at least a monthly basis. Be wary when using disinfectants with reptiles. it must be ensured that they are suitable for use with reptiles. Seek advice if unsure.

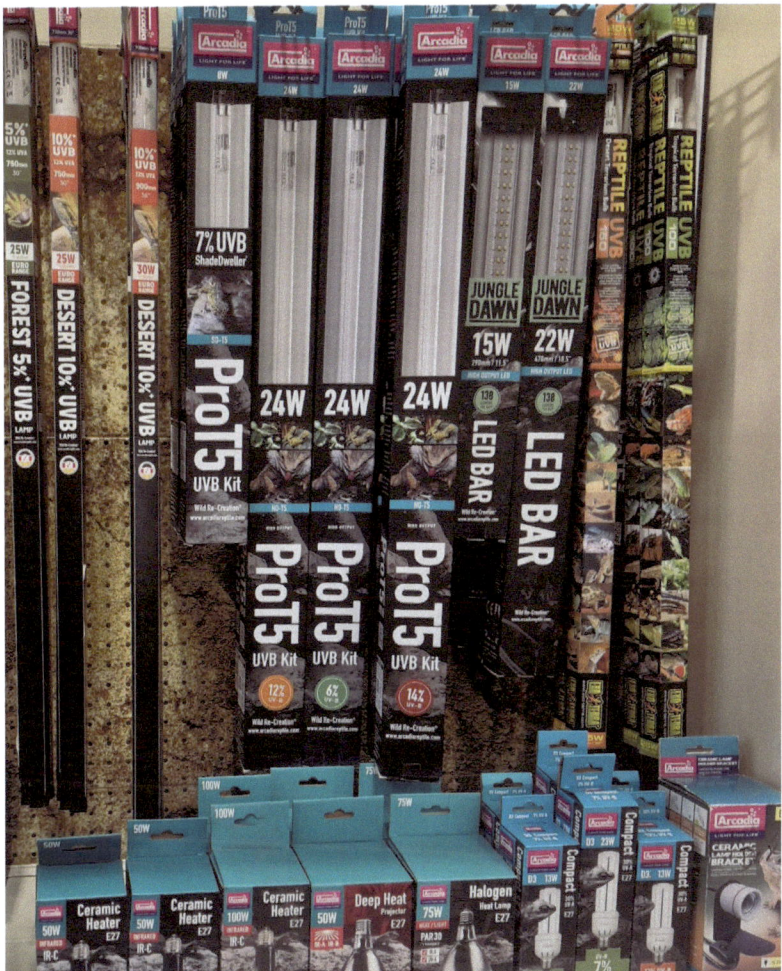

Figure 24.25 Lighting options for reptiles.

Feeding reptiles

The diet required will depend on the species of animal kept. Many lizards are insectivorous, and this will mean keeping live food such as crickets, locusts and mealworm to be fed to the animal. This live food will have specific care requirements to keep it alive to feed to the reptile. It is also important to ensure that the live food is provided with a vitamin/mineral supplement on their own food to increase the nutritional value of the food to the reptile. Vitamin/mineral deficiencies are common problems in captive reptiles. Advice should be sought on the best supplement to give the species being kept.

Some reptiles are omnivorous and require a small amount of plant matter in their diet, and others are herbivorous and only feed on plant matter. Many reptiles are carnivorous and require vertebrate food.

Invertebrates such as crickets, locusts and mealworms can be fed live to those animals that require them. For animals that require small mammals such as mice, rats and gerbils in their diet, it is illegal to feed these animals when they are alive. Any vertebrate food source must be dead when provided to the reptile, and this type of food can be purchased from specialist suppliers and certain pet stores as frozen products that must be thoroughly defrosted before being fed. The feeding habits of the animal being fed should be researched so that the food can be provided in a similar way. With snakes, it is recommended to remove them from their normal accommodation into a separate feeding container, secured with a lid. Snakes should also not be handled for 2–3 days after feeding to avoid regurgitating their food which can cause feeding problems subsequently.

Fresh water should always be available in a reptile enclosure. The container in which it is provided must be suitable for the species and should be cleaned on a regular basis as the heat and humidity in a vivarium can encourage algal and fungal growth which can be detrimental to the health of the reptile and the owner/carer/keeper. Some species will also defaecate in their water bowl, and this should be cleaned as soon as possible.

Handling reptiles

For many reptiles, handling can be a stressful experience, and so care must be taken to observe the behaviour of the species and recognise signs of stress. Some reptile species will acclimatise more to handling than others. Short, regular sessions of handling will aid this process. During the handling process, it is important to let the animal move freely between hands rather than trying to restrain them in a certain position. Take care with some snakes however as they can coil around parts of the body such as hands, arms, necks etc., to secure themselves, and this can constrict the blood flow in the handler. Handling should be a positive experience for both animal and handler (See Chapter 21).

Summary of Other Animals Kept as Pets

As can be seen in this chapter, there are many animals that may be kept as pets in addition to the ever-popular cats and dogs. This chapter only covers some species, but there are others, such as tortoises, that have their own specific husbandry requirements.

When owning or working with different animals, it is the owner/carer/keepers' responsibility to find out about the husbandry requirements for that species along with the behaviour that is usually seen in the species, so that the five welfare needs can be met.

Section 4

The Animal Industry

25

The Animal Industry

Learning goals

In this chapter, the learning goals are:

- To raise awareness of the animal industry in the United Kingdom
- To identify possible careers within the animal industry in the United Kingdom

The animal industry is varied and diverse. From sole traders to global organisations, it is a multifaceted industry looking at many different aspects relating to animals. The animal industry offers a wide range of career opportunities in different sectors, such as animal health, animal welfare, farm livestock, wildlife, and zoological conservation to list a few. Within each sector, there can be specialities relating to the animals that are being focused on, e.g. companion animal species, aquatics, exotics, equine, farm livestock, and wildlife (Table 25.1). This chapter aims to provide a basic awareness of the animal industry in the United Kingdom.

The Diversity of the UK Animal Industry

Animal health care and veterinary services

Animal health care and veterinary services are a critical part of the animal industry for all species. The sector includes private veterinary practices, animal hospitals, and research facilities. The importance of animal health care and veterinary services is emphasised by the fact that over 60% of animal medicine sales are now for companion animals. In 1985, over 70% of animal medicine sales were for farm livestock. This demonstrates how the companion animal care sector continues to grow due to a increased focus on pet health and wellness. This sector is also continuing to grow due to cutting-edge technological developments in the veterinary industry, such as the inclusion of virtual reality education, stem cell therapies, 3D bioprinting, and wearable health monitors for animals.

Since the COVID pandemic in 2020/2021, there has been an increase in the need for services from animal behaviourists as pandemic puppies reach maturity. The lack of early socialisation for these puppies has had a lasting impact on their behaviour.

More owners are now aware of services, such as animal physiotherapy, hydrotherapy, and chiropractic for their pets, and referrals to these services continue to grow.

Animal Biology and Care, Fourth Edition. Emily Jewell.
© 2026 John Wiley & Sons Ltd. Published 2026 by John Wiley & Sons Ltd.
Companion Website: https://www.wiley.com/go/animal/biology4e/jewell

Examples of careers in this sector could include:

- Animal behaviourist
- Animal healthcare assistant
- Animal physiotherapist
- Animal scientists/research specialists
- Practice managers
- Veterinary nurse
- Veterinary receptionists
- Veterinary surgeon

Animal welfare organisations

There are many animal welfare and charitable organisations, both in the United Kingdom and globally, as identified in Chapter 6. These organisations represent the interests of animals and may be interested in the welfare of all animals or specific animals only.

Activities carried out by animal welfare organisations may include rescue and rehabilitation services, lobbying Parliament for changes to animal legislation, educating the public, or providing veterinary care for animals.

Despite the growth in the animal health and pet care sectors, few owners appear to be aware of the Five Animal Needs as reported in the PAW report, 2024. This is disappointing when the Animal Welfare Act has been in existence since 2006.

Examples of careers in this sector could include:

- Animal behaviourist
- Animal inspectors
- Animal welfare officer
- Dog handler
- Educational roles
- Health and welfare technician
- Rehoming and welfare assistant/manager
- Support service roles, such as marketing, HR, fundraising, and receptionist

Table 25.1 **Summary of the animal industry.**

Animal industry

Animal health care and veterinary services	Animal welfare organisations	Farming and livestock	Pet care and retail	Wildlife conservation and zoological collections
Aquatics	Aquatics	Farm livestock	Aquatics	Aquatics
Companion animals	Companion animals		Companion animals	Wildlife and zoological species
Equine	Equine		Exotic species	
Exotic species	Exotic species			
Farm livestock	Farm livestock			
Wildlife and zoological species	Wildlife and zoological species			

Farm livestock

The farm livestock sector in the United Kingdom includes livestock farming for dairy, meat, and fibre products across a range of livestock species. Similar to traditional farms, smaller farm parks fall under this sector. Farmers in the United Kingdom contribute significant amounts to the animal health sectors by using preventative medicines such as vaccines and anthelmintics (wormers). Smaller farm parks may keep a range of mixed livestock, e.g. Pygmy goats, Suffolk sheep, Kune Kune pigs and Highland cattle, or they may choose to focus on a specific sector, e.g. rare breeds such as Golden Guernsey goats, Gloucester Old Spot pigs, Cotswold sheep and White Park cattle.

Examples of careers in this sector could include:

- Animal inspectors
- Animal nutritionist
- Animal scientist
- Breeding technicians
- Business support staff
- General farm worker
- Farm manager
- Veterinary advisor

Pet care and retail

The pet care industry in the United Kingdom is significant, with an estimated annual expenditure of £8 billion in 2025. The 2024 PDSA Animal Wellbeing (PAW) report published by the PDSA indicates that 51% of households in the United Kingdom own one or more pets. There are approximately 36 million non-aquatic pets in the United Kingdom with dogs remaining the most popular pet.

This sector includes pet food and treats, grooming, pet sitting, and dog walking services. There are many pet stores (approximately 3000) across the United Kingdom (independent and part of global organisations), and the demand for personalised pet products and services is predicted to grow further in the next decade. An anticipated area of growth in the pet care market is the sales of smart pet devices (connect to owners' phones via Bluetooth or WiFi) and GPS trackers for cats and dogs.

The UK pet care industry is expanding due to an increased focus on pet health and well-being. Some owners are becoming more aware of the importance of correct diets, exercise levels, and prophylactic health treatments for their animals.

Examples of careers in this sector could include:

- Animal insurance specialist
- Digital content creator
- Dog walker
- Groomer
- Pet sitter
- Pet product developer
- Pet store assistant
- Pet store manager

Wildlife conservation and zoological collections

This sector includes charitable organisations such as the RSPB, county wildlife trusts, and zoological collections that work to educate the public, conserve animals, protect and preserve wildlife habitats, and promote animal welfare.

Examples of careers in this sector could include:

- Animal biologist
- Conservation officer
- Ecologist
- Environmental educator
- Park ranger
- Sustainability officer
- Wildlife assistant
- Zookeeper

Summary of the Animal Industry

As previously mentioned, the animal industry is varied and diverse and can be split into sectors that cover all animal species. Sectors continue to grow with the development of technology and with improved knowledge about animal health and welfare. From direct contact with animals to business support services, there is a wide range of career paths available.

26

Employability Skills in the Animal Industry

Learning goal

In this chapter, the learning goal are:

- To identify key employability skills for the animal industry

Employability Skills

Whatever career is entered in the animal industry, good employability skills are essential. Often referred to as 'soft skills', these skills are far from soft. They are crucial as they underpin all roles and careers. Employability skills are transferable across all industries. Employers can often teach you the knowledge required for a particular role, but they require you to demonstrate good employability skills from the start.

Employability skills relevant to the animal industry include:

- *Attention to detail*
  - Attention to detail when working with animals is essential. Imagine providing the wrong dose of medication at the wrong time to an animal. There could be serious consequences to the animal, and it could affect the business' reputation. Diluting disinfectants and antiseptics at an incorrect ratio could cause health consequences for all animals if pathogens are able to establish themselves and cause disease.
- *Communication*
  - Being open and honest with colleagues is essential to build trust in each other's abilities and ensure the smooth running of the business.
  - Being able to explain processes and procedures to customers is crucial to ensure they understand what is happening.
  - Being able to hold a telephone call is crucial as messages may need to be taken, information may need to be given, orders may need to be placed, bookings may need to be taken, etc., and this needs clear, polite communication.
  - Being able to write clearly, concisely, and professionally in emails and letters using plain English is another key skill relating to communication.
- *Customer service skills*
  - Being able to talk to and work with customers is essential in many roles, such as in veterinary practices, grooming businesses, boarding establishments, and rescue centres.

Animal Biology and Care, Fourth Edition. Emily Jewell.
© 2026 John Wiley & Sons Ltd. Published 2026 by John Wiley & Sons Ltd.
Companion Website: https://www.wiley.com/go/animal/biology4e/jewell

- Building positive customer relationships by being friendly, polite, and professional will ensure a customer returns to the business.
- **Digital skills**
  - Being able to use software packages and social media is becoming more important in today's world. A greater amount of business is being conducted in the online world and employees should know how to use software, maintain confidentiality, and be aware of cybersecurity procedures to protect the business.
  - More and more businesses are using social media platforms and employees that use platforms confidently and professionally are an asset to the business.
- **Empathy**
  - Being able to demonstrate empathy to customers or clients when they are explaining their situations or when they have recently had a pet euthanised is key, otherwise they will think that you do not care.
- **Flexibility**
  - Having an employee who is willing to take on different roles and responsibilities as required and to adjust to new situations that the business encounters is a key asset.
- **Initiative**
  - Being proactive to solve issues before they become a problem shows leadership and dedication.
  - Being able to find creative solutions for a business can be a very useful skill, for example, improving animal habitats or improving business processes.
- **Organisational skills**
  - Employers need staff who can manage multiple tasks efficiently. Keeping accurate records and storing them in an organised way helps everyone in the business to locate information when required.
- **Physical fitness**
  - Some roles in the animal industry require physical fitness. For example, veterinary nurses, kennel assistants, and zookeepers are on their feet for long periods of time during their work shift, and this requires strength. Safe lifting and carrying applies to roles in pet stores, veterinary practices, and animal rescue centres. Using incorrect lifting and carrying techniques can potentially cause injury to staff and animals.
- **Problem solving**
  - As you gain experience in a role, employers will expect that any problems that arise can be solved effectively. Quick decisions may need to be made to resolve emergency situations that arise.
- **Punctuality**
  - Being on time for work and for appointments demonstrates reliability as an employee. It shows customers and colleagues that you respect the time that they are taking to work with you.
  - Being punctual demonstrates to your employer that you are committed to your role and take it seriously.
- **Professionalism**
  - Maintaining a professional appearance is vital to uphold a positive business reputation. Any uniforms need to be clean, footwear needs to be safe and appropriate, and dress codes relating to not wearing jewellery or false nails need to be stuck to.

- Being aware of demonstrating positive body language, such as making eye contact (where possible) and having a friendly demeanour, helps to build trust with customers and colleagues. Smiling goes a long way with everyone.
- Knowing your own skills and recognising where they need developing helps you to contribute better to the team that you work in.
- Being aware of your own emotions is important, as well as understanding the emotions of customers and colleagues. Staying calm and collected helps to manage difficult situations.
- Treating all colleagues and customers with respect and dignity is a big part of professionalism. Remember to use your manners at all times.
- Maintaining confidentiality about the business ensures compliance with data protection regulations.
- *Teamwork*
  - Being able to work with all colleagues is essential to the smooth running of a business.
- *Time management*
  - Managing your time efficiently enables colleagues to build trustful relationships otherwise colleagues will feel that they cannot rely on you.
  - Completing tasks on time at the right time can be crucial in animal businesses, otherwise animal welfare can be compromised.
- *Willingness to learn*
  - No employee knows everything and demonstrating a willingness to learn and develop knowledge on a personal level shows the employer your commitment to the role.
  - It is important to stay up to date with the latest developments in the sector that you work in, and demonstrate to customers that skills are kept current and up to date in the business.

Summary of Employability Skills

Having good employability skills makes an employee valuable to an organisation. There are many employability skills, and all can have an impact on the business and its reputation.

Employability skills develop over time, but being able to recognise strengths and aspects for development is a key part of an employee's own personal development.

Further Reading

SECTION 1

Aspinall, V. & Cappello, M. (2015) *Introduction to Veterinary Anatomy and Physiology Textbook*, 3rd edition. Butterworth-Heinemann, UK.

BBC Bitesize (2024) *Acids, Bases and Salts* [Online]. Available at https://www.bbc.co.uk/bitesize/guides/zmjyqp3/revision/2. Accessed October 2024.

Beckett, B. & Gallagher, R. (2001) *New Coordinated Science: Biology Students' Book: For Higher Tier*, 3rd edition. OUP, Oxford, UK.

Bell, J.S. (2007) *Common Genetic Disorders of the Dog and Cat* [Online]. Available at https://www.vin.com/apputil/content/defaultadv1.aspx?pid=11243&id=3861465. Accessed November 2024.

BD Editors (2020) *Osmosis* [Online]. Available at https://biologydictionary.net/osmosis/. Accessed October 2024.

Biology Insights (2024) *Pineal Gland: Anatomy and Function across Species* [Online]. Available at https://biologyinsights.com/pineal-gland-anatomy-and-function-across-species/. Accessed October 2024.

Boden, E. & Andrews, A. (2016) *Black's Student Veterinary Dictionary*, 22nd edition. Bloomsbury, London, UK.

Brookes, M. (1999) *Get a Grip on Genetics*. Weidenfeld and Nicolson, London, UK.

Clegg, C.J. (2007) *Biology for the IB Diploma*. Hodder Education, UK.

Cleveland Clinic (2022) *Adipose Tissue* [Online]. Available at https://my.clevelandclinic.org/health/body/24052-adipose-tissue-body-fat. Accessed September 2024.

Cooper, B. (2020) *BSAVA Textbook of Veterinary Nursing*, 6th edition. British Small Animal Veterinary Association (BSAVA), Gloucester, UK.

England, G. (2012) *Dog Breeding, Whelping and Puppy Care*. Wiley Blackwell, UK.

GCSE Bitesize (2024) *Cell Structure* [Online]. Available at https://www.bbc.co.uk/bitesize/guides/z84jtv4/revision/7. Accessed August 2024.

Gov.UK (2025) *Standards of Modern Zoo Practice for Great Britin* [Online]. Available at https://assets.publishing.service.gov.uk/media/681494272de62f4a103a828d/standards-of-zoo-practice-2025.pdf. Accessed 15 June 2025.

Hollings, P. (2011) *Breeding Dogs: A Practical Guide*. The Crowood Press Ltd., UK.

Jones, A., Reed, R. & Weyers, J. (2021) *Practical Skills in Biology*, 7th edition. Pearson, UK.

Jones, S. & van Loon, B. (2011) *Introducing Genetics: A Graphic Guide*, 4th edition. Icon Books Ltd., London, UK.

Animal Biology and Care, Fourth Edition. Emily Jewell.
© 2026 John Wiley & Sons Ltd. Published 2026 by John Wiley & Sons Ltd.
Companion Website: https://www.wiley.com/go/animal/biology4e/jewell

Lane, D.R., Guthrie, S. & Griffith, S. (2016) *Dictionary of Veterinary Nursing*, 4th edition. Elsevier, Edinburgh, UK.

MacKean, D.G. (2002) *Biology*, 3rd edition. Hodder Education, UK.

Macobi, F. (2024) *Animal Cell* [Online]. Available at https://animal-cell-definition-structure-parts-functions-and-diagram/. Accessed September 2024.

Masters, J. & Martin, C. (2001) *BVNA Pre-Veterinary Nursing Textbook*. Butterworth-Heinemann, UK.

McLaughlin, K. (2020) *Active Transport* [Online]. Available at https://biologydictionary.net/active-transport/. Accessed October 2024.

Murato, C. (2012) *Tumours of the Pineal Region in Principles of Neurological Surgery*, 3rd edition. Elsevier Inc Drs. Richard G. Ellenbogen, Saleem I. Abdulrauf and Laligam N. Sekhar.

Nicholas, F.W. (2009) *Introduction to Veterinary Genetics*, 3rd edition. Wiley Blackwell, Oxford, UK.

Ojha, T.R. (2024) *White Blood Cells* [Online]. Available at https://microbenotes.com/white-blood-cells/. Accessed September 2024.

Robbins, H. (2024) *Researchers Map Genome for Cats, Dolphins, Birds, and Dozens of Other Animals* [Online]. Available at https://phys.org/news/2024-01-genome-cats-dolphins-birds-dozens.html. Accessed November 2024.

Robinson, R. (2016) *Companion Animal Fluid Therapy Part 2* [Online]. Available at https://www.vettimes.co.uk/app/uploads/wp-post-to-pdf-enhanced-cache/1/companion-animal-fluid-therapy-part-2-planning-and-monitoring.pdf. Accessed October 2024.

Royals, J.W. (2024) *Royal Python Genetics* [Online]. Available at https://www.jwroyals.co.uk/genetic. Accessed November 2024.

Sapkota, A. (2023a) *Connective Tissue* [Online]. Available at https://microbenotes.com/connective-tissue/. Accessed August 2024.

Sapkota, A. (2023b) *Epithelial Tissue* [Online]. Available at https://microbenotes.com/epithelial-tissue/. Accessed August 2024.

Sichting. F., Holowka, N.B., Ebrecht, F. & Lieberman, D.E. (2020) Evolutionary anatomy of the plantar aponeurosis in primates, including humans, *Journal of Anatomy* 237, 185–104 [Online]. Available at https://onlinelibrary.wiley.com/doi/10.1111/joa.13173. Accessed September 2024.

Study Rocket (2024) *Cells* [Online]. Available at https://studyrocket.co.uk/revision/gcse-biology-triple-aqa/triple-cell-biology/cells. Accessed September 2024.

Sturtz, R. & Asprea, L. (2012) *Anatomy and Physiology for Veterinary Technicians and Nurses: A Clinical Approach*. Wiley-Blackwell, UK.

Tamang, S. (2024a) *Fat Cells* [Online]. Available at https://microbenotes.com/fat-cells-adipocytes. Accessed September 2024.

Tamang, S. (2024b) *Muscle Cells* [Online]. Available at https://microbenotes.com/musclecells/. Accessed September 2024.

Tamang, S. (2024c) *Nerve Cells* [Online]. Available at https://microbenotes.com/nerve-cells/. Accessed September 2024.

Taylor, D. (1986) *You and Your Dog*. Dorling Kindersley, London, UK.

VCA Animal Hospitals (2023) *Stem Cell Therapy* [Online]. Available at https://vcahospitals.com/know-your-pet/stem-cell-therapy. Accessed 28 August 2024.

SECTIONS 2 and 3

Agar, S. (2001) *Small Animal Nutrition*. Butterworth Heinnemann, London, UK.

Alderton, D. (1997) *The Reptile Survival Manual*. Ringpress Books, Gloucestershire, UK.

Alderton, D. (2011) *The Ultimate Encyclopedia of Caged & Aviary Birds*. Southwater, UK.

Alderton, D. (2005) *Encyclopedia of Aquarium & Pond Fish.* Dorling Kindersley, London, UK.

Alderton, D. (2008) *The Illustrated Practical Guide to Small Pets & Pet Care.* Southwater, UK.

Alderton, D., Edwards, A., Larkin, P. & Stockman, M. (2015) *Encyclopedia of Pets & Pet Care.* Hermes House, London, UK.

Aldridge, P. & O'Dwyer, L. (2013) *Practical Emergency and Critical Care Veterinary Nursing.* Wiley-Blackwell, Chichester, UK.

Anderson, R.S. & Edney, A.T.B. (1990) *Practical Animal Handling.* Pergamon Press, Oxford, UK.

Andrews, A., (2022) *Overview of Coccidiosis in Animals* [Online]. Available at https://www.msdvetmanual.com/digestive-system/coccidiosis/overview-of-coccidiosis-in-animals. Accessed 26 January 2025.

Aspinall, V. (2019) *Clinical Procedures in Veterinary Nursing,* 4th edition. Elsevier, Amsterdam.

Aspinall, V. & Ackerman, N. (2016) *The Complete Textbook of Veterinary Nursing,* 3rd edition. Elsevier, Edinburgh, UK.

AVMA (nd) *Antimicrobial-Resistant Pathogens Affecting Animal Health* [Online]. Available at https://www.avma.org/resources-tools/one-health/antimicrobial-use-and-antimicrobial-resistance/antimicrobial-resistant-pathogens-affecting-animal-health. Accessed 16 February 2025.

Bayshore Veterinary Hospital (2024) *Veterinary Glossary* [Online]. Available at https://www.bayshorevethospital.com/veterinary-glossary. Accessed 16 February 2025.

Boldrick, L. (2010) *Essential First Aid for Dog Owners.* All Publishing Company, Orange, CA.

Bradshaw, J., Brown, S.L. & Casey, R. (2012) *The Behaviour of the Domestic Cat,* 2nd edition. CABI Publishing, Oxfordshire, UK.

Broom, D.M. (1991) Animal welfare: Concepts and measurements, *Journal of Animal Science* 69 (10): 4167-75.

Brown, M. & Richardson, V. (2000) *Rabbitlopaedia: A Complete Guide to Rabbit Care.* Ringpress Books, Dorking, UK.

BSAVA (nd) *Drug Storage and Dispensing* [Online]. Available at https://www.bsavalibrary.com/content/formulary/frontmatter/canine-and-feline/drugstorageanddispensing. Accessed 16 February 2025.

Burger, I. (1993) *The Waltham Book of Companion Animal Nutrition.* Pergamon Press, Oxford, UK.

Cannon, M. & Forster-van Hijfte, M. (2006) *Feline Medicine: A Practical Guide for Veterinary Nurses and Technicians.* Butterworth-Heinemann, London, UK.

Chapman, S. (2017) *Safe Handling and Restraint of Animals: A Comprehensive Guide.* Wiley-Blackwell, UK.

Cherian, G. (2019) *III. Carbohydrates, Structures and Types: A Guide to the Principles of Animal Nutrition* [Online]. Available at https://open.oregonstate.education/animalnutrition/chapter/chapter-3/. Accessed 09 February 2025.

Colville, J. & Berryhill, D. (2007) *Handbook of Zoonoses: Identification and Prevention.* Mosby, St. Louis, MO.

Colville, J. & Oien, S. (2013) *Clinical Veterinary Language.* Mosby, St. Louis, MO.

Cooper, B., Mullineaux, E. & Turner, L. (2020) *BSAVA Textbook of Veterinary Nursing,* 6th edition. British Small Animal Veterinary Association (BSAVA), Cheltenham, UK.

Dallas, S. & Simpson, G. (1999) *Manual of Veterinary Care.* BSAVA, Gloucester, UK.

Dallas, S., North, D. & Angus, J. (2006) *Grooming Manual for the Dog and Cat.* Wiley-Blackwell, Oxford, UK.

Divers, S.J. (2020) *Viral Diseases of Reptiles* [Online]. Available at https://www.msdvetmanual.com/exotic-and-laboratory-animals/reptiles/viral-diseases-of-reptiles#Retroviruses_v3309402. Accessed 15 January 2025.

Ducommum, D. (2011) *Rats: Practical, Accurate Advice from the Expert (Complete Care Made Easy)*. Bow Tie Press, Irvine, CA.

Edney, A. (2006) *RSPCA Complete Cat Care Manual*. Dorling Kindersley, London, UK.

Edney, A.T.B. & Hughes, I.B. (1986) *Pet Care*. Blackwell Science, Oxford, UK.

Elward, M. & Ruelokke, M. (2003) *Guinea Piglopaedia: A Complete Guide to Guinea Pigs*. Interpet Publishing, London, UK.

England, G. & von Heimendahl, A. (2010) *BSAVA Manual of Reproduction and Neonatology*, 2nd edition. British Small Animal Veterinary Association, Gloucester, UK.

Evans, J.M. & White, K. (1994a) *Book of the Bitch*. Henston, Guildford, UK.

Evans, J.M. & White, K. (1994b) *The Catlopaedia*. Henston, Guildford, UK.

Evans, J.M. & White, K. (1994c) *The Doglopaedia*. Henston, Guildford, UK.

Ferret-World (2025) *Ferret Breeds* [Online]. Available at https://www.ferret-world.com/ferret-facts/types-of-ferrets/. Accessed 27 February 2025.

Fogle, B. (1995) *First Aid for Dogs*. Pelham, London, UK.

Fogle, B. (2006) *RSPCA Complete Dog Care Manual*. Dorling Kindersley, London, UK.

Fogle, B. (2011) *Complete Cat Care: What Every Cat Owner Needs to Know*. Mitchell Beazley, London, UK.

Gay, J. (2005) *The Perfect Aquarium: The Complete Guide to Setting up and Maintaining an Aquarium*. Hamlyn, London, UK.

Girling, S.J. (2013) *Nursing of Exotic Pets*, 2nd edition. Wiley-Blackwell, West Sussex, UK.

Girling, S. & Raiti, P. (eds) (2019) *BSAVA Manual of Reptiles*, 3rd edition. BSAVA, Cheltenham, UK.

Gov.UK (2019a) *Notifiable Diseases in Animals* [Online]. Available at https://www.gov.uk/government/collections/notifiable-diseases-in-animals. Accessed 15 December 2024.

Gov.UK (2019b) *Put Your Pet in Rabies Quarantine* [Online]. Available at https://www.gov.uk/guidance/put-your-pet-in-rabies-quarantine. Accessed 15 February 2025.

Gov.UK (2024) *Taking Your Pet Dog, Cat or Ferret Abroad* [Online]. Available at https://www.gov.uk/taking-your-pet-abroad. Accessed 28 November 2024.

Gull, T. (2023) *Candidiasis in Animals* [Online]. Available at https://www.msdvetmanual.com/infectious-diseases/fungal-infections/candidiasis-in-animals. Accessed 25 January 2025.

Gunn, A. & Pitt, S.J. (2012) *Parasitology: An Integrated Approach*. Wiley Blackwell, Chichester, UK.

Gurney, P. (2011) *Guinea Pig (Collins Family Pet Guide)*, Relaunch edition. HarperCollins.

Hall, E. (2021) Keeping your cool monitoring body temperature, *Veterinary Nursing Journal* 26, 19–23.

Harkness, J.E. & Wagner, J.E. (1985) *The Biology and Medicine of Rabbits and Rodents*. Lea & Febiger, Philadelphia, PA.

Harvey, A. & Tasker, S. (2013) *BSAVA Manual of Feline Practice: A Foundation Manual*. British Small Animal Veterinary Association, Gloucester, UK.

Hoppes, S.M. (2021) *Mycotic Disease of Pet Birds* [Online]. Available at https://www.msdvetmanual.com/exotic-and-laboratory-animals/pet-birds/mycotic-diseases-of-pet-birds. Accessed 25 January 2025.

Horwitz, D. & Mills, D.S. (2010) *BSAVA Manual of Canine and Feline Behavioural Medicine*. BSAVA, Gloucester, UK.

Hotston-Moore, P. & Hughes, A. (2007) *Manual of Practical Animal Care*. British Small Animal Veterinary Association, Gloucester, UK.

International Cat Care (2024a) *Feline Immunodeficiency Virus* [Online]. Available at https://icatcare.org/articles/feline-immunodeficiency-virus-fiv. Accessed 30 November 2024.

International Cat Care (2024b) *Feline Infectious Enteritis* [Online]. Available at https://icatcare.org/articles/feline-infectious-enteritis-feline-parvovirus-panleukopenia-virus. Accessed 30 November 2024.

International Cat Care (2024c) *Feline Infectious Peritonitis* [Online]. Available at https://icatcare.org/articles/feline-infectious-peritonitis-fip. Accessed 30 November 2024.

International Cat Care (2024d) *Feline Leukaemia Virus* [Online]. Available at https://icatcare.org/articles/feline-leukaemia-virus-felv. Accessed 30 November 2024.

Keeble, E. & Meredith, A. (2009) *BSAVA Manual of Rodents and Ferrets*. BSAVA, Gloucester, UK.

Knetsch, C.W., Kumar, N., Forster, S.C., Connor, T.R., Browne, H.P., Harmanus, C., Sanders, I.M., Harris, S.R., Turner, L., Morris, T., Perry, M., Miyajima, F., Roberts, P., Pirmohamed, M., Songer, J.G., Weese, J.S., Indra, A., Corver, J., Rupnik, M.W., Ren, B.W., Riley, T.V., Kuijper, E.J. & Lawley, T.D. (2018) Zoonotic transfer of clostridium difficile harboring antimicrobial resistance between farm animals and humans, *Journal of Clinical Microbiology* 56(3), e01384-17 [Online]. Available at https://journals.asm.org/doi/10.1128/jcm.01384-17. Accessed 16 February 2025.

Laber-Laird, K., Flecknell, P. & Swindle, M. (1996) *Handbook of Rodent and Rabbit Medicine*. Butterworth-Heinemann, London, UK.

Lane, D.R., Guthrie, S. & Griffith, S. (2007) *Dictionary of Veterinary Nursing*, 3rd edition. Butterworth-Heinemann, London, UK.

Legislation.gov.uk (2024) *The Animal Welfare (Licensing of Activities Involving Animals)(England) Regulations 2018* [Online]. Available at https://www.legislation.gov.uk/uksi/2018/486/contents. Accessed October 2024.

Leicester, D. (2023) *How to: First Aid for Pet Burns* [Online]. Available at https://www.vets-now.com/pet-care-advice/how-to-first-aid-for-pet-burns/. Accessed 15 February 2025.

Logsdail, C., Logsdail, P. & Hovers, K. (2003) *Hamsterlopaedia*. Ringpress Books Ltd., Dorking, UK.

McBride, D.F. (1996) *Learning Veterinary Terminology*. Mosby, St. Louis, MO.

Mercer, A. (2024) *Ferret Focus: Dealing with a Unique Species*. VN Times, Volume 24, issue 2.

Meredith, A. & Johnson Delaney, C. (2010) *BSAVA Manual of Exotic Pets*, 5th edition. British Small Animal Veterinary Association, Gloucester, UK.

Moriello, K.A. (2025) *Dermatophytosis in Dogs and Cats* [Online]. Available at https://www.msdvetmanual.com/infectious-diseases/fungal-infections/candidiasis-in-animals. Accessed 25 January 2025.

Morris, D. (1986) *Animal Watching*. Jonathan Cape, London, UK.

Morrisey, J.K. (2024) *Breeding and Reproduction of Ferrets* [Online]. Available at https://www.msdvetmanual.com/all-other-pets/ferrets/breeding-and-reproduction-of-ferrets. Accessed 27 February 2025.

Orpet, H. & Welsh, P. (2010) *Handbook of Veterinary Nursing*, 2nd edition. Wiley-Blackwell, UK.

Pellett, S. & Varga, M. (2013) *Reproductive Management of Ferrets*, Vet Times [Online]. Available at https://www.vettimes.co.uk/app/uploads/wp-post-to-pdf-enhanced-cache/1/reproductive-management-of-ferrets.pdf. Accessed 27 February 2025.

Rich, G. & Axelson, R. (2022) *Psitaccine Beak and Feather Disease in Pet Birds* [Online]. Available at https://vcahospitals.com/know-your-pet/psittacine-beak-and-feather-disease-in-pet-birds. Accessed 25 January 2025.

RSPCA (nd) *Ferrets* [Online]. Available at https://www.rspca.org.uk/adviceandwelfare/pets/ferrets. Accessed 27 February 2025.

RVC (2016) *Pasteurella in Rabbits* [Online]. Available at https://www.rvc.ac.uk/Media/Default/small-animal/documents/Rabbits_pasturella_30.11.16.pdf. Accessed 19 January 2025.

RVC (2017) *Viral Haemorrhagic Disease in Rabbits* [Online]. Available at https://www.rvc.ac.uk/Media/Default/small-animal/documents/Rabbit-Viral-Haemorrhagic-Disease%20rabbit-VHD%20Updated%204.9.17.pdf. Accessed 19 January 2025.

RVC (2021) *Myxomatosis in Rabbits* [Online]. Available at https://www.rvc.ac.uk/Media/Default/small-animal/documents/Rabbit_myxomatosis_2021.pdf. Accessed 19 January 2025.

RVC (nd) *Ferret Vaccinations* [Online]. Available at https://www.rvc.ac.uk/small-animal-vet/general-practice/practice-services/routine-pet-healthcare/vaccinations/ferret.

Sandford, G. (2004) *Mini Encyclopaedia of the Tropical Aquarium*. Interpet Publishing, Dorking, UK.

Smith, J. (2012) *Rats – Pet Friendly*. Magnet & Steel Publishing Ltd., London, UK.

Sullivan, P. (nd) *Dental Disease in Domestic Ferrets* [Online]. Available at https://www.mspca.org/angell_services/dental-disease-in-domestic-ferrets/. Accessed 27 February 2025.

Taylor, D. (1986) *You and Your Cat*. Dorling Kindersley, London, UK.

Taylor, D. (2002) *Collins Small Pet Handbook: Looking After Rabbits, Hamsters, Guinea pigs, Gerbils, Mice and Rats*. Collins.

Tynes, V. (2010) *Behavior of Exotic Pets*. Wiley-Blackwell, Chichester, UK.

UKFMC, (2022) *How can you manage Notifiable Diseases in Animals?* [Online]. Available at https://ukfmc.co.uk/manage-notifiable-diseases-animals-apha-defra/. Accessed 15 December 2024.

UK Pet Food Association (2025) *UK Pet Population* [Online]. Available at https://www.ukpetfood.org/industry-information/statistics-new/uk-pet-population.html. Accessed 28 February 2025.

Vanderlip, S. (2003) *The Guinea-Pig Handbook*. Barron's Educational Series, New York.

Varga, M., Lumbis, R. & Gott, L. (2012) *BSAVA Manual of Exotic Pet and Wildlife Nursing*. British Small Animal Veterinary Association, Gloucester, UK.

Warren, D. (2009) *Small Animal Care and Management*, 3rd edition. Delmar, CA.

Witola, W.H. (2024) *Cryptosporidiosis in Animals* [Online]. Available at https://www.msdvetmanual.com/digestive-system/coccidiosis/overview-of-coccidiosis-in-animals. Accessed 26 January 2025.

SECTION 4

Carter Robb, M. (2023) *Truly Cutting Edge Tech Developments in Pet Health Care* [Online]. Available at https://www.linkedin.com/pulse/truly-cutting-edge-tech-developments-pet-health-care-carter-robb/. Accessed 28 February 2025.

Indeed (2024) *What are Valuable Job Skills* [Online]. Available at https://www.indeed.com/career-advice/resumes-cover-letters/valuable-job-skills. Accessed 28 February 2025.

NOAH (2025) *Industry Facts and Figures* [Online]. Available at https://www.noah.co.uk/about/industry-facts-and-figures/. Accessed 28 February 2025.

PDSA (2025) *The PAW Report 2024* [Online]. Available at https://www.pdsa.org.uk/what-we-do/pdsa-animal-wellbeing-report/paw-report-2024. Accessed 28 February 2025.

P£t Money Saver (2023) *5 of the Hottest Smart Tech Pet Products* [Online]. Available at https://www.petmoneysaver.co.uk/blog/best-smart-pet-products/. Accessed 28 February 2025.

UK Pet Food Association (2025) *UK Pet Population* [Online]. Available at https://www.ukpetfood.org/industry-information/statistics-new/uk-pet-population.html. Accessed 28 February 2025.

Williams, J. (2023) *Behaviour Management in a Post-pandemic World* [Online]. Available at https://www.veterinary-practice.com/article/post-covid-behaviour-management. Accessed 28 February 2025.

Index

Note: Page numbers in *italics* refer to Figures; those in **bold** to Tables.